Ergometry

Ergometry

Basics of Medical Exercise Testing

Harald Mellerowicz, Berlin
Vojin N. Smodlaka, New York

With Contributions by

Kurt Maidorn
Fritz Matzdorff
Paul Nowacki
Hans-Friedmund Rittel
Horst Schmutzler

Fritz A. Schön
Hans Stoboy
Elmar Waterloh
Hans Zapfe

Translated by Allan L. Rice

Urban & Schwarzenberg
Baltimore – Munich 1981

Urban & Schwarzenberg, Inc.
7 E. Redwood Street
Baltimore, Maryland   21202
USA

Urban & Schwarzenberg
Pettenkoferstrasse 18
D-8000 München 2
Germany

Printed in the United States of America

Library of Congress Cataloging in Publication Data

Mellerowicz, Harald.
   Ergometry: basics of medical exercise testing.

   Translation of Ergometrie.
   Includes index.
   1. Function tests (Medicine)   2. Work—Physiological   aspects.
3. Physical fitness—Measurement.   4. Work measurement.
I. Smodlaka, Vojin N., joint author.   II. Title.
[DNLM: 1. Exertion.   2. Physical fitness—Heart function tests.
3. Respiratory function tests. WG141.5.F9 M525e]
RC71.8.M4413   1980   616.07'54   80-11140
ISBN 0-8067-1241-4

ISBN 0-8067-1241-4 (Baltimore)

ISBN 3-541-71241-4 (Munich)

Contents

Foreword

While the recorded history of mankind can be considered in terms of thousands of years, the serious study of physical exercise has occurred only during the last fifty years. It was not until the twentieth century that the average person had time to devote to competitive and recreational sport; for this reason, little attention was given the physiological responses of persons participating in organized sport activities or general physical exercise. Few published reports of the controlled investigation of exercise appeared before 1900.

Serious study of exercise was initiated in the 1930s, but the use of exercise as a procedure in clinical testing, disease prevention, or rehabilitation long went unrecognized. The interest of the medical community in exercise was not aroused until the 1960s when it was realized that graded exercise represented a powerful tool for intervention, diagnosis and treatment.

The last twenty years represent a boom period in the interest of the general public in physical activity, the growth of both amateur and professional sport, and the use and prescription by scientists and clinicians of graded exercise testing. In order to employ exercise as a precision tool, ergometers of a wide variety of models have been designed and constructed in scientific and clinical laboratories around the world.

The appropriateness of ergometric devices for their intended applications, the accuracy of calibration, and the selection of proper protocols represent issues that deserved far more attention than they have received. Only too often, the specificity that the human body's functional capacities have for different forms and intensities of exercise and the precision with which exercise could be controlled have been overlooked. It was, therefore, of great importance that the German-speaking community of the world received *Ergometrie* in 1962. No such treatment of the subject was available at that time in any other language nor has any comparable publication appeared during the intervening years.

In the original German publication and now in the English edition, important consideration has been given to the relationships between the aspects of basic physics involved with ergometric performance and the physiological capacities of the human organism. Detailed discussions of the basic cardiovascular, ventilatory, and respiratory responses to ergometric exercise are presented. Additional information is presented on the physiological measurements themselves, as well as on the use of computers with ergometry testing. Such complete coverage will provide clinicians and investigators with provocative approaches and a wealth of information.

As editor of the original version, Dr. Harald Mellerowicz deserves great praise for both his personal initiative and the quality of the original work. The contributions of Dr. Vojin Smodlaka as the collaborating editor of this English edition deserve an equal share of praise. Scientists and clinicians of the English-speaking community will find this book both a rich reference and a powerful stimulus to constructive planning as regards the use of ergometry in research and health care.

Spring, 1981

HOWARD G. KNUTTGEN
Boston, Massachusetts

Preface to the First German Edition

In internal medicine, industrial medicine and sportsmedicine, in insurance and compensation cases, and even pre- and postoperative cardiac and pulmonary surgery there are many fields of application for ergometry. The importance of ergometric methods of examination in preventive medicine for early diagnosis of even pre-morbid conditions of the heart and circulatory system and in rehabilitory medicine for the prescription of rehabilitory exercise has also been described in the literature.

In our mechanized civilization the value of physical performance and physical ability is generally underestimated even by the medical profession. Yet these stand in close reciprocal relationships with health and the laws of Nature, as is being recognized once more to an increasing degree.

Ergometry has, in the course of recent decades, enjoyed steadily increasing attention in Germany and various other European countries. The disciples of Knipping, among them Bolt, Valentin, Venrath and Hollman; Reindell, Roskamm and associates; Lehmann and E. A. Müller, as well as Bartels, Bücherl, Hertz, Rodewald and Schwab; in Scandinavia Christensen and Åstrand, and in Switzerland Fleisch, Rossier, Bühlmann and Wiesinger have all contributed important basic work to the establishment and practical application of ergometry. In the last seven years our group in Berlin with Peterman, Lerche, Dransfeld, Schmutzler, Dressler, Stoboy, Maidorn and others have actively engaged in filling many remaining gaps in our knowledge and throwing light on many unresolved problems in this relatively new field of medicine.

But still the methodology of ergometric examination suffers many inadequacies. It has not yet been fully standardized. There is therefore considerable divergence in the data from different authors. Experiments aimed at determining average values and ranges of variation in functions of performance for particular age and sex groups are not yet completed and in some cases have been carried out on insufficiently large populations. Thus the factual knowledge presented herein cannot be considered complete. For this and other shortcomings may the authors be forgiven. We have conscientiously indicated the still-open questions and problems insofar as we have been aware of them.

The aim of this book is to provide a comprehensive and in many respects newly established presentation of our current knowledge of ergometry. In its form, we have made an effort to keep the text as concise and clear as possible yet as comprehensive as necessary. We have made a point of using the most striking graphic presentations and illustrations possible. These, in tune with the purpose of the book, actually form the main part of the work. The presentation of the methodological parts and the range of physiological variation in performance have been given more space as compared with the physiological and pathogenetic contexts, which can be found in more complete form in other books. Preponderantly non-invasive bloodless methods have been presented, which should be those of preference in practical ergometry.

On practical grounds we have been able to present only the "basics of ergometry," in no way a complete coverage. It is intended to provide the physician with the opportunity to work his way into ergometry without too much expenditure of time and/or extensive pursuit of the literature.

I should like to thank all my collaborators and especially our technical assistant, Mrs. L. Kabisch, for her reliable and faithful cooperation.

The publishers, Urban & Schwarzenberg, and in particular Dr. Urban have contributed much to the creation of this book through their generous readiness to further the work with willing support. We must also thank them for the elegant craftsmanship represented in the physical format of the book.

Spring, 1974

HARALD MELLEROWICZ
Berlin

Preface to the English Edition

Since the appearance of the first edition, ergometry has won still wider application, especially in preventative and rehabilitative cardiology, pulmonology, pre- and postoperative diagnosis, surgery and orthopedics, as well as internal medicine, industrial and sportsmedicine and rehabilitation. Three international seminars on ergometry have been held in Berlin, attracting many "ergologists" from research institutes around the world. There has been wide publication of new experimental results in ergometry and we have included here those that are of significance for the "basics" of ergometry. This is also true for the development of ergometric apparatus, a matter to which numerous firms have addressed themselves successfully during the past ten years. Although it is unfortunate that neither standardization in ergometer construction nor application of ergometric methodology has yet been achieved, new initiatives toward a more exact comparability and reproducibility of ergometric data are in prospect.

This edition contains new chapters on the ergometric EKG (Matzdorff), arterial blood gases and acid balance in ergometric performance (Schön and Waterloh) and treadmill versus ergometry (Smodlaka). We have also added sections on criteria of quality in ergometry and contraindications to ergometric measurements. Many errors and insufficiencies from the previous editions have been corrected and earlier data have been revised in the light of newer knowledge. Data on conversion to international SI units for force (newtons), work (joules) and power (watts) are included in Chapter I while Chapter VIII contains data for converting arterial pressure measurements. The reader is referred to Lippert: *SI Units in Medicine,* Urban & Schwarzenberg, Baltimore, 1978, for data and problems concerning conversion to SI units.

We believe that this English translation of the third German edition will provide the English-speaking community with a comprehensive reference and guide to the ever broadening field of ergometry.

Spring, 1981

HARALD MELLEROWICZ
Berlin

VOJIN N. SMODLAKA
New York

Contributors

Harald Mellerowicz, M.D., Director, Institut für Leistungsmedizin, Forckenbeckstr. 20, 1000 Berlin 33, Germany;

Kurt Maidorn, M.D., Pädagogische Hochschule, Abt. f. Sportmedizin, Malteser Str. 74, 1000 Berlin 46, Germany;

Fritz Matzdorff, M.D., Director of Taunus-Clinic of DFA Goethesh. 4–6, 6350 Bad Nauheim, West Germany;

Paul Nowacki, M.D., Director, Institut für Sportmedizin der Universität, Kugelberg 22, 6300 Giessen, West Germany;

Vojin N. Smodlaka, M.D., Sc.D., Clinical Professor of Rehabilitation Medicine, State University of New York, College of Medicine and Director of the Department of Rehabilitation Medicine at The Methodist Hospital, 506 Sixth St., Brooklyn, New York 11215, USA;

Hans Rittel, Science Collaborator, Sportmedizinisches Institut, Rhein-Westfälische Technische Hochschule, Roermonder Str. 7–9, 5100 Aachen, West Germany;

Horst Schmutzler, M.D., Director of the Cardiologic Department, Westend Clinic of the Free University, Spandauer Damm 130, 1000 Berlin 19, Germany;

Fritz Andreas Schön, Science Collaborator, Sportmedizinisches Institut, Rhein-Westfälische Technische Hochschule, Roermonder Str. 7–9, 5100 Aachen, West Germany;

Hans Stoboy, M.D., Director of the Department of Physiological Performance, Institut für Leistungsmedizin, Forckenbeckstr. 20, 1000 Berlin 33, Germany;

Elmar Waterloh, M.D., Director, Sportmedizinisches Institut, Rhein-Westfälische Technische Hochschule, Roermonder Str. 7–9, 5100 Aachen, West Germany;

Hans Zapfe, M.D., Medical Director, Krankenhaus am Mariendorfer Weg, Abteilung für Chronischkranke, Mariendorfer Weg 48 u. 74, 1000 Berlin 44, Germany.

I. Physical and Biological Fundamentals of Ergometry

1. Physical and Biological Performance

An ergometer is a device for measuring power in watts (1 watt $=$ 1 joule/s $=$ 1 newtonmeter/s) and physical work in joules.

Newtons (N), joules (J) and watts (W) are SI units (SI-Système International d'Unités).

1 Newton is the force which imparts an acceleration of 1 m/s^{-2} to a body having a mass of 1 kg.

1 Joule is the work performed when the point of application of a force of 1 N is displaced 1 m in the direction of the force.

1 Watt is the power with which 1 J of energy is converted during 1 s of time.

Force—Work—Power

Force	$=$ mass $\times$ acceleration
1 dyne	$=$ the force which imparts unit acceleration (1 cm/s^{-2}) to 1 gram of mass
1 pond (p)	$=$ 981 dynes
1 kp	$=$ 9.81 newtons (N)
Work	$=$ force $\times$ distance
1 erg	$=$ the work performed by 1 dyne in displacing a body 1 cm in the direction of the force
10^7 ergs	$=$ 1 joule (J)
1 kpm	$=$ 9.81 joules ($\approx$10 joules) $=$ 9.81 newtonmeters ($\approx$10 Nm)
1 Nm	$=$ 1 joule

Power   = Work/time, i.e., work per unit of time
  1 Joule/s   = 1 watt
  1 kpm/s   = 9.81   watts   ($\approx$10   watts) = 9.81   newtonmeters/s
                  ($\approx$10 Nm/s)
  1 HP (metric) = 75 kpm/s = 736 watts

For an equal physical performance, a different "biological performance" may be required, because the efficiency (degree of effectiveness) of biological performance is determined by the mechanical properties of the ergometer as well as by numerous endogenous and exogenous factors. Biological performance on the ergometer and its efficiency are influenced by:

1. Cranking speed, crank height and cranking radius
2. Whether the cranking is being done by hand- or foot-power, and whether the subject is standing, sitting or reclining
3. The individual variables of motion economy
4. Constitutional factors, age and sex
5. The subject's physical and mental state at the time of the test, both of which depend on degree of training, life style, working conditions, diet, etc.
6. Ambient temperature, humidity, barometric pressure and other climatic conditions
7. Time of day and time of year.

This biological background must be taken into consideration whenever obtaining ergometric performance data, just as, in general, in any medical examination where comparative measurement is being undertaken. The most precise possible knowledge of the effects of these conditioning factors on biological performance is therefore an essential prerequisite for the evaluation of ergometric data.

Performance capacity must be distinguished from biological performance. It can be defined as the physical and mental capacity of an individual to reach an individual *maximal achievement* (performance limit under normal conditions) which is greatly influenced by environmental conditions. Performance capacity is highly dependent on physical conditions and the willpower to achieve (ambition), which may to a greater or lesser extent call up available *reserves of power*. *Total* reserve power can be called forth only in certain emergency situations. The maximal powers of achievement attainable under normal conditions by great application of willpower must therefore be distinguished from peak achievement attainable only under stress of emergency.

For any maximal power the conditions under which it was achieved must be recorded. For comparative ergometric measurements, the standardization of all conditions possible is a prime requisite. The dependence of maximal achievement on imponderables of motivation injects a significant factor of uncertainty into the evaluation. However, in measuring the functions of performance at various levels of submaximal achievement and in comparing them with physiological regularities and the physiological range of variation of various functions, this factor of uncertainty is of practically no importance.

2. Cardiac, Pulmonary and Other Organic Factors of Physical Performance

In any testing of performance, we are measuring a physical power that depends on numerous partial organic factors, such as the heart, vascular system, lungs, blood, endocrine glands, vegetative system, liver, kidneys, locomotor apparatus and nervous system. The ergometric findings must always be viewed in the light of data from the total clinical examination. The employment of special methods of examination during the ergometric performance also makes possible a direct measurement and comparative evaluation of the performance functions and performance maxima of individual organic factors, especially of the heart, vascular system and lungs. Thus, for example, the measurement of the respiratory minute-volume, the respiratory equivalent and O_2 consumption at submaximal and especially at maximal power permits an evaluation of the performance functions and achievement maxima of the respiratory system. From the more difficult measurement of the cardiac output and the arterial pressure during ergometric performance, we can calculate cardiac performance and evaluate it on a comparative basis. Methodological difficulties may arise from individual performance factors, e.g., O_2 consumption, respiratory and circulatory performance, O_2 capacity of the blood, as well as from vegetative and endocrine factors and the like.

With the means currently available, ergometry is less suitable for measurement of the partial organic performances. However, it gives satisfactory results if we pose the more practically oriented question: How capable of performance is the subject, even in view of his heart damage, his pulmonary disease, his anemia or his vegetative dystonia? The most exact qualitative clinical diagnosis possible is therefore a prime requisite for ergometric measurement of performance and evaluation of any given case. While the specific diagnosis is of a qualitative nature, the measurement of performance affords quantitative conclusions. As in all fields of biology and medicine, all the individual and especially all the psychological factors must be considered. In this area lie the problems and methodological difficulties of this as well as all other medical testing methods.

3.   The Relationship of Physical Power on the Ergometer to Cranking Speed, Cranking Length, Crank Height and Motion Economy

At equal power on the ergometer, the biological performance may vary as a function of cranking speed, cranking radius, the crank height selected and individual differences in the economy of motion. The differences in biological performances at equal physical power depend on the degree of efficiency of muscular action, or, as the case may be, the metabolic economy with regard to the rapidity of contraction and the amount of isometric or isotonic muscular action. Thus, for every ergometric power, depending on constitutional factors, there are optimal cranking speeds, cranking radii and crank heights with relatively minimal biological performance at maximal efficiency of the muscles involved. The problem of optimal economy is relatively complex, since relationships to constitution, sex, age and numerous exogenous influences must also be assumed. To achieve greater accuracy in diagnosis through ergometric performance, further study of this problem is essential; available data show a wide range of optimal economy.

3.1   Optimal Cranking Speed

The optimal economies of ten untrained men aged 27 and over, at various cranking speeds and powers of 50, 100, 150 and 200 watts, are seen in Figure 1. The experiments were carried out with six-minute hand-cranking exercises on a Dargatz ergometer on different days during morning hours. Between test sessions, the subjects had 30- to 60-minute breaks, to allow heart rate (HR) values to return to normal. In order to obviate a possible influence on the subsequent exercise bout by its predecessor, some of the trials were carried out at increased cranking speeds, some at decreased cranking speeds. During the exercise bouts, we measured the HR by means of an elongated stethoscope attached precordially and a stopwatch, ascertaining the total HR of the performance. In all experiments the cranks were 1/3 meter in length. The average values were calculated from 200 experiments in 40 series and entered on a coordinate system.
The curve in Figure 1 shows that:

1. At equal physical power the biological power varies as the cranking speed on the hand-cranked ergometer.
2. For each ergometric power there are too-high, optimal and too-low cranking speeds as regards performance economy.

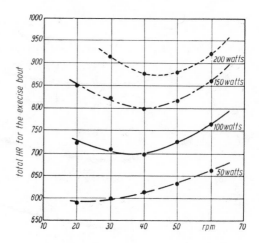

Fig. 1. Total HR at varying cranking speeds of 20, 30, 40, 50 and 60 rpm on a manually operated ergometer at 50-, 100-, 150- and 200-watt power (average values for ten subjects).

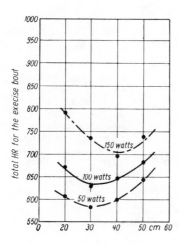

Fig. 2. Total HR at varying cranking radii of 20, 30, 40 and 50 cm on the manual ergometer at 50-, 100- and 150-watt powers (average values for 11 subjects).

3. The optimal cranking speed increases with power.
4. The following optimal cranking speeds are for men of average age, stature and weight:

At 50 watts: ≈20 to 30 rpm	At 150 watts: ≈40 rpm
At 100 watts: ≈35 to 40 rpm	At 200 watts: ≈40 to 50 rpm

Experiments by Atzler, Herbst, Lehmann and E. A. Müller on cranking efficiency at varying exertions and varying cranking radii (19.4, 28.4 and 36.6 cm) also gave optimal cranking speeds (that is, the cranking speeds with greatest efficiency) at about 30 to 50 rpm.

Similarly, in the case of foot-pedaling while seated, at the same physical power, the total HR for the power varied as a function of the biological power, depending on the rpm. Experiments by Wolff (1978) gave the following results with ten untrained men aged 18 to 30 (Fig. 3):

1. At 50 watts: ≈40 rpm
   At 100 watts: ≈40 to 50 rpm
   At 150 watts: ≈50 to 60 rpm

   At 200 watts: ≈55 to 65 rpm
   At 250 watts: ≈65 rpm

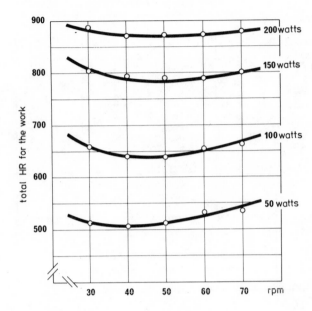

Fig. 3. Total HR during 6-minute work at various speeds of 30, 40, 50, 60 and 70 rpm on bicycle ergometers at powers of 50, 100, 150 and 200 watts. Curves connect average values for ten subjects.

2. The optimal rpm in manual cranking while standing increases with an increase in power.
3. As the power increases, the difference between maximal and minimal total HR decreases at different rpms; the correlation between physical and biological power becomes closer.

Grosse-Lordemann and E. A. Müller found, in the case of foot-pedaling performances of 6 to 20 kpm/s, that the maximal performance was achieved with 40 to 50 rpm. Stegemann and associates demonstrated the highest efficiency rate in the range of 40-60 rpm in foot-pedaling experiments of 2 to 7.9 kpm/s.

Experiments by Isreal et al. showed an increase of the regression lines for HR, O_2 consumption, systolic pressure, blood lactate and respiratory quotients with equal physical power of 100, 200 and 300 watts at speeds increasing from 50 to 100 rpm. Likewise, comparative measurements of cardiopulmonary function in 50- to 350-watt power at 60 rpm resulted in lower values for HR and O_2 consumption than at 90 rpm (Schürsch et al.). Also Ulmer found in comparative studies of one-hour maximal power at 60, 90 and 120 rpm an increased heart rate and O_2 consumption at higher rpm. The average maximal power was little less at 90 rpm and considerably less at 120 rpm than at 60 rpm (Fig. 4).

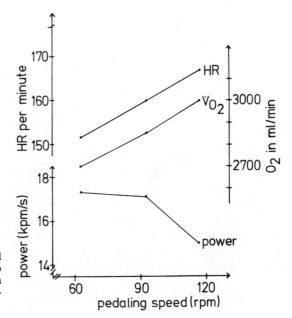

Fig. 4. Average power, HR and O₂ consumption (converted to perminute values) during a one-hour maximal foot-cranking (after *Ulmer*).

3.2 Optimal Crank Length (Radius)

To determine the optimal crank length, eleven healthy males (average age 24 years, average weight 71 kg and average height 176 cm) performed 132 individual six-minute experiments at ergometric powers of 50, 100 and 150 watts in 33 separate series on various days. We allowed 30- to 60-minute rests between individual performances, at least until complete restoration of normal heart rate. Some of the performances were with progressively longer cranking radii, some with progressively shorter, on a Dargatz eddy-current ergometer with constant crank height of one meter. The results of the experiments are shown by the curves in Figure 2. Tables and curves reveal that:

1. At 50- to 100-watt exertion the optimal crank length lies between 30 and 35 cm.
2. At 150 watts it approaches 40 cm.
3. The 33 individual curves agree in showing that the optimal crank length increases with an increase of power, higher power levels being easier to achieve with a longer crank radius.
4. The experiments lead to the assumption that at equal power, a greater crank radius is preferable for taller subjects.

Atzler, Herbst and Lehmann likewise found an increase in optimal cranking radius as the power increased.

In experiments using foot pedaling while seated, with crank lengths of 14, 18 and 22 cm, Grosse-Lordemann and E. A. Müller showed that at average performances between 8 and 40 kpm/s the efficiency is not essentially dependent on the crank length.

At higher powers, however, efficiency increases with the crank length. Thus, the same regularity regarding optimal crank length is revealed with foot pedaling as with hand cranking. The agreement becomes more clear if the crank lengths of the two foot pedals are added together.

For better comparability of experimental results, and to simplify the practical experimental methodology, it is necessary to standardize the crank length of the ergometer. To this end a hand-crank length, or as the case may be, a double foot-crank length (cranking radius) of 1/3 meter (33.33 cm), seems suitable. With this cranking radius, the steady-state powers of 30 to 200 watts most commonly met with in practice with short, average and tall men can be achieved with relatively minor variations in efficiency. For special purposes, a crank of adjustable length can be employed.

The maximal power in foot pedaling is achieved, especially with short or medium periods of time, at rpm above the optimal economy already mentioned. At speeds of around 90 rpm the efficiency is actually lower. However, higher spurts of energy and improved performance of short duration can be obtained. Higher rpm at the same power level are felt subjectively to be less stressful, especially in subjects with moderately strong leg muscles. The amount of force required for each turn of the pedal here naturally becomes less. In ergometric studies at submaximal levels of power, the economical range of rpm must be taken into account for purposes of comparability and reproducibility. In vita-maxima measurements they may be exceeded to individually altered degrees within the range of maximal power (see Chapter III, 1.5).

3.3   Optimal Crank Height in Hand Cranking

In the case of seven subjects (average age 27 years, average height 179 cm, average weight 69 kg) the heart rate was determined during performance and recovery at a uniform power of 100 watts and with uniform crank length of 30 cm but variable crank heights of 80, 90, 100, 110 and 120 cm. The average values for seven subjects show a high degree of agreement at all crank heights, as is seen in Figure 5. Small, relatively insignificant differences also occur in the several subjects' HR during performance and during recovery. In the shortest subject, height 163 cm, the performance HR reached the highest value with a crank height of 120 cm, the lowest value at 90 and 100 cm. In the case of the tallest subject (186 cm), however, the HR during exertion was lowest with the crank at 120 cm and highest with a height of 90 cm.

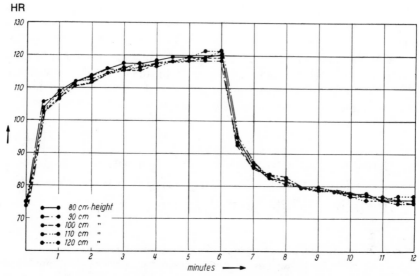

Fig. 5. Average HR in seven subjects, 163 to 186 cm tall, during and after 100-watt power on the hand-crank ergometer with crank heights ranging from 80 to 120 cm.

Summarizing the above, we may draw some conclusions: The influence of crank height on exercise HR and recovery HR at an equal average power of 100 watts and a uniform crank length of 30 cm is relatively slight within a range of 80 to 120 cm crank height. On the average, in different subjects of medium height there is no significant difference at these crank heights. Short individuals, however, probably work more economically at lower crank levels and taller individuals at higher levels.

Atzler, Herbst and Lehmann found, too, that optimal crank height was subject to relatively little variation at a greater cranking radius in experiments with a male subject 171.5 cm tall, a cranking radius of 36.6 cm, crank height between 100 and 120 cm at various powers. They also concluded from their studies that optimal crank height decreases with increasing resistance.

An average crank height of 100 cm may be suggested as standard. It is less suited for extremely tall individuals but is quite satisfactory even for younger people and children 10–12 years of age, as the crank height can be reduced through the use of platforms 10 to 20 cm high. For special applications, ergometers are available with adjustable heights. However, it can be assumed that more than 90 per cent of the usual ergometric experiments can be carried out with approximately optimal efficiency at a crank height of 100 cm. The differences in efficiency, compared with that at crank heights of 110 to 120 cm, are practically negligible except for a small percentage of very tall men, because the subject can readily adapt himself to various crank heights by changing the angle of his body position to suit the height of the crank.

In contradistinction to hand cranking, foot pedaling calls for adjustable seat heights. Experience indicates that the adjustment should be such that when the foot is extended farthest in pedaling, the angle between the foot and the shin is between 90 and 120 degrees.

4.   Biological Comparison of Ergometric Hand Cranking While Standing with Foot Pedaling While Seated and Reclining

O_2 consumption and degree of efficiency at the same rate of physical exertion differ between hand cranking while standing and foot pedaling while seated and reclining.

In 36 healthy male subjects aged 20 to 40, we carried out comparative ergometric experiments with the subjects standing, sitting and reclining. During and after a session at 100 watts lasting ten minutes, we read the HR, respiratory minute-volume, O_2 consumption, CO_2 production, and O_2 pulse (cranking speed 35 rpm, hand-crank length and foot-cranking diameter 33.3 cm, crank height when standing 1 meter). There were rests between workouts until complete return to initial HR. The series of exercise sessions was varied for the individual subjects, so that one-third of the series started with the standing session and a third each seated and reclining. The HR was determined by stopwatch with the aid of an extended stethoscope attached in front of the heart, the respiratory minute-volume was measured with a dry-gas meter and steady-state O_2 consumption and CO_2 production with the "Magnos" and "Uras" instruments, respectively, from Hartmann & Braun. We took running control readings by the Micro-Scholander method (Figs. 6–15; see also p. 243). If we designate steady-state O_2 consumption in hand cranking while standing as 100%, then the O_2 consumption with foot pedaling while seated rates 89% and with foot pedaling while reclining 90.5%.

These figures make it possible to compare the three most common exercise forms on the cranking ergometer with regard to steady-state O_2 consumption and relative efficiency.

Figures 8 through 15 (after Mellerowicz and Nowacki) show the behavior of HR, O_2 consumption, respiratory minute-volume and CO_2 production during a 100-watt ergometric session while standing, sitting and reclining (36 male subjects aged 20 to 40).

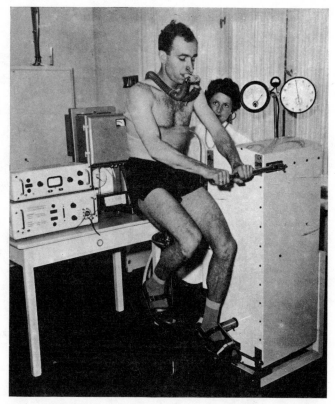

Fig. 6. Experimental setup for ergometric foot pedaling while seated, using the Lauckner Universal ergometer plus "Uras" and "Magnos" instruments from Hartmann & Braun.

In hand cranking while standing, the HR, respiratory minute-volume, O_2 consumption and CO_2 production are significantly greater than in foot pedaling while seated and reclining. With approximately equal O_2 consumption, all average values for HR are greater while seated than while reclining. On the other hand, the average values for respiratory minute-volume verified statistically and for CO_2 production in the steady state are definitely greater in foot pedaling while reclining than in foot pedaling while seated.

At maximal power, approximately equal values are obtained in hand cranking while standing and foot pedaling while seated. In foot pedaling while reclining, values roughly 15% lower were observed for maximal O_2 consumption (Mellerowicz and Galle).

An overview of the behavior of various cardiac and pulmonary functions in foot pedaling while seated and reclining is given in Table 1 (after Valentin and Holzhauser).

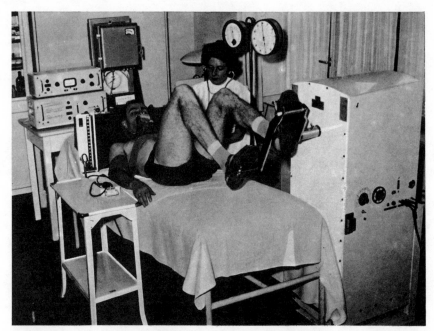

Fig. 7. Experimental set-up for reclining ergometric foot-pedaling workout, using Lauckner Universal ergometer and "Uras" and "Magnos" instruments from Hartmann & Braun.

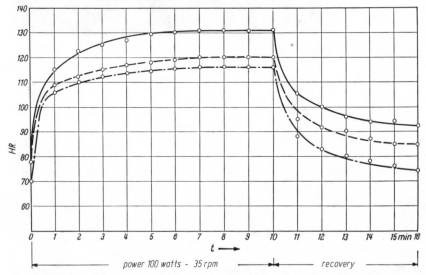

Fig. 8. Behavior of the average HR in comparative studies of hand cranking while standing ——, foot pedaling while seated — — — and foot pedaling while reclining —·—·— at equal powers (100 watts) during a ten-minute workout and six-minute rest in 36 untrained male subjects aged 20 to 40 (after *Mellerowicz* and *Nowacki*).

Fig. 9. Average steady-state HR in hand cranking while standing and foot pedaling while seated and reclining at equal powers of 100 watts in 36 untrained male subjects aged 20 to 40. Statistically verified difference between standing and sitting, and standing and reclining (after *Mellerowicz* and *Nowacki*).

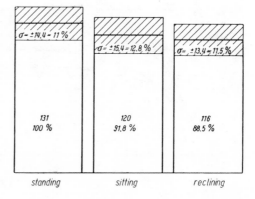

Fig. 10. Behavior of the average O_2 consumption (standard temperature pressure dry—STPD) in comparative studies of hand cranking while standing ———, and foot pedaling while seated — — — and reclining —·—·— during equal 100-watt sessions lasting ten minutes and six-minute rests in 36 untrained male subjects aged 20 to 40 (after *Mellerowicz* and *Nowacki*).

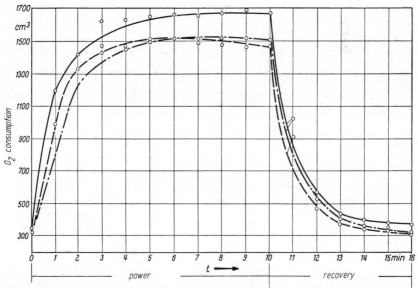

Fig. 11. Average (STPD) steady-state O_2 consumption with hand cranking while standing and foot pedaling while seated and reclining during equal sessions of 100 watts on the part of 36 untrained male subjects aged 20 to 40. Statistically verified difference between standing and sitting, and standing and reclining (after *Mellerowicz* and *Nowacki*).

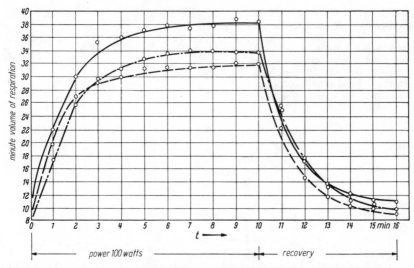

Fig. 12. Behavior of the average respiratory minute-volume in studies of hand cranking while standing ———, and foot pedaling while seated — — — and reclining —·—·— at equal powers of 100 watts during ten-minute exercise sessions and six-minute rests in 36 untrained male subjects aged 20 to 40 (after *Mellerowicz* and *Nowacki*).

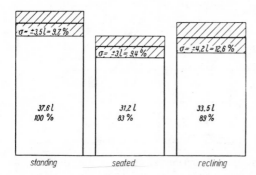

Fig. 13. Average steady-state respiratory minute-volume during hand cranking while standing and foot pedaling while seated and reclining with equal powers of 100 watts in 36 untrained male subjects aged 20 to 40. Statistically verified difference between standing and sitting, standing and reclining, and reclining and sitting (after *Mellerowicz* and *Nowacki*).

Table 1. Differing behavior of individual cardiovascular parameters in seated and reclining bicycle ergometer performance. + = greater, − = less (after *Valentin* and *Holzhauser*).

Function	Sitting	Reclining
HR	+	−
Arteriovenous O_2 difference	+	−
O_2 consumption	+	−
O_2 pulse	approximately equal	
Cardiac volume	−	+
Stroke volume	−	+
Cardiac output	−	+
Systolic and diastolic blood pressure	+	−

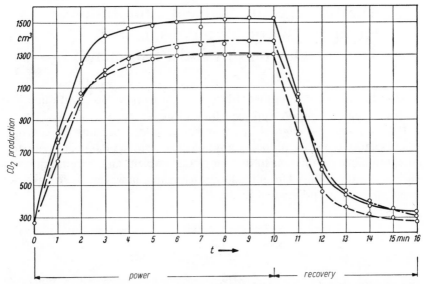

Fig. 14. Behavior of the average CO_2 production (STPD) in comparative studies of hand cranking while standing ——————, and foot pedaling while seated — — — and reclining —·—·— at equal powers of 100 watts lasting ten minutes, followed by a six-minute rest, in 36 untrained male subjects aged 20 to 40 (after *Mellerowicz* and *Nowacki*).

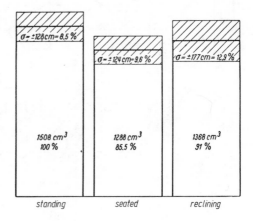

Fig. 15. Average steady-state CO_2 production (STPD) with hand cranking while standing and foot pedaling while seated and reclining at equal powers of 100 watts in 36 untrained male subjects aged 20 to 40. Statistically verified difference between standing and sitting, and sitting and reclining (after *Mellerowicz* and *Nowacki*).

σ = ±128 cm = 8.5 %

σ = ±124 cm = 9.6 %

σ = ±177 cm = 12.9 %

1508 cm³
100 %

1288 cm³
85.5 %

1368 cm³
91 %

standing   seated   reclining

5. The Influence of Ambient Temperature, Humidity, Barometric Pressure and Time of Day on Physical Performance

Physical performance is influenced by ambient temperature, heat radiation, humidity, barometric pressure and time of day.

For all types and degrees of performance, and depending on constitutional factors, there are probably physiological optima of ambient temperature, humidity (in relation to motion of the ambient air), barometric pressure and time of day. Up until the present time, however, these have not been pinpointed and studied in detail.

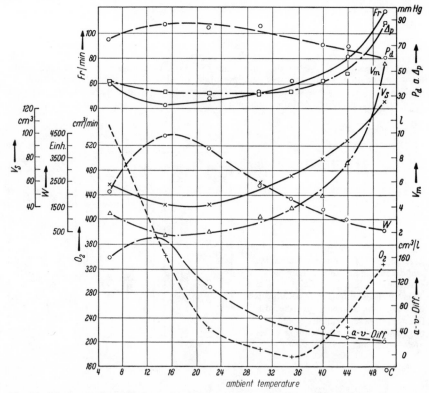

Fig. 16. Circulatory data and O_2 consumption in a young, healthy subject as a function of an ambient temperature of 6°C to 50°C (relative humidity 50 per cent). Pd = diastolic pressure; Fr = HR/minute; Δp = blood pressure amplitude; Vs = stroke volume; Vm = cardiac output; W = effective peripheral circulatory resistance; a-v Diff. = arteriovenous O_2 difference; O_2 = O_2 consumption/minute. All data after 2-1/2 hours excercise (after experiments by *Wezler* and *Thauer*).

Figure 16, after Wezler and Thauer, shows the effect of ambient temperature on HR, stroke volume, cardiac output, amplitude of arterial pressure and arteriovenous O_2 difference in a healthy subject at rest. Qualitatively quite similar but quantitatively differing temperature effects are to be anticipated in human subjects during bodily exertion. Herxheimer found a great increase in HR in the case of equal steady-state exercise when the ambient temperature is increased. Figure 18, after E. A. Müller, makes apparent the very great differences in HR during the same work by the same individual, with and without excessive ambient temperature. Temperatures and humidities above the comfort range can lead to an extra load on the organism during ergometric performance, depending on movement of the ambient air. They cause a rise in HR, cardiac output, and amplitude of arterial pressure during equal powers as expressions of increased regulatory functions. During the performance, the organism generates considerable amounts of heat. This excess can amount to ten or twenty times the basal metabolic rate, depending on the degree of exertion.

The excessive overheating due to exertion leads to increased internal temperature, in spite of intensive heat-regulatory functions on the part of the organism. Depending on constitutional factors, this temperature generally increases with greater and more prolonged exercise (Fig. 17). As internal temperature rises, the HR and cardiac output increase, accompanied by decreased arteriovenous O_2 difference, in order to distribute and dissipate the increased muscular heat.

Comfort zones of ambient temperature, humidity and air movement for the individual at rest differ very greatly from the physiological optima for exertion of various intensities and durations. For example, the studies by Hasse on the rowing ergometer showed a drop in exercise capacity with exertion at effective temperatures of 18°C to 24°C (Fig. 19), which correspond approximately to the comfort zone for a fully clothed individual at

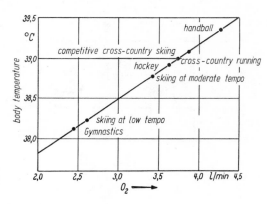

Fig. 17. Body temperature as prolonged exertion increases (after *Christensen,* as cited by *Nöcker*).

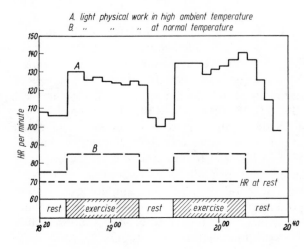

Fig. 18. HR during same exercise with and without ambient temperature overload (stoker in a rolling mill) (after *E. A. Müller*).

rest. Long-standing experience in sports is in agreement with this, in that cooler temperatures (below 20 °C) have a favorable effect on endurance performance whereas higher temperatures favor sprints. For all practical purposes it must be borne in mind that most ergometric studies are carried out at "normal" temperatures of 18 °C to 24 °C and relative humidities between 30 and 70%. These are probably not optimal temperatures and humidities for protracted physical power, but they are the standard exogenous conditions under which the norms have been established in ergometric studies. At higher ranges of temperature and humidity the further increase in HR and cardiac output must be taken into account in evaluating results. An important field for further research would be investigating the effects of

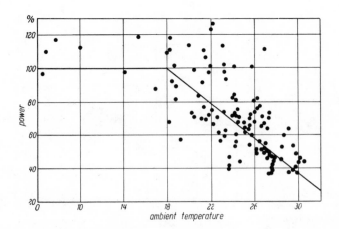

Fig. 19. Dependence of the capacity to exercise with the ergometric rowing machine on ambient temperature (after *A. Hasse*).

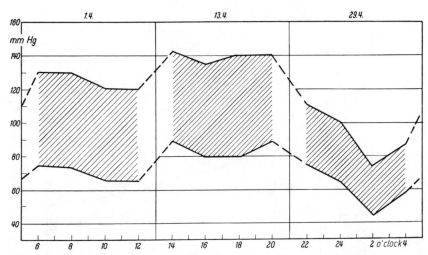

Fig. 20. Course of the systolic and diastolic pressures in a 24-hour period (after *W. Menzel*).

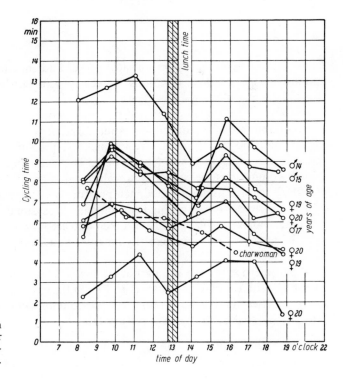

Fig. 21. Circadian rhythms of power capacity (after *Lehmann* and *Michaelis*).

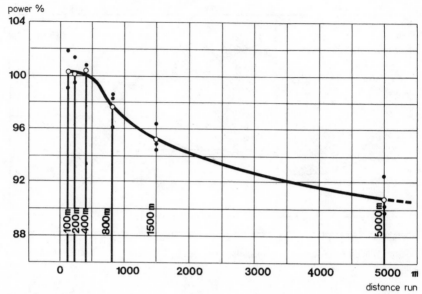

Fig. 22. Relative drop in power in percentages on the part of 15 untrained 100-5000 meter runners in relation to distance run (after *Mellerowicz* and *Meller*).

temperature and humidity on physical power and the various circulatory and respiratory functions at various degrees of ergometric exertion in larger age and sex populations.

The data for O_2 consumption and CO_2 production obtained under ambient conditions must be reduced for standardization purposes to values based on $0°C$ and 760 mm Hg (standard temperature pressure dry—STPD) with the aid of conversion tables (see p. 408). The data for tidal volume and minute-volume must be converted to values based on $37°C$ and 760 mm Hg and 100% relative humidity (body temperature pressure saturated—BTPS). Also, the increase from morning to evening in HR, systolic pressure (Fig. 20) and other biological factors must be taken into account. Likewise, allowance must be made for the circadian rhythms of physical capacity for performance (Fig. 21).

As barometric pressure and partial O_2 pressure fall, the endurance capacity for physical exercise decreases (Fig. 22). In the case of submaximal exercise intensities, the HR, respiratory minute-volume and respiratory equivalent all rise as the barometric pressure falls.

6. Sex and Performance

The capacity for exercise performance per kg of body weight in women is, on the average, considerably below that of men in short-, middle- and

Table 2. Comparative table of constitutional factors and performance functions in men and women.

	Women	Men
Bodily structure:	size and weight smaller, pelvis broader and heavier, body relatively longer, more fat tissue, lower specific weight	size and weight greater, shoulders broader, extremities longer, less fat tissue, greater specific weight
Musculature:	$\approx$30–35% of body weight, less favorable balance between mass and strength	$\approx$40% of body weight, more favorable balance between mass and strength
Skeleton:	skeletal weight relatively and absolutely less	skeletal weight relatively and absolutely greater
Blood: volume hemoglobin red blood cells (in mm³)	less, absolutely $\approx$13–14 g/100 cc fewer	five liters $\approx$15–16 g/100 cc 4.5–5 million/mm³
Cardiovascular: heart volume heart weight greatest heart performance	absolute: $\approx$65–75% relative: (per kg) over $\approx$65–75% absolute: $\approx$65–75% relative: (per kg) over $\approx$65–75% probably: $\approx$65–75% relative: (per kg) over $\approx$65–75%	$\approx$800 ml $\approx$300 g 100 %
Respiration: vital capacity O_2 consumption	absolute: $\approx$70% relative: (per kg) $\approx$80–85% absolute: 70% relative: (per kg) $\approx$80–85%	$\approx$4000–4500 ml $\approx$3000 ml $\approx$50 ml/kg
Hormonal system:	menstrual cycle can affect performance	
Nervous system and psychology:	differences in motor details and attitudes toward performance	
Performance: endurance > 6 min average 1–6 min brief < 1 min strength	absol: rel: (per kg) record: $\approx$60–80% over $\approx$60–80% $\approx$90% $\approx$60–80% over $\approx$50–80% $\approx$80% $\approx$50–80% over $\approx$50–80% $\approx$90% $\approx$60–80% over $\approx$60–80%	 100% 100% 100% 100%

Based on the results of studies by *Astrand, Bausenwein, Hettinger, Hoffmann, Hollmann, Klaus, Král, Mellerowicz, Nöcker, Reindell* and *Stoboy.*

long-endurance performance, both relatively speaking and absolutely. Results of studies by various authors on the relative muscular strength of women as compared with men vary between ≈60 and ≈80% (Hettinger; Ufland; Reijs; and Cullumbine et al.). According to Åstrand, the O_2 consumption of women as well as their other performance capacities is 25–30% less than those of men, but in relation to body weight they are only 15–20% less. Lehmann says that the maximal power capacity in women is 20–25% lower than in men. A systematic comparative survey of six specific factors and performance functions according to the results of studies by numerous authors is presented in Table 2.

Women's average ergometric power can be assumed to be ≈20–30% absolutely and ≈15–20% relatively lower than that of men.

7. Age and Power

Studies by Åstrand, Bengtsson, Mellerowicz and Lerche indicate that, on the average, the maximal steady-state power and recovery capacities in young people of both sexes ranging from 6 to 18 years of age increase roughly in proportion to body weight (Figs. 23, 24, 43). Bengtsson writes, "Both the increase of capacity from one weight group to another and the linear rela-

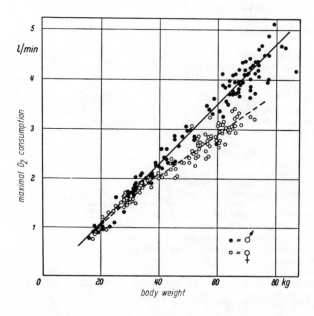

Fig. 23. Maximal O_2 consumption in men and women in relation to body weight.

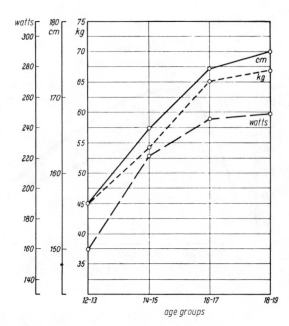

Fig. 24. Maximum three-minute performance capacity on the handcrank ergometer in 160 males aged 12–19 (after *Mellerowicz* and *Lerche*).

tion were just as regular as in the case of the older groups." Åstrand found in males aged 7 to 33 years an approximately equal maximal O_2 consumption per kilogram of body weight at all age levels: "For males the maximal O_2 consumption showed a high correlation with the body weight."

Up to age 9 or 10, young girls are—relatively (per kg of body weight)—approximately the equals of boys in power. However, their absolute endurance in both brief and protracted performances is somewhat less (Åstrand and Bach). From about age 13 or 14, the sex differentials in relative and absolute physical power increase up to age 18 or 19.

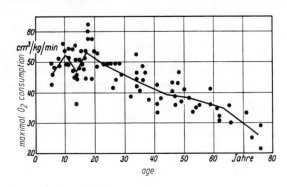

Fig. 25. Maximal O_2 consumption capacity per kg of body weight for males relative to age (after *Robinson*).

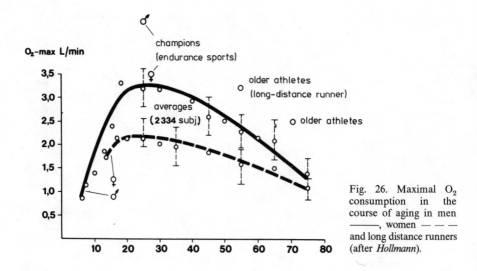

Fig. 26. Maximal O₂ consumption in the course of aging in men ———, women — — — and long distance runners (after *Hollmann*).

The highest achievements in strength and speed performance can be maintained only up to about age 30, but the endurance maxima can be maintained up to age 30–40, according to data now available. After that age, a progressive diminution in performance capacity sets in. However, considerable individual differences are found, depending on inherited constitution as well as life style and other exogenous influences. Robinson studied O_2 consumption in 95 untrained males of ages 6 to 91 (Fig. 25). A continuous diminution of relative O_2 consumption became evident from ages 25–30 on. Data for maximal O_2 consumption in 81 brewery employees aged 50–64, as reported by I. Åstrand, show good agreement with those of Robinson (Åstrand: 2.48 liters/min of O_2 for men 50 to 64; Robinson: 2.63 to 2.351 liters/min of O_2 for men 51 to 63). Figure 26, after Hollmann, shows in schematic form the age pattern for maximal O_2 consumption.

The decrease in maximal O_2 consumption and maximal endurance capacity with advancing years is caused by morphological aging processes in the vascular system, respiratory organs and skeletal musculature. Among important causative factors are the following:

1. Aging processes in the capillaries and the intercellular tissue between the capillaries and cells (Henry), which reduce O_2 permeability (Bürger, Ries) and probably the O_2 utilization
2. Age-induced atrophy of the myocardium and progressive sclerotic processes in the heart, coronaries, heart capillaries and the large vessels, leading to progressive diminution of power reserves and of maximal cardiac output

3. Decrease in vital capacity and maximal voluntary ventilation of the lungs with advancing years. Also, the O_2 consumption of inhaled air decreases in both maximal and submaximal power (Robinson)
4. Morphological aging processes of the alveolar membranes and alveolar capillaries may also cause decreased O_2 saturation of the blood in older individuals (Dill et al.; Robinson)
5. Progressive atrophy with aging in the skeletal musculature, which goes hand in hand with an increase in the amount of connective tissue (Botelho). With decreasing muscular mass, the maximal O_2 consumption must naturally also decrease.

Available data indicate that in consequence of these aging processes the range of power in ergometric studies is

at ages 20–30	to	100%
at age 40	to	≈80–90%
at age 50	to	≈75–80%
at age 60	to	≈70%
at age 70	to	≈60%

At equal chronological age, biological age can vary considerably. It is possible to maintain a higher performance level for a longer period, especially through exercise and healthful life style.

8.   State of Training and Ergometric Performance

Any performance is highly dependent on the state of training of the individual; this must be taken into consideration in evaluating ergometric results. Any diminution in performance can be the result of a more or less pronounced deterioration in training habits. Specific improvements in performance can be achieved through training in strength, speed, flexibility, endurance and coordination. In most forms of exercise, these are combined in various proportions. Any endurance training, especially, has the effect of increasing maximal ergometric steady-state power. Specialized training— e.g., bicycle racing—increases especially the power in ergometric foot pedaling while seated and reclining.

All training consists basically of the use of functional above-threshold practice stimuli of increasing intensity. These have morphological and functional effects on the organism, leading to increases in both general and particular performance capabilities.

The performance-heightening effects of training are dependent on:

1. Amount of exercise (intensity, duration and frequency)

2. Nature of the exercise (forms calculated to enhance strength, speed and endurance have different effects on the individual)
3. Endogenous factors (e.g., constitution, age and sex)
4. Exogenous factors (e.g., ambient temperature, diet, etc.).

Depending as they do on these controlling factors, all training effects are very complex. Functional exercise stimuli demand development and growth of the skeletal and muscular structure; in fact, the muscles are subject to hypertrophy from strength- and speed-oriented exercise. In various sports and motor activities the total motor apparatus adapts itself in particular ways and undergoes very special morphological, biochemical and physiological changes.

Many demonstrable effects of training, especially effects of protracted exercise, make possible an increased O_2 supply to the organism and the organs and tissues involved in the exercise. Not only the performance capacity, but also the health of the organism depends heavily on abundant O_2 supply.

The capillarity of exercised tissues is enhanced. Petrén et al. found in exercised skeletal muscles of experimental animals a 40 to 50% increase in the number of capillaries. The internal capillary surface area increases with exercise. The utilization of O_2 of the blood is consequently much greater in the exercising individual (>6 to 8% by volume). The O_2 supply and removal of metabolic end-products are thus improved. These are essential prerequisites for decreasing fatigue and increasing physical capacity in the trained organism. Training stimuli encourage erythropoiesis in the red marrow and increase the total number of red cells. The blood's O_2 transport capacity improves, especially in endurance training. The improved O_2 supply in the trained organism also serves to enhance the vital capacity of the lungs, to expand their maximal voluntary ventilation, respiratory economy and O_2 consumption of the inhaled air. Lack of training worsens the O_2 supply situation, impairs power and has a deleterious effect on health in general.

The exercised heart grows proportionally. A large athletic heart develops. Its musculature is strengthened. Its ventricles and atria expand commensurately. While the organism is at rest, the heart beats very slowly; it works very economically and has great power reserves (up to 35 liters/min cardiac output). It needs less O_2 for the same ergometric performance. Its maximal O_2 supply is, however, much increased. This training effect is of great importance for maintaining cardiac health.

Exercise on a regular prolonged basis—i.e., training—attunes the cardiovascular system to very economic high-gear operation. The trained heart in the trained organism needs to do considerably less work in the course of a day. Early wear and tear and abuse phenomena in the heart and vascular system are therefore not found in athletes and not even in heavy laborers, but rather in the sedentary, the office workers, intellectuals and the like. Lack of physical labor and exercise leads to small, underdeveloped, morbid "civilization hearts," such as are encountered in caged rabbits and other domestic animals living in enclosures. Such hearts operate on a very uneconomic basis. They are subject to great toil and stress in their daily work and their O_2 supply is curtailed.

Physical exercise also has pronounced effects on the endocrine glands. It brings about hypertrophy of the adrenal cortex, which plays an important role in determining performance capacity. It is probable that the comparatively small hypoplastic adrenal cortex of exercise-starved civilized man plays a causative role in curtailment of development, health and achievement. Training also enhances the regulatory potency of the vegetative system. This is especially demonstrable in the circulatory functions, which favor predominance of its economizing recuperative parasympathetic portion. In bradycardia and bradypnea, this exercise adaptation of the vegetative system becomes clearly evident.

These biological effects of training are prerequisite to any real enhancement of performance. They are also important in human bodily development and health. Because of these effects, training is one of the most effective measures in preventive and rehabilitative medicine.

Insufficient training (at less than a third of maximal power) leads to rapid loss of capacity. But too much exercise can also lead to loss of capacity and a negation of the beneficial effects of exercise. The same can happen, even with maintenance of a course of exercise, if there is an excess of stressful business and mental activity and upsetting trivia that interfere with the serenity of well-being. Early signs of excessive training fatigue are loss of the joy of living, of appetite and of sound sleep habits. Objectively there comes about an impairment of power despite more and more determined exercise, loss of weight, decreased metabolic economy, disturbances in the regulatory functions of the vascular system, and a tendency to extrasystoles and the like.

Regular ergometric testing allows:
1. Precise comparative evaluation of the state of training of the body and its performance
2. Comparison with the norms for one's age and sex groups
3. Early recognition of factors which reduce physical condition.

Regular and balanced exercise schedules also have rehabilitative effects on the abused organism favoring improved fitness, for example in cases of damage incurred by the heart, lungs, locomotor functions, etc. Comparative ergometric testing of one's performance makes it possible to prescribe exact dosages of exercise and control the success of a rehabilitative program.

9. Absolutely or Relatively Equivalent Performance as a Basis for Ergometric Comparison

Ergometric measurement of power at submaximal levels can be carried out either at absolutely equal powers or at relatively equal powers (such as one, two, or three watts per kg of body weight). Both are possible from a methodological standpoint. However, in comparative studies, the use of absolutely equal submaximal power levels is less satisfactory in the case of very small, light individuals and tall, heavy ones, and especially with children and teenagers at various stages of their development. A power of 100 watts ($\approx$10 kpm/s) represents relatively much greater exertion for a person weighing 50 kg than for a person of the same age weighing, say, 80 kg.

On the basis of presently available studies, there exist high correlations between performance capacity (Bengtsson), maximal O_2 consumption (Åstrand), HR under stress (Mellerowicz and Lerche; Dransfeld and Mellerowicz), and body weight. Additional governing factors to be considered are natural endowment, age and sex.

In most athletic sports and types of exercise, and also, for example, in knee-bending and stair-climbing activities, the individual has to lift his own body weight. The load-strength ratio and that of cardiac performance to body weight is crucial to maximal power production. For these reasons, for comparative ergometric studies at submaximal power levels, especially in children and teenagers and other persons weighing less than 50 or over 100 kg, the relatively equal power level based on body weight is preferable. However, the relative values can also be calculated when using absolutely equal submaximal power.

References

Åstrand, I.: Acta Physiol. Scand.: 42, (1958) 73.

Åstrand, P. O.: Acta physiol. Scand. 42, (1958) 73; Experimental studies of physical working capacity in relation to sex and age. Kopenhagen: Munksgaard, 1952.

Åstrand, P. O.: Progress in Ergometry. In: Ergebnisse der Ergometrie. Berlin: Ergon-Verlag, 1974.

Atzler, E., R. Herbst, G. Lehmann and E. A. Müller: Pflügers Arch. Physiol. 208, (1925) 212.

Bach, F.: Ergebnisse von Massenuntersuchungen über die sportliche Leistungsfähigkeit und das Wachstum Jugendlicher in Bayern. Frankfurt/Main: Limpert, 1955.

Bar-Or, O.: Arm ergometry vs. treadmill running and bicycle riding in men with different conditioning levels. In: 3. Internationales Seminar für Ergometrie. Berlin: Ergon-Verlag, 1973.

Bengtsson, E.: Acta med. Scand. II, (1956) 91.

Bolt, W., H. W. Knipping, H. Valentin and H. Venrath: in: Lehrbuch der Sportmedizin. Leipzig: Barth, 1956.

Botelho, S., L. Cander and N. Guiti: J. Appl. Physiol., Wash. 7, (1954) 93.

Bürger, M.: Altern und Krankheit, III. Aufl. Leipzig: Thieme, 1957.

Christensen, E. H.: after Nöcker: Grundriß der Biologie der Körperübungen. Berlin: Sportverlag, 1955.

Cullumbine, H., S. W. Bibile, T. W. Wikramanajake and R. S. Watson: J. Appl. Physiol., Wash. 2, (1950) 488.

Dill, D. B. et al.: Arbeitsphysiologie 4, (1931) 508.

Dransfeld, B. and H. Mellerowicz: Zschr. Kreisl.forschg. 48, (1959) 901.

Eckermann, P. and H. P. Millahn: Int. Z. angew. Physiol. 23, (1967) 340.

Ekelund, L.-G.: Rapid determination of work load at a heart rate of 170 beats/min with a heart-rate controlled ergometer. In: 3. Internationales Seminar für Ergometrie. Berlin: Ergon-Verlag, 1973.

Grosse-Lordemann, H.; and E. A. Müller: Arbeitsphysiologie 9, (1937) 119 and 454.

Hasse, A.: Arbeitsphysiologie 8, (1935) 455.

Henry, F. M.: The influence of the aging process on physiological ability to exercise. Gerontology Session, Amer. Acad. of Physical Education. Los Angeles, Calif., 1952.

Herxheimer, H.: Arbeitsphysiologie 7, (1933/34) 181; Grundriß der Sportmedizin. Leipzig: Thieme, 1933.

Hettinger, Th.: Arbeitsphysiologie 15, (1953) 201.

Hollmann, W., H. Valentin and H. Venrath: Münch. med. Wschr. 39, (1959) 1680.

Israel, S., D. Junker and D. Mickein: Sportarzt u. Sportmedizin 1, (1976) 272.

Komi, P. V.: A new electromechanical ergometer. In: 3. Internationales Seminar für Ergometrie. Berlin: Ergon-Verlag, 1973.

Kubicek, F.: Wien. klin. Wschr. 85, (1973) 1.

Lehmann, G. and H. Michaelis: Arbeitsphysiologie 11, (1941) 376.

Lehmann, G.: Praktische Arbeitsphysiologie. Stuttgart: Thieme, 1953.

Löllgen, H. and H.-V. Ulmer: Zum Problem der Tretgeschwindigkeit in der Ergometrie. In: 3. Internationales Seminar für Ergometrie. Berlin: Ergon-Verlag, 1973.

Mellerowicz, H. and B. Dransfeld: Arbeitsphysiologie 16, (1957) 464.

Mellerowicz, H. and L. Galle: Der Sportarzt 10, (1962) 332.

Mellerowicz, H. and D. Lerche: Zschr. Kinderhlk. 81, (1958) 36.

Mellerowicz, H. and W. Meller: Sportarzt u. Sportmedizin 12, (1967) 496.

Mellerowicz, H. and P. Nowacki: Zschr. Kreisl.forsch. 50, (1961) 1002.

Menzel, W.: Arbeitsphysiologie 14, (1950) 304.

Müller, E. A.: Arbeitsphysiologie 14, (1950) 271.

Nowacki, O. P.: Der Wirkungsgrad bei ergometrischer Leistung. In: Ergebnisse der Ergometrie. Berlin, Ergon-Verlag 1974.

Ogawa, K.: A new Japanese ergometer. In: 3. Internationales Seminar für Ergometrie. Berlin: Ergon-Verlag, 1973.

Petrén, T. et al.: Arbeitsphysiologie 9, (1936) 376.

Reijs, J.: Pflügers Arch. Physiol. 191, (1921) 234.

Ries, W.: Zschr. Altersforsch. 10, (1956) 153 and 160.

Robinson, S.: Arbeitsphysiologie 10, (1938) 251.

Schmidt, F. L.: Über den Einfluß der Umdrehungszahl auf verschiedene Parameter des kardio-pulmonalen Systems während Tretkurbelarbeit bei submaximaler Belastung. In: 2. Internationales Seminar für Ergometrie. Berlin: Ergon-Verlag, 1967.

Schochrin, W. A.: Arbeitsphysiologie 8, (1934) 251.

Schürsch, P. M., J. Hesch, M. D. Fotescu and W. Hollmann: Sportarzt u. Sportmedizin 1, (1976) 7.

Schwalb, H., P. Schwendemann: Der Einfluß der Übergewichtigkeit auf einige Parameter der kardialen und körperlichen Leistungsfähigkeit bei 20- bis 70jährigen Männern. In: 3. Internationales Seminar für Ergometrie. Berlin: Ergon-Verlag, 1973.

Selye, H.: Einführung in die Lehre vom Adaptionssyndrom. Stuttgart: Thieme, 1953.

Sjöstrand, T.: Acta physiol. Scand. 18, (1949) 324.

Skranc, O.: Vergleich der Leistungsfähigkeit von Männern und Frauen verschiedenen Alters. In: Ergebnisse der Ergometrie. Berlin: Ergon-Verlag, 1974.

Stegemann, J., H.-V. Ulmer and K. W. Heinrich: Z. angew. Physiol. 25, (1968) 224.

Ufland, J. M.: Arbeitsphysiologie 7, (1933) 251.

Ulmer, H.-W.: Zur Methodik, Standardisierung und Auswertung von Tests für die Prüfung der körperlichen Leistungsfähigkeit. Deutscher Ärzte-Verlag, Köln 1975.

Usami, M.: Erfahrungen mit einer ergometrischen Standardleistung von 1 Watt/kg Körpergewicht in Japan. In: 3. Internationales Seminar für Ergometrie. Berlin: Ergon-Verlag, 1973.

Valentin, H. and K. P. Holzhauser: Funktionsprüfungen von Herz u. Kreislauf. Deutscher Ärzte-Verlag FT. Nr. 17 Köln 1976.

Wezler, K. R., K. Thauer and K. Greven: Zschr. exper. Med. 107, (1940) 751.

Wolff, R.: Deutsche Zschr. Sportmed. 2, (1978) 52.

Wright, G.: Science 112, (1950) 423.

II. Technical Development of the Ergometer

1. Development of Mechanically Braked Ergometers

As early as 1883, Speck was using performance done with a crank in his studies on the physiology of exercise. He had seated subjects turn an iron crank, its friction being controlled by tightening or loosening a screw. By measuring this frictional resistance, Speck tried to calibrate this hand-cranking device. He hung weights of increasing mass on the horizontal crank axle until they began to sag. Although this procedure was simple and fundamentally exact, changes in the frictional resistance at various cranking speeds could not be pinpointed.

Zuntz, at the close of the last century, used Gärtner's "ergostat" for measuring human performance. This machine may be regarded as the forerunner of the present-day ergometer. A wheel, turned by the subject by means of a crank, was braked by a bar along which a weight could be slid. The amount of braking effect was in this device dependent on the size and position of the braking weight along the bar and the frictional resistance between the under surface of the bar and the top of the wheel. With this device, steady work of various intensities could be performed. However, the work and power could not be measured accurately. Katzenstein later attempted to calibrate Gärtner's ergostat more accurately with a spring scale.

In 1891, a very simple, practical, readily calibrated, mechanically braked ergometer was described by Fick. In this device, a braking strap was applied around the periphery of a wheel being turned by the patient. This strap was attached elastically to a second strap by means of a metal spring. When the wheel was turned, the straps braked its rotation. The braking effect was equal to the tension in the spring which in turn could be measured in meter-kilograms. In order to render the rotation of the wheel more uniform,

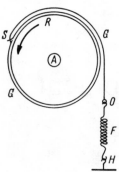

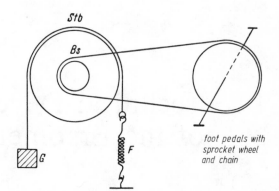

foot pedals with sprocket wheel and chain

Fig. 27. Fick's ergometer.   Fig. 28. Frictional bicycle ergometer (after *Holzer* and *Kalinka*).

Fick used a belt transmission to drive a flywheel at double the speed of the main wheel (Fig. 27).

Exercise done with the crank can be measured by multiplying the braking force (in kp) by the braking distance on the circumference of the wheel, which amounts to $2\pi r$ per full turn. The exercise performed in cranking equals kp · $2\pi r$.

The cranking power is the performance accomplished per unit of time (one second). For example, the cranking power in kpm/s at 30 rpm (revolutions per minute) equals:

$$\frac{kp \cdot 2\pi r \cdot 30}{60}$$

In this manner cranking performance and cranking power at constant speed can be calculated on Fick's simple ergometer. In basically this same way, performance and power can be calculated on any other ergometer, with minor differences in methodology. The performance can be varied on Fick's ergometer only by varying the speed of cranking. Here great differences between physically measured and actual biological performance can result if low or high speeds lie beyond the subject's economical range of speed of revolution.

In 1901, Johannson, in his studies on the formation of CO_2 in muscular activity, used a form of ergometer which made it possible to measure the exercise done and the performance in lifting, holding and lowering weights. The subject sat with his chest in contact with the machine and pulled, held or lowered weights of various mass by means of a pulley, using a handle sliding on a horizontal rail. The number of times the weight was moved, the total height traversed by the weights and the total elapsed time were recorded. A speed indicator permitted the setting of five different cranking speeds. With the aid of a spring scale, the frictional losses at various cranking speeds were ascertained and the ergometer was calibrated accordingly. The device was suitable for carrying out studies of these specialized forms of movement.

To measure physical exercise and performance, Fick's "work collector" has also been widely employed. By turning a hand crank, a weight is raised on a rope wound around the drum of a windlass. The considerable frictional losses in the bearings of the windlass, in the hand grips of the crank, and the friction of the rope against itself are difficult to pinpoint, however, and are not taken into account.

A simple frictional bicycle ergometer was constructed by Holzer and Kalinka and described in 1935 (Fig. 28). A steel band (Stb) was applied around the circumference of a brake disc (Bs) of Siemens-Martin steel substituted for the rear wheel of a bicycle. One end of the steel brake band was attached to the base plate by means of a spring scale (F). At its other end hung a counterweight (G), whose size could be varied according to the desired ergometric performance rating. When the subject turned the brake disc, a frictional force (R) worked on its circumference and was equal to the difference of the reading on the spring scale and the weight of the counterweight. At n revolutions per minute, the performance L amounted to:

$$L = 2\pi r \cdot \frac{n}{60} R$$

If a radius of $\frac{60}{2\pi} = 9.549$ is used, then

$$L = R \frac{n}{100}.$$

In this case, the authors reported the inherent frictional resistances (bearing friction and wind resistance in the bicycle) at various powers and pedaling speeds.

A simple, inexpensive frictional hand-crank ergometer constructed on the principle of the Prony bridle has been marketed by the Dargatz Co. (Fig. 29a). It is, however, difficult to maintain approximate uniformity of cranking speed and rpm, since the device has no flywheel and no revolution counter. This deficiency limits its practical usefulness.

An improved frictional ergometer was built by Fleisch. With it, it is possible to maintain a definite, constant braking effect, thanks to a special mechanical braking system. A speed regulator makes it easier for the subject to maintain a given pace in rpm and a particular power. Fleisch therefore referred to it as an "ergostat." This ergometer is calibrated with the aid of an electric dynamometer, and is simple in construction and operation. It is exclusively for use while seated, there being no possibility of operating it

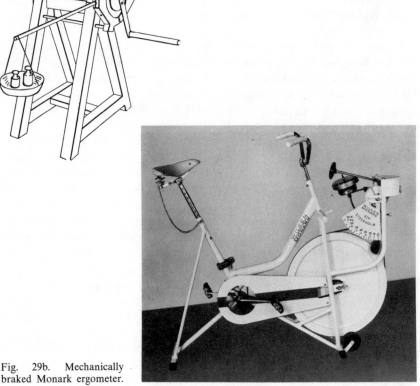

Fig. 29a. Dargatz frictional ergometer.

Fig. 29b. Mechanically braked Monark ergometer.

while standing or reclining. It can be set for only three different speeds: 30, 60 or 90 rpm. These speeds do not permit the subject to maintain an economical speed for all levels of power.

A mechanically braked ergometer which has proved practical for use in ergometric studies has been developed by Åstrand with the cooperation of Monark (bicycle manufacturers) of Stockholm (Figure 29b). It has a brake band in contact with the greater part of the periphery of the flywheel. This is attached to a pendulum balance at the axle of its oscillation system which consists of an oscillating drum, an oscillating beam and an oscillating weight. The pendulum hangs straight down when the machine is at rest and is displaced by the pull of the brake band when the machine is in operation. The displacement and thus the pulling force can be read on a scale calibrated in kiloponds and newtons.

A mechanically braked ergometer for use with foot pedaling while seated or reclining has been developed by Bosch, a German manufacturer, and this machine permits setting powers as small as 10 watts.

2. Development of the Electrodynamic Ergometer

A new development in the construction of medical devices for measuring physical power was introduced by Atwater and Benedict in 1903. They were the first to use a bicycle ergometer electrically braked by a small dynamo generator. They made the rear wheel of the bicycle turn the driving wheel of the generator, and read the current generated with an ammeter. In this contrivance, however, the inherent frictional resistances of the bicycle were ignored. Moreover, the mechanical contact between the rear wheel and the generator proved unreliable, especially at high pedaling speeds. This apparatus, therefore, still failed to read accurately the amount of exercise performed.

Benedict and Carpenter (1909), and Benedict and Cady (1912) replaced the rear wheel of the bicycle with a copper disc revolving between the two poles of an electromagnet. By varying the excitation current in the magnet, they controlled the braking effect of the eddy currents in the copper disc. By changing the rpm, registered on a revolution counter, and the braking current, the power level could be preset. Benedict's suggestion of calibrating his ergometer calorimetrically, however, was beset by considerable practical obstacles which militated against wider acceptance of this first eddy-current ergometer.

On the basis of Benedict's device, Krogh constructed (1913) an ergometer (Fig. 30) which could in practice be satisfactorily calibrated. He left the electromagnet free to revolve about the axis of the copper disc. As the disc revolved, the electromagnet moved with it in the same direction. The force of the induced co-revolution was measured by counterweights which just prevented corevolution of the electromagnets. Not measured along with these were frictional losses in the crank, the transmission and the axle of the disc. Variations in the house current led to aberrations in the braking power. However, when these were eliminated and the losses in efficiency were measured and accounted for, Krogh's ergometer was capable of high accuracy in measuring power.

In 1928, Knipping described an ergometer which consisted of a transmission for 0 to 100 rpm with a hand crank and adjustable handle, a wheel for foot pedaling while reclining, a DC-shunt generator, a field regulator (up to

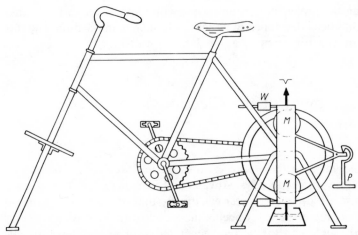

Fig. 30. Krogh's eddy-current bicycle ergometer. MM are the two freely revolving electromagnets. P is the weight pan, whose own weight can be counterbalanced by the counterweights W. To damp vibrations of the frame supporting the scales and electromagnets during operation of the bicycle, a vertical hydraulic plunger attached to its lower extremity works in a chamber filled with a high-viscosity fluid. The work represented by one revolution (disregarding friction) equals x kpm · 2πr. To facilitate calculation, the distance from the axle to the fulcrum of the scales is 1/π or 0.3183 m, making the work function 2x kpm. Exercise and performance can thus easily be found.

5 amps) with ammeter for reading the field current, a load resistance in series for canceling out the power, a wattmeter or voltmeter and ammeter, and a revolution counter. The number of revolutions and of watts could be indicated on a running basis during the exercise with the aid of a revolution recorder or a drop-gimbal wattage recorder. By varying the field current, the load resistance and the rpm, any desired performance level up to 1.5HP (metric) could be set. The wiring diagram is shown in Figure 31.

In 1934, Kelso and Hillebrandt described an electrodynamic bicycle ergometer. The armature of the generator was turned directly by the pedals through a chain drive. A 12v storage battery independently supplied the field current. In the secondary circuit derived from the armature were a resistance and a voltmeter for measuring the current induced by the bicycle exercise. The apparatus was calibrated in such a way as to take into account the frictional resistance.

Grosse-Lordemann and E. A. Müller published in 1936 the description of a bicycle ergometer which monitored the maintenance of a certain constant power level and pedal rpm. The rear wheel rolled on a belt running on two rollers which could be driven by a three-phase electric motor. A transmission permitted infinitely variable regulation of the belt speed between 0 and

48 km/h. The weight of the rear wheel was supported by eight rollers arranged under the belt on which the wheel turned. The front wheel was fixed in a carriage movable on casters. On the carriage was attached a contact shoe with six laminations connected to a corresponding series of lights. This arrangement permitted the subject to keep the bicycle and carriage in situ, thus assuring a constant power level. When the subject began to pedal the bicycle, he delivered an added output at the preset, constant belt speed and motor output. Since a three-phase motor has the property of keeping its rpm very nearly constant with varying power, it automatically reduces its power output until the sum of the power output of the motor and that of the subject have adapted themselves to the power required for the desired pulley speed. The power is measured by measuring the roller resistance at a particular belt speed. Monitoring with a measuring motor mounted on the bicycle at various pedaling speeds gave relatively great deviations (up to 15%) from the indicated power readings, however; for ergometric studies, greater accuracy than this and less cumbersome apparatus are required. At high power rates and low pedal speeds, furthermore, the frictional contact between the rear wheel and the belt proved unsatisfactory.

E. A. Müller in 1940, using the Prony principle and the slight variation in the rpm of a three-phase motor at varied power levels, described a hand-crank and foot-pedal ergometer that was a considerable improvement both in construction and precision and which forced the subject to maintain a given cranking speed and a given exercise level per revolution.

The construction, calibration and use of a bicycle-generator ergometer, modified from that of Kelso and Hellebrandt, were described in 1945 by

Fig. 31. Wiring diagram of the Knipping dynamo ergometer of 1928. The field current from the line is fed to the generator at binding posts A and B. Cut into the field current are the field regulator at S and T and an ammeter. The current generated by the subject is fed in at A and B. The load on the generator can be controlled by a variable resistance at R and L. The wattage or kpm/s of physical power from the subject cannot, however, be read directly with this apparatus, but must be worked out by means of the following formula, which has been arrived at empirically:

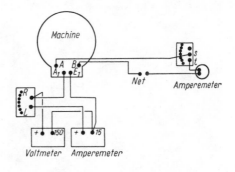

$$L = J \cdot E J^2 \cdot 3.1 + 2.J + \text{friction loss} + \text{iron loss}$$

The value $J \cdot E/100$ corresponds to the additional losses in the machine; $J^2 \cdot 3.1$ are copper and heat losses; J^2 brush losses. Frictional losses and iron losses can be obtained from a chart. The percentage of error in measurement and calculation of power is given as $<1\%$. The formula and the chart do not make allowance for variations in frictional resistance arising at various performance levels or from progressive wear and tear during the life of the ergometer.

Tuttle and Wendler. In place of the 12-volt battery, they used house current at 110 volts AC, a rectifier unit and a transformer. The voltage produced by exercise on the part of the subject was continuously recorded graphically. From the voltage curve and the calibration curve of the ergometer, it was possible to read at any given moment the amount of exercise being done at each phase of a non-uniform exercise.

Holmgren and Mattsson (1954) built a bicycle ergometer which made it possible to maintain a given power level independently of the cranking speed. The braking resistance was provided by a DC generator with outside magnetization. The generator was controlled by a regulator and delivered its output to a ballast resistance. The regulator was regulated by rpm and turning moment in such a way that the product of braking effect times rpm was kept constant at varying speeds. This was accomplished by conducting the voltage differences between a reference voltmeter and the generator voltage to an electronic intensifier. The greater the voltage difference at increased

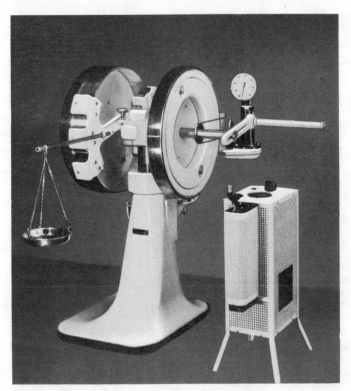

Fig. 32. The Dargatz eddy-current ergometer, type 171.

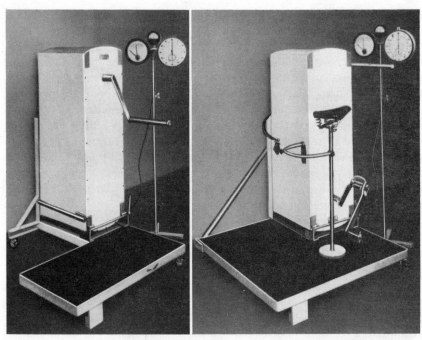

Fig. 33a. Universal ergometer (after Lauckner) with power regulation either dependent on or independent of cranking speed.

Fig. 33b. The hand crank can be replaced with foot pedals by turning the ergometer housing 180°.

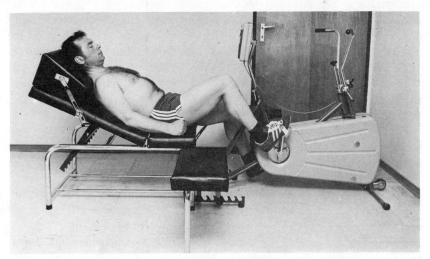

Fig. 33c. Foot-pedaling exercise while reclining with a bicycle ergometer (Bosch ERG 301, with mechanical braking and electronic measurement). This type of machine is adapted for measuring arterial pressure and for the use of invasive methods.

rpm, the further the field current of the generator was diminished. The voltage difference between voltmeter and generator was thus regulated to 0. Calibration was achieved with the aid of a calibrating pendulum generator, taking into account the mechanical frictional resistances.

The Dargatz Co. developed a transmissionless crank ergometer without sprocket and chain, usable for either hand cranking or foot pedaling while reclining. Any power level can be coordinated with any desired cranking speed. Frictional losses on the axle with its two ball bearings are not accounted for in its calibration, but are minimal. Eddy-current braking and ergometer power can be monitored at any time on the Prony bridle. The device has a large gearless flywheel. The absence of gearing and the large, slow-moving flywheel assure greater continuous precision but do call for relatively massive construction (Fig. 32).

The Lannoy ergometer (1956) (Lode Co., Oosterstraat 38, Groningen, Netherlands), which is suitable for cranking exercise while standing, sitting, or reclining, employs a special form of eddy-current braking. It permits the maintenance of constant power at varied cranking speeds.

Lauckner's Universal ergometer (Franzke, Ritterfelddamm 105, Berlin, Germany), is a very simple and practical dynamo ergometer with outside current excitation, suitable for cranking while standing, sitting, or reclining. The wattage (or kpm/s) achieved can be read directly from the meter. A built-in revolution counter enables the average power per minute to be read from the calibration curve even when the subject does not exercise at a perfectly uniform rate. The three stages of resistance in the ergometer are appropriate to the most common range of power levels and economical cranking speeds. The power level, which increases along with the cranking speed, is ergometrically practical, since the economical cranking speed increases along with performance level. Since the ergometer is attuned to three fixed resistances, it is possible in the calibration curve and meter dial to account with precision for all frictional losses. The apparatus is also available with power regulation independent of cranking speed (Figs. 33a, b and c).

The Jäger Co. (Röntgenring 5, Würzburg, Germany) manufactures a universal ergometer called the Ergotest, which offers infinitely variable regulation of power level, either independent of or dependent on cranking speed.

A special bicycle ergometer (after E. A. Müller) permits an increase in power levels by increments of 1 kpm/s for determination of the performance pulse index. It shows the increase in the performance HR which accompanies an increase in power of 1 kpm/s (see p. 84, Fig. 61).

During the last decade various manufacturers (Siemens, Hellige, Jäger, etc.) have offered the medical profession electromagnetically braked ergometers intended for foot pedaling while seated or reclining.

3. Medical and Technological Requirements in Ergometry

Today several practical and useful ergometers are on the market. Friction ergometers, dynamo ergometers and eddy-current ergometers can be produced, all fairly equal in quality. All possible advantages and disadvantages for use in practical and scientific ergometry should be considered. Further improvements in construction and refinements in the methodology of ergometric examination are still possible, provided all the following medical and technological points are taken into account:

1. The ergometer should be suitable for foot pedaling while seated and reclining and if possible also for hand cranking while standing. Conversion of the machine from one use to the other must be easy and quick.
2. The ergometer must include the following measuring equipment:
   a) Devices for measuring power level, reading directly in kpm/s or watts
   b) A speed counter showing rpm at any given moment
   c) Counters to record each individual full revolution, the total number of complete strokes for individual time periods, and the total elapsed time for the work
   d) For scientific purposes, it must be possible to record power and number of strokes at any given moment.
3. Any power level from 0 to 500 watts must be performed at an economical cranking speed. For special scientific purposes, types of construction may be required which permit any power rate to be preset at any physically possible speed.
4. The product of the flywheel mass and its speed of revolution (i.e., its angular momentum) must be kept as great as possible but at the same time the structure of the ergometer must not become too massive and the unavoidable frictional resistance must not be excessive. The greater the angular momentum of the flywheel, the easier it is to maintain a uniform speed of performance. A standardization of the flywheel mass is necessary because physical and biological power levels differ with differences in flywheel mass (see Chapter III, 1.4).
5. In addition, an electrical control should be included to hold constant the product of electrodynamic braking effect times cranking speed. Such a control would increase the braking effect as the rpm count falls and reduce it as the rpm rises. Such a device is necessary for fine adjustment of constant power. It would also enable subjects who can not maintain a uniform rpm to perform at a set level.
6. It is advisable to standardize the height of the cranking axle from the floor at one meter. This height is practical for short, medium and tall

individuals and even for children down to the age of 10 without undue effect on their output efficiency. Comparative studies using subjects of various statures at equal power exercising at crank heights ranging from 80 to 120 cm produced no significant differences in the total HR. Provision for altering the crank height may be required for special scientific purposes. The seat height must be adjustable.

7. On the basis of studies by Atzler, Herbst, Lehmann and Mellerowicz, a standard crank length of 1/3 meter (33.3 cm) appears to be best. It fits short, medium and tall persons and teenagers from 12 to 18 at the levels of power normally encountered in practice. For special scientific purposes, the crank length must be adjustable, as optimal crank length is directly proportional to exertion and stature. For pedals, a double crank length of 33.3 cm is also suitable.

8. The calibration of the ergometer can be achieved most practically with the aid of a Prony bridle or a calibrating dynamo in the reciprocal work procedure, taking into account all frictional resistances. More precise, though more difficult, is the calibration procedure that uses the Deprez balance (see textbooks on physics).

9. Frictional resistances in the bearings should be kept to a minimum and should vary as little as possible during a particular exercise. The ergometer should operate quietly enough to allow auditory monitoring of HR and blood pressure during performance. Power transmission should involve as little use of sprocket chains as possible. Inclusion of freewheeling of the crank is a practical feature. When using house current, it is necessary to include a device to compensate for possible voltage fluctuations, and differences in the standard voltages available in different localities must be taken into account.

10. The complete ergometer must be as light and portable as possible, yet heavy enough for steadiness at higher levels of power.

4.   Calibrating the Ergometer

1. In mechanically braked ergometers, work and power level can be calculated from:
   a) The braking force, which can be measured in kp with calibrated spring balances
   b) The braking distance on the periphery of the wheel, which in one revolution amounts to $2\pi r$
   c) The revolutions per minute, for calibration of the braking distance per second.

Accordingly, the measurements necessary for calibration are (per revolution):

cranking exercise (kpm) = kp (braking force) · $2\pi r$

cranking performance (kpm/s) = kp (braking force) · $2\pi r \cdot \dfrac{rpm}{60\ sec}$.

These do not account for friction in the bearings and the handles or pedals, being only measurements of net work and power output. Therefore, the frictional losses in the bearings must be measured additionally if precision calibration of various rpm and braking forces is required (see below).

2. In calibrating *electrodynamic ergometers,* the same basic methods are used as with mechanical braking. In measuring the power level and calibrating it, a Prony bridle is used with a brake band applied around an extension of the shaft (or as the case may be, a brake disc mounted on the shaft) (Fig. 34). The friction of the brake band on the turning brake disc or shaft creates a turning moment which can be measured by means of the scales attached to the lever arm of the Prony bridle. From braking force, breaking distance and rpm, exercise and amount of energy expended can be calculated according to the same formulae used with mechanically braked ergometers (see above), and the measured values can be used for calibration.

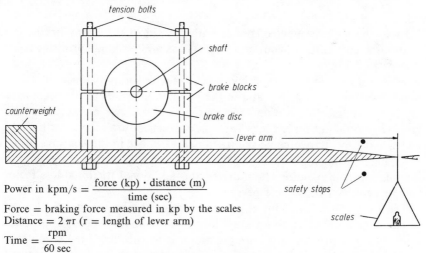

Power in kpm/s = $\dfrac{\text{force (kp)} \cdot \text{distance (m)}}{\text{time (sec)}}$

Force = braking force measured in kp by the scales

Distance = $2\pi r$ (r = length of lever arm)

Time = $\dfrac{rpm}{60\ sec}$

With a lever arm 95.5 cm long, the following formula applies:

power (in kpm/s) = $\dfrac{kp \cdot rpm}{60\ sec}$

With a lever arm 97.4 cm long, the formula is:

power (watts) = kp · rpm

Fig. 34. Dynamometer on the principle of the Prony bridle for calibrating electrodynamically braked ergometers.

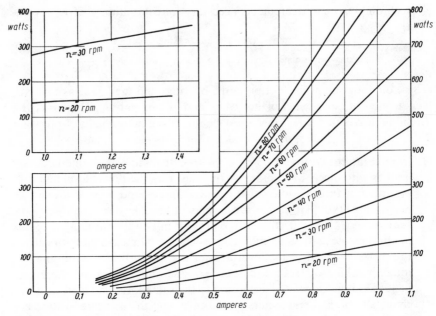

Fig. 35. Calibration curves for the Dargatz ergometer, type 171.

From the measurement of power with the aid of the Prony bridle, the calibration curves for various cranking speeds and braking currents can be drawn (Fig. 35).

When calibrating with the Prony bridle, as with spring balances, the frictional losses in the bearings and in the handles or pedals of the ergometer are not included. In addition to the amount of exercise measured on the ergometer (braking force times $2\pi r$), the subject must also put forth slight additional effort to overcome the frictional resistance in the bearings of the machine. By using high-quality bearings, keeping the number of bearings to a minimum and avoiding chain drives, this additional frictional loss factor can be kept well below one percent.

The total of frictional losses in the bearings can be ascertained by the so-called reverse exercise procedure for various cranking speeds and power rates. For this purpose, a calibrating motor is used to drive the ergometer. The frictional losses are equal to the difference between the performances of the calibrating motor and of the ergometer. As a matter of principle, they are to be taken into account in the calibration curve of the ergometer if they amount to more than one per cent.

The frictional resistance in the ergometer can be measured directly using the methods given by Wereschtschagin in 1930, in which calculations are made on the basis of the retardation of the free fall of various weights. The delay in the free fall of a weight is directly proportional to the frictional resistance in the apparatus.

Holzer and Kalinka determined the inherent frictional resistance in the ergometer from a curve starting with free turning at a given rpm. The curve, which can be recorded on a kymograph, is determined by the magnitude of the frictional resistances. From its shape it is possible to calculate the frictional forces.

However, it must not be overlooked that the frictional resistance in the bearings when the ergometer is under load are greater than when it is running free at the same rpm. It is not possible to ascertain this difference by either the Wereschtschagin or the Holzer-Kalinka procedure. Calibration of an ergometer to include its inherent frictional resistances, varying from load to load and rpm to rpm, can be achieved most efficiently with the aid of the calibration motor.

The calibration of an ergometer must at all times be readily supervised. It must be checked at frequent intervals and this must invariably be done before any scientific studies.

References

Atwater, W. and F. G. Benedict: U.S. Dept. Agr. Office Exp. Sta. Bull. 136 (1903).

Benedict, F. G. and T. M. Carpenter: U.S. Dept. Agr. Office Exp. Sta. Bull. 208 (1909).

Benedict, F. G. and W. G. Cady: Carnegie Inst. Washington, Pub. No. 167 (1912).

Blasius, W.: Med.-Markt. 412, (1957) 11.

Fick, A.: Pflügers Arch. Physiol. 50, (1891) 189.

Fleisch, A.: Pflügers Arch. Physiol. 212, (1936) 81.

Gärtner: after Fick and Katzenstein.

Große-Lordemann, H. and E. A. Müller: Arbeitsphysiologie 9, (1937) 454.

Holmgren, A. and K. H. Mattsson: Scand. J. Clin. Laborat. Invest. 6, (1954) 2.

Holzer, W. and N. Kalinka: Arbeitsphysiologie 9, (1936) 778.

Johannson, J. E.: Skand. Arch. Physiol. 11, (1901) 273.

Katzenstein, G.: Pflügers Arch. Physiol. 49 (1891) 330.

Kelso, L. A. E. and F. A. Hellebrandt: J. Laborat, Clin. Med. 19, (1934) 1105.

Knipping, H. W.: Zschr. exper. Med. 66, (1929) 517.

Krogh, A.: Skand. Arch. Physiol. 30, (1913) 375.

Mellerowicz, H. and P. Nowacki: Zeitschrift für Kreislaufforschung 50, (1961) 1002.

Müller, E. A.: Arbeitsphysiologie 14, (1950) 271; Radmarkt 4, (1952) 514.

Speck, M.: Dtsch. Arch. klin. Med. 45, (1889) 461.

Tuttle, W. and A. J. Wendler: J. Laborat. Clin. Med. 301, (1945) 173.

Wereschtschagin, N. K.: Arbeitsphysiologie 2, (1930) 427.

Zuntz, N.: Pflügers Arch. Physiol. 42, (1889) 189.

III. Suggestions for Standardization of the Ergometric Measurement of Performance

At equal physical power on the ergometer, biological performance may vary depending on numerous factors (type of cranking work, cranking radius, height of the crank above the floor, mass of the flywheel, exogenous factors, etc.). In order to achieve comparability of data obtained on the ergometer, standardization in methodology is essential.

At the meeting of the International Council of Sports Medicine and Physical Education (ICSPE) Research Committee for International Standardization in Ergometry during the 16th World Congress on Sports Medicine in Hannover, Germany, June 14, 1966, the following compromise proposals were accepted:

1. ICSPE Agreements

1.1 Type of Ergometer Exercise

For ergometric measurement, foot pedaling while seated is employed, or if preferred, foot pedaling while recumbent or hand cranking while standing.

Conversion values based on comparative studies of these three different types of ergometric work have been established (see pp. 12-15).

1.2 Crank Length

A double foot-pedal crank length and a single hand-crank length of 33.3 cm is suggested as standard.

This crank length favors the most common power levels of from 3 to 30 kpm/s on the part of short, medium as well as tall persons, with relatively minor resultant differences in efficiency.

For special purposes, however, adjustable-radius cranks may be employed.

1.3 Height of Cranking Axis from the Floor

The standard height of the cranking axis for hand cranking while standing shall be one meter.

Varying the crank height from 80 to 120 cm has a relatively slight effect on the exercise and resting HR at equal, average exertion rates of 10 kpm/s and equal crank lengths of 33.3 cm.

In foot pedaling, the seat height shall be adjustable to such an extent that when the pedal is at its lowest point, the foot forms an angle of from 90° to 120° with the shin.

1.4 Flywheel (Rotating mass)

In order to ensure completely uniform ergometric exercise, the flywheel shall be as large as possible without making the exercise too strenuous. For standardization purposes, the following specifications are suggested by available ergometric data and personal experience: a round flywheel weighing 100 kg with a radius of 33.3 cm, flywheel and ergometer both turning at the same rpm. Flywheels of smaller radius and weight may be used but there must be a correspondingly higher rpm and the same kinetic energy.

1.5 Revolutions per Minute (rpm)

For various ergometric powers, the following rpm are suggested:

0–10 kpm/s	30 (25–35) rpm
10–20 kpm/s	40 (35–45) rpm
20–30 kpm/s	50 (45–55) rpm
>30 kpm/s	60 (55–65) rpm

For practical reasons, it is not possible to select one optimal rpm for all individuals and all power levels. It seems satisfactory for practical purposes to stick to a range of 25 to 50 rpm at the usual power levels of 3 to 30 kpm/s. The ICSPE suggestions as of 1965 on rpm for ergometry are based chiefly on measurements made with hand cranking while standing. Studies by Wolf (1978) gave somewhat higher optimal rpm for foot pedaling while seated:

5 kpm/s	40 rpm
10 kpm/s	$\approx$40–50 rpm
15 kpm/s	$\approx$50–60 rpm
20 kpm/s	$\approx$55–65 rpm
>25 kpm/s	>65 rpm

Wolf's figures agree quite well with data from Grosse-Lordemann and E. A. Müller; Hess; Eckermann and Millahn; and F. L. Schmidt.

For ergometric foot-pedaling exercise in the maximal range, higher speeds (ranging up to 60 to 90 ($\pm$10) rpm) can be used for subjects of various strengths and degrees of training, regardless of the optima (see Chapter I, 3.1).

Since biological efficiency at a given power varies with rpm, it is not possible to choose just any rpm for an ergometric study.

Taking into account the available study data and personal experience, the following rpm might be suggested for ergometric measurements with foot-pedaling exercise.

At submaximal powers: 50 ($\pm$10) rpm
At maximal powers: 60–90 ($\pm$10) rpm
($> -2\sigma$ of HR max; $\sigma =$ standard deviation)

The rpm (ideal as well as actual value) should be given in the data report of the study (in agreement with Israel, Hollmann, Hüllermann, Keul, Kubisek, Valentin, Waterloh, et al.).

2. Metabolic Requirements in Ergometric Examinations

a) Diet should be altered as little as possible prior to the day of the test. On the day of the test, a small carbohydrate meal is permissible at least three hours before the test itself (two slices of bread and butter, and one glass of a beverage such as water, fruit juice, or milk).

b) On the day before the test, heavy mental and physical exertion should be avoided, and on the day of the test even slight physical or other stresses should be ruled out, because they can alter the performance metabolism in ergometric tests.

c) The testing program should be explained to the subject in advance. He should be reassured as much as possible. External stimuli such as noise, drafts, sight of heavy street traffic and the presence of superfluous by-standers should, insofar as possible, be eliminated.

d) Before starting the test, the subject should relax for at least ten minutes seated or—better—lying down.

e) Room temperature should be as close as possible to 18-22°C (not under 16° nor over 24°C), with a relative humidity of not over 60%. At higher temperatures and humidities respective correction factors are necessary. Ergometric testing should be avoided if possible on hot, humid days.

f) For thermoregulatory reasons, only shorts should be worn during the test.

g) All medication and all stimulants such as coffee, tea, tobacco and alcohol, are to be avoided on the day of the test, and medications having a prolonged effect should be discontinued even on preceding days. Any indispensable medication must be mentioned on the test report.

h) The time of day of the ergometric test is to be reported. Any repetition of tests for comparative or corroborative purposes should take place at the same time of day if possible, since functional performance changes as the day progresses.

i) Any uncommon circumstances are to be entered on the test report.

Research Committee of the ICSPE for International Ergometric Standardization, Berlin, 1967.

3.   Power Increments in Ergometric Studies

a) Power increments of 5, 10 or 25 watts are desirable when working with patients, starting at 25, 30, or 50 watts.

b) With subjects in whom an average performance capacity is to be expected, start at 50 watts. In female subjects, the power should increase 25 watts every two minutes: e.g., 50, 75, 100 watts. In male subjects, 50-watt increments may be used from the outset, but on approaching the limits of performance capacity the changes should be held to 25 watts, e.g., 50, 100, 125 or 50, 100, 150, 175 watts, etc.

c) In individuals of either sex in whom great endurance in power is anticipated, a starting level of 100 watts may be used, with subsequent increments of 50 watts each, or in the case of very powerful individuals, 100 watts each from the start, e.g., 100, 150, 200, or 100, 200, 250, 300 watts. On approaching the limits of performance capacity, however, the increments should be held to 25 watts.

Use at least three power levels with all subjects. The final power should lie in the border range of attainable power under the prevailing conditions (see below).

If tests on the same individual are planned as a follow-up, e.g., before and after a training period, or before and after cardiac surgery, the same power should be used both times for comparability.

4. The Duration of Individual Power Increments

The power increments should last as long as necessary but yet be as brief as possible. Exercises lasting one or two minutes are generally sufficient for increments of 10 or 25 watts, three to six minutes being necessary with 50 or 100 watt increments.

In the case of comparative determinations of the pulse working capacity 170 (PWC_{170}; see Chapter XX, 5.2) on 65 subjects, with increments of 10 watts for one minute, 25 watts for two minutes, 1 watt/kg for three minutes, and 50 watts for six minutes, no clear-cut differences became apparent according to Franz and Chintanaseri. The maximal differences in the averages amounted to 4%.

5. Determination of Maximal Values in Measuring Ergometric Performance

It is suggested that in determining maximal ergometric power, increments of 25 watts and one minute duration or 50 watts and two minutes duration generally be used. To get the maximal values, increments of 25 and 50 watts lasting three minutes or more, requiring increasing time and exertion, are not necessary for healthy, robust individuals (Maidorn and Mellerowicz). The total duration of all the exertion stages must last to from six to twelve minutes. For subjects or patients of sharply reduced fitness, increments as low as 10 watts for one minute or 25 watts for two minutes may be necessary.

5.1 Criteria of "vita maxima" conditions

a) The HR must exceed the -2σ threshold of the maximal values compatible with age. The following HR can be considered valid for healthy persons as criteria for maximal stress according to available experimental data:

Subject's age (years)	HR/min
10–20	200–180
20–30	170
30–40	160
40–50	150
50–60	140
60–70	130

b) The respiratory quotient should attain or exceed a value of approximately one.

c) The respiratory equivalent, $\dfrac{\text{RMV (BTPS)}}{\text{O}_2 \text{ (STPD)}}$, should exceed the -2σ threshold of maximal value compatible with age (RMV = respiratory minute-volume).

d) The lactate level and the pH must exceed certain threshold values that are yet to be defined and agreed upon (lactate $> \approx 7$ mmol/1; pH ≈ 7.2).

6. Criteria of Quality in Ergometry

Observance of the following criteria must be required if ergometry is to be a scientific method of measurement:

a) The mechanical and methodological margin of error in ergometric measurement should be held within a range of $\pm 2\%$ if possible and must never exceed $\pm 5\%$. This demands precise and repeated calibration of apparatus as well as careful attention to the methodology of measuring.

b) The reproducibility of the data must be highly reliable. For test-and-retest reliability, deviations of $\pm 2\%$ are tolerable, more than $\pm 5\%$ unacceptable. In checking reproducibility in double or (better) multiple tests, the conditions of exercise metabolism (see Chapter III, 2) must be precisely maintained. The retests are to be performed insofar as possible at the same times of day and under the same exogenous and endogenous conditions.

c) The ergometric data should be highly comparable; i.e., comparability must be at least above 95 and if possible exceed 98%. To this end, it is necessary that:

1. Standard ergometers be employed, having flywheels of equal weight, equal crank radius, and equal crank height (see Chapter III, 1)

2. Equal rpm be maintained within a range of not over ±10
3. Equal methodological standards be observed as to power and duration of performance levels.

The comparability of measurement methods is to be tested in double or multiple test-and-retest experiments with the same subjects under the same exogenous and endogenous conditions.

d) High validity is to be demanded of ergometric measurements; the ergometric data must coincide with or at least be representative with great accuracy of the ostensible corporeal (e.g., cardiac or pulmonary) function. The validity of an ergometric testing is high if, for example, the maximal cardiac pressure and volume performance is to be determined through measurement of arterial pressure and cardiac output at top ergometric exertion. The validity is low if the avowed goal is to determine the vitality of cardiac performance through measurement of maximal O_2 consumption.

e) The ergometric results are to be objective; i.e., they must not be subjectively altered by the examining party or any others present on the occasion of the test.

f) Economic principles are to be observed in ergometric measurement; i.e., the tests should be performed with the least possible expenditure of time and wear-and-tear on apparatus. It is irrational and unnecessarily time-consuming to take, for example, 24 minutes (e.g., four stages at 25 watts of six minutes duration) if comparable, reproducible and valid data are obtainable in eight minutes (e.g., four stages at 25 watts of two minutes duration). It is inexcusably wasteful to use high-cost (thousands of dollars) apparatus for certain routine ergometric studies if the same results can be obtained on apparatus costing less than a tenth as much. Regarding waste of time and machinery in ergometry, the motto should be "as little as possible but as much as necessary."

References

Eckermann, P. and H. P. Millahn: Int. Z. angew. Physiol. 23, (1967) 340.

Franz, I. and Ch. Chintanaseri: Sportarzt und Sportmedizin 2, (1977) 35.

Grosse-Lordemann, H. and E. A. Müller: Arbeitsphysiol. 9, (1937) 119+454.

Hess, P. and J. Seusing: Int. Z. angew. Physiol. 19, (1963) 468.

Larson, L. A.: Fitness, Health, and Work Capacity: International Committee for the Standardization of Physical Fitness Tests. New York: Macmillan Publishing Co., Inc., 1974.

Maidorn, K. and H. Mellerowicz: Der Sportarzt 11, (1962) 355.

Schmidt, F. L.: Sportarzt und Sportmedizin 19, (1968) 354.

Wolff, R.: Deutsche Zschr. Sportmed. 2, (1978) 52.

IV. Measurement and Evaluation of Maximal Ergometric Power

1. Measurement

The measurement of maximal power of various durations is the simplest ergometric method, but it demands great stress and considerable willpower on the part of the subject. Therefore, it is often not applicable (for example, in compensation cases).

Experience teaches that in addition to the less essential one-minute maximal power test, the three- and six-minute maximal power tests are well-suited for standardization. These are the approximate equivalents of the 400-, 1000-, and 2000-meter dashes. Briefer tests tell us less about the performance of organs, especially the vascular and respiratory systems. Performances of longer duration are for practical reasons less feasible.

The maximal endurance power is dependent on the maintenance of as uniform a power production as possible. In male subjects of average age and of about average performance capability, the standard power is set at 4 watts per kg for the three-minute test and 3.3 watts per kg for the six-minute test. In older persons the effect of age on performance capacity must be taken into consideration and a correspondingly lower standard must be set (see Chapter I, 7). In a pathological case with obviously reduced ability, it is necessary to estimate a power standard.

The patient is asked at first to maintain the standard power level for one or two minutes, and then to increase the rpm and power level as far as possible, or, if despite maximum effort it proves impossible to keep this up, to slack off gradually. Since, however, the optimal rpm is greater at maximal than at submaximal power, the resistance for the expected power must be preset for about 40–60 rpm in hand cranking and 60–90 for foot pedaling.

In a brief preliminary experiment, hints can be given pointing toward the most efficient technique of motion. Here we must pay particular attention to the optimal use of leg, hip and body muscles in hand cranking. Errors in motion technique which obviously reduce performance levels can be corrected even during the exercise. During the exercise, the HR should be measured in order to be able to judge the degree of exertion on the part of the patient.

This method is indicated:

a) In healthy individuals with a will to perform, especially athletes. In the course of repeated tests, the results afford a comparative evaluation of the performance capacity and current physical condition.
b) In persons with permanent organ damage who will not be harmed by maximal effort.
c) In persons with purely functional defects.

This method is contraindicated:

a) In patients who may be harmed by maximal effort. This is especially true of those suffering from acute and chronic conditions still developing or who show advanced degenerative age-changes in the vascular system.
b) For people who cannot or do not want to perform maximal physical effort. In this group belong many compensation cases in which the subject is interested in demonstrating his inability to work. Also, people who have become unaccustomed to physical exercise apparently may become incapable of mustering up their reserve energy to a sufficient degree.

A relatively simple and very reliable way of checking up on performance in such cases is afforded by measuring the HR during or immediately after the exercise. On the basis of available data and experience, a HR of 170 to 200 in subjects 20–30 years old indicates a maximal effort. A HR below 170 does not permit us to assume maximal effort. There are exceptions in the

Table 3. Absolute and relative maximal power in 1-, 3-, and 6-minute maximum tests on the hand-crank ergometer (one-meter crank height, 33.3 cm cranking radius) in 100 healthy untrained males aged 20–30.

	1-min maximum	3-min maximum	6-min maximum
Average performance in watts	404	278	233
σ	±60.9	±48.3	±41.3
Watts/kg	5.80	3.97	3.35
σ	±0.87	±0.69	±0.59
Max. average HR	185	190	190
σ	±5	±7	±7
Body weight in kg	70	70	70
Height in cm	177	177	177

Table 4. Results of 3-minute maximum tests in 160 male teenagers, aged 12–19 (after *Mellerowicz* and *Lerche*).

Group	Age	n	kg	cm	watts	σ	watts/kg	kpm/min	rpm	HR max.	σ
I	12–13	40	45	156	161	41	3.60	2952	36.9	193	10.6
II	14–15	40	54	166	222	49	4.10	4114	37.8	195	11.1
III	16–17	40	65	174	246	46	3.80	4520	41.2	195	12.4
IV	18–19	40	67	176	249	49	3.70	4388	41.2	194	7.8

case of hearts with pronounced hypertrophy, coronary insufficiency, inflammatory conditions, "old-man's heart" or extreme vagotonia. The physiologically maximal HR drops by about 10 beats/minute with each ten years of age.

A point of reference in evaluating the one-minute, three-minute and six-minute tests is afforded by the studies of Dransfeld and Mellerowicz on 100 healthy, untrained men between the ages of 20 and 30 (Table 3).

HR measured during or immediately following a maximal effort enables us to evaluate the "exertion level" on the basis of the maximal values found for healthy male subjects of average age and their standard deviations (Figs. 45, 46, and 47). Lower maximal HR are not to be assumed for women; in teenagers they tend to be higher and drop with advancing years (see p. 75).

Among teenagers (10–19), the younger age brackets have lower absolute performance capacity at maximal ergometric power. In their relative power production (watts per kg of body weight), however, no significant differences are apparent as compared with 20–30 year olds. Relatively, i.e., based on body weight, they show just about equal capacity for physical performance in the three- as in the six-minute maximum tests (Tables 4 and 5).

Age-regression has not yet been determined with large enough populations nor with satisfactory methodology. According to our present knowledge (especially Robinson and Reindell) (Table 6), it may be assumed that the maximum power and O_2 consumption, considering 20–30 year old values as 100%, would be about as follows:

At age 40   ≈80–90%
At age 50   ≈75–80%
At age 60   ≈70%
At age 70   ≈60%

Table 5. Results of 6-minute maximum tests in 161 male teenagers (after *Mellerowicz* and *Lerche*).

Group	Age	n	kg	cm	watts	σ	watts/kg	kpm/min	rpm	HR max.	σ
I	12–13	40	47	158	157	37	3.30	5760	38.0	196	10.6
II	14–15	40	54	166	180	39	3.30	6006	35.4	193	13.1
III	16–17	40	65	175	195	40	3.00	7128	40.4	204	7.7
IV	18–19	41	65	176	193	35	3.00	7112	40.1	198	7.3

Table 6. Maximal O_2 consumption, maximal ergostasis, 6-minute duration of power in each wattage stage (foot pedaling while reclining) at various age levels (after *Reindell, König, Roskamm* and *Keul*).

Age	No. of subjects max.	O_2 consumption	Percent
20–30	50	2373	100
30–40	50	2008	85
40–50	31	1848	78
50–60	30	1643	70

Women should score about 20–30% absolutely and about 15–20% relatively (per kg of body weight) below men in maximal-performance tests. The same proportions hold for O_2 consumption in short-duration tests (see Chapter I, 6).

When evaluating the one-, three- and six-minute maximal power, the following must be borne in mind:

1. The one-minute maximum test is overwhelmingly dependent on muscular power and the neutralization and buffer capacities of the blood, and to a lesser extent on the performance of the vascular and respiratory systems.
2. The six-minute maximum test depends overwhelmingly on the performance of the vascular and respiratory systems, the O_2 transport capacity of the blood and the biochemical capacity of the suprarenal gland. The aerobic and anaerobic capacity and capillarity of the musculature are also of importance.
3. The three-minute maximum test is influenced by components 1 and 2.

2. Evaluation of Data

On the basis of available study results (Wahlund; Sjöstrand; Bolt, Knipping, Valentin and Venrath; E. A. Müller and Karrasch; Bransfeld and Mellerowicz; and others) and over 10,000 outpatient performance studies on the healthy and performance-deficient vascular system (Table 7), the following schematic distinctions were drawn up:

1. In the case of medium to severe limitation of circulatory performance (definitely pathological), the maximal long-duration (>6 minutes) power is less in watts than the simple kg figure for body weight (or one tenth in kpm/s of the kg body weight); e.g., if the body weight is 75 kg: power $<$ 75 watts ≈ 7.5 kpm/s (≈ 0.1 metric HP). The power (in watts)–weight (in kg) quotient is <1.

2. In the case of minor to medium power limitation, the maximal long-duration power in watts is less than twice the body weight in kg (or 0.2 of the body weight in kg expressed in kpm/s); e.g., if the body weight is 75 kg: power < 150 watts ≈ 15 kpm/s (≈0.2 metric HP). The power-weight quotient ≈ 1–2.

3. In the case of average vascular performance capacity, the maximal long-duration power in watts amounts to two or three times the body weight in kg (or 0.2 to 0.3 of the kg figure for body weight in kpm/s); e.g., if the body weight is 75 kg: power is from 150 watts ≈ 15 kpm/s (≈0.2 HP) to 225 watts ≈ 22.5 kpm/s (≈0.3 HP). The power-weight quotient ≈2–3 (in persons of average age).

4. In the case of a very robust vascular system, the maximal long-duration power in watts is more than three times the body weight in kg (or 0.3 of the kg body weight in kpm/s); e.g., if the body weight is 75 kg: power > 225 watts ≈ 22.5 kpm/s (≈0.3 metric HP). Power-weight quotient: >3.

This simple evaluation of relative power capacity of the body and vascular system can also be used in the case of women, teenagers and the aged by using special correction factors (see Chapter I).

Table 7. Summary of the evaluation of performance in the vascular system.

Nomenclature	Vascular system of greatly limited capacity (pathological cases)	Vascular system of average to slightly limited capacity	Vascular system of average capacity	Robust vascular system
Endurance (W) > 6 min weight (kg)	≈0–1	≈1–2	≈2–3	≈3→
Maximal bodily endurance (cranking) at ≈75 kg body weight	HP ≈0–0.1 W ≈0–75 kpm/s ≈0–7.5 kpm/min ≈0–450	≈0.1–0.2 ≈75–150 ≈7.5–≈15 ≈450–≈900	≈0.2–0.3 ≈150–225 ≈15–≈22.5 ≈900–≈1350	≈0.3→ ≈225→ ≈22.5→ ≈1350→
Reduction in capacity according to *Knipping, Bolt, Valentin* and *Venrath*	100–75%	75–30%	0%	
Capacity for sports (*Mellerowicz*)	at low exertion levels	low to average exertion levels	greater exertion levels	maximal performance
Classification by Criteria Committee N.Y. Heart Assoc., based on functional capacity of vascular system (4th ed.) 1947	vascular problems cause moderate to severe limitation of performance (class 3)	vascular problems cause slight to moderate limitation of performance (class 2)	vascular problems no limitation to performance capacity (class 1)	

The reports of American, English, French and Belgian researchers seem to agree quite well with this classification, which also agrees with our personal schematic guidelines at average weights.

Wahlund takes a maximal endurance power of 1200 kpm/min ($\approx$200 watts) as normal. The lower threshold, according to his studies, lies at about 900 kpm/min ($\approx$150 watts).

E. A. Müller and Karrasch report PPI performance pulse index rates in average workers of from nearly 3 up to 6 (see p. 66). That is approximately maximal physical power (on a bicycle) in HR range of 150 to 300 watts.

Düntsch found an average endurance power of 199 watts with 10-minute maximal hand-cranking exercise in 80 athletically untrained radio-factory employees aged 20 to 30 and weighing an average of 68.7 kg. The average HR was 198 and the power-weight quotient was 2.9.

He also studied 20- to 30-year old female employees in the same plant, also untrained in athletic sports, and weighing on the average 61.5 kg. Their average maximal endurance power in ten-minute cranking exercises was 123 watts, the average HR 178, and the average power-weight quotient 2.0.

Mellerowicz made calculations from numerous studies including his own, on O_2 consumption, energy expenditure, exercise performance and intensity of exercise. He found powers of 75 to 100 watts in minor to average athletic performances, as for example cycling 12 to 15 km per hour, rowing 4 to 6 km per hour, hiking 5 to 6 km per hour, cross-country skiing 5 to 7 km per hour and ice skating 8 to 12 km per hour. These are loads achievable even in the face of slight or moderate limitation of performance capacity. With average vascular capacity (and average body weight), the maximal endurance power tops these figures (150 watts).

In youthful persons weighing 20 to 80 kg and aged 5 to 35, a general, regular dependence of maximum O_2 consumption on weight can be recognized. Since the maximal O_2 consumption is also dependent on vascular performance, according to studies by Åstrand, the relationship of the (relative) vascular performance to body weight is justified. The absolute physical power and vascular performance, which up until now were used only as points of reference, are definitely of much less importance for the evaluation of performance capacity of the circulatory system than the relative performance, which places performance in relation to body weight. This is especially true in view of the fact that in most exercise the weight of the body itself has to be moved as well.

For persons of average weight, maximal endurance power of 150 to 225 watts is to be regarded as average power. But the same power cannot be demanded of persons of lesser weight or greater age. For 50-kg persons, a maximal endurance power of 200 watts will not in general be attainable, even when their circulatory systems are healthy and can certainly not be designated as limited in power capacity. The declining endurance power capacity that accompanies advancing age can be taken into consideration to an approximate degree using Robinson's data (see Chapter I, 7).

According to Åstrand, for women we must reckon with a relative power capacity 10 to 20% lower (based on kilograms of body weight) than that of men. The absolute power (according to the maximal O_2 consumption) is on the average ≈20 to 30% lower (see Chapter I, 6).

References

Åstrand, P. O.: Experimental studies of physical working capacity in relation to sex and age. Kopenhagen: Munksgaard, 1952.

Bolt, W., H. W. Knipping, H. Valentin and H. Venrath: Untersuchung und Beurteilung des Herzkranken, S. 180. Stuttgart: Enke, 1955.

Dransfeld, B. and H. Mellerowicz: Internat. Zschr. angew. Physiol. einschl. Arbeitsphysiol. 16, (1957) 465.

Düntsch, G.: Diss. Berlin 1960.

König, K.: Med. Klin. 10, (1952) 308.

Mellerowicz, H. and D. Lerche: Zschr. Kinderhk, 81, (1958) 36.

Müller, E. A.: Arbeitsphysiologie 14, (1950) 271.

Müller, E. A. and E. Karrasch: Zbl. Arbeitsmed. 2, (1953) 37.

Reindell, H., K. König, H. Roskamm and J. Keul: M.kurse ärztl. Fortbild. Nr. 4 (1959).

Robinson, S.: Arbeitsphysiologie 10, (1938) 251.

Sjöstrand, T.: Acta physiol. scand. 18, (1949) 324; Svenska läkartidn. 7, (1950) 349; Dtsch. med. Wschr. 24, (1955) 963.

Wahlund, H.: Acta med. Scand. 215 (1948).

V. Heart Rate in Ergometric Performance

1. Methodology of Measurement and Registration of the HR During and After Ergometric Performance

The HR can be measured during ergometric pedaling while seated and reclining by auditory or palpation methods with the aid of a stopwatch. It has proved effective to time ten cardiac periods and calculate from that the per-minute frequency (or read it from a table). Likewise, the number of heart beats in six seconds can be counted; then simply multiplying by ten gives the rate per minute. Over longer periods, however, any alteration in HR during performance is less easy to ascertain with precision.

To determine the HR during performance of hand-cranking exercise while standing, a wide elastic band is applied around the thorax of the subject and the microphone of a stethoscope is placed over the heart and attached to a meterlong plastic tube (as in Fig. 4). In this manner it is simple to monitor the heart during the exercise and measure the HR with the aid of a stop watch.

An even simpler way is to interrupt the hand-cranking exercise at one-minute intervals for either ten heart beats or six seconds and read the number of heart beats by either auditory or palpation methods. The readings will lie more or less below the actual performance HR depending on how quickly the HR drops after the cessation of the performance. This error is relatively slight and decreases with increased performance.

The performance HR can thus be determined at intervals of one minute during or immediately after the exercise. The comparison of the resulting performance HR with normal values graphically recorded (Figs. 48 and 49) makes possible a statistically based evaluation of the cardiac and physical endurance power.

Another method of investigation is to determine the physical work capacity 170 (PWC_{170}; see Chapter XX, 5.2). In three to six submaximal stages of performance at ten watts for one minute or 25 watts for two minutes or 50 watts for three to six minutes, the performance HR is measured during the last ten seconds of each stage. These three different stages of performance result in no significant differences in the PWC_{170} (according to Franz and Chintanaseri). The HR of the lowest level of power should here exceed a value of 100 per minute and that of the highest level of power an age-dependent value of 130 to 150 per minute. If the readings are entered on a coordinate system, they will lie in a straight line which cuts the coordinate for HR 170 at a point characterizing the PWC_{170} in watts or kpm/s. The normal value is 3 watts per kg for men aged 20–30 (± 0.5 watts per kg) and ≈ 2.5 watts per kg (± 0.5 watts per kg) for women of like age.

With advancing age (in the case of a healthy cardiovascular system), the theoretical PWC_{170} seems to change only slightly or not at all, just as comparative studies of the HR at relatively equal power levels of one watt per kg in subjects aged 20–40 and 40–60 showed no significant differences (Domnick, 1966). However, in the evaluation of the PWC_{170} of older people,

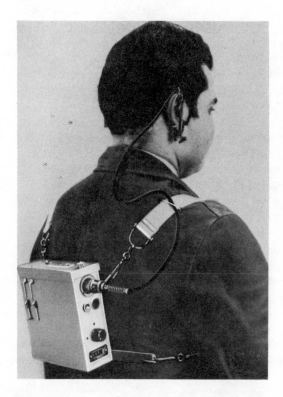

Fig. 36. Photoelectric pulse counter (after *E. A. Müller*).

it must be borne in mind that maximal HR decreases with advancing age, the average rate of decrease being about 10 beats per minute per decade. The actual PWC for a given age is therefore to be assumed to be relatively lower with increasing age, for example, $\approx$150 for persons about 50 years old.

The maximal HR range in various groups of subjects (trained and untrained, men and women, teenagers and adults), shows varying levels, which are yet to be more precisely defined both experimentally and statistically (see Chapter V, 4.1 and 4.2).

When there are reasons, in the presence of changes in the cardiovascular system, to exercise caution in approaching the limits of power production, it will suffice to determine the HR at two or three smaller wattages. The probable HR of borderline performance can be ascertained graphically by assuming a regular rise in performance HR through intermediate ranges; that is, by extrapolation. In many pathological cases, however, a maximal HR less than 160–130 can be assumed (coronary insufficiency, stressed and highly hypertrophic hearts, etc.).

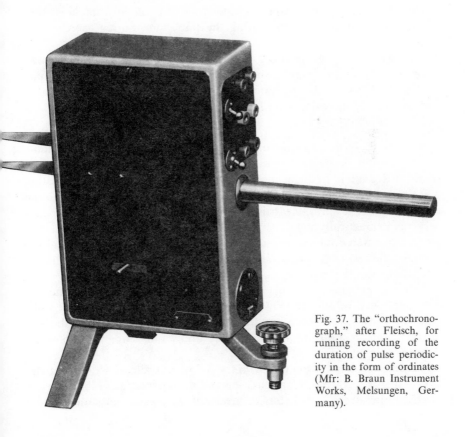

Fig. 37. The "orthochrono-graph," after Fleisch, for running recording of the duration of pulse periodicity in the form of ordinates (Mfr: B. Braun Instrument Works, Melsungen, Germany).

In such cases, it is useful to determine the performance pulse index (PPI) according to E. A. Müller and Karrasch. This gives the average increase in frequency for the performance increase of 1 kpm/s (≈ 10 watts). However, it is worthwhile in evaluating the PPI to take into account the body weight and the product of PPI times body weight. A PPI that indicates limitation of the capacity of the vascular system of a person weighing 80 kg may indicate an average performance ability in a person weighing 50 kg.

To verify the results of the study, whenever that seems necessary, additional ergometric studies should be called upon, such as measurement of O_2 consumption, the O_2 pulse, etc.

A running record of the performance HR can be accomplished by the following methods:

1. By use of a photoelectric pulse counter, as developed by E. A. Müller and J. J. Reeh (manufactured by W. Himmelmann, of Dortmund, Germany). This method uses a principle first employed by Matthes in biological studies. The alterations in light absorption in the earlobe occurring with each pulse beat are picked up photoelectrically, amplified and automatically registered by means of a counter (Fig. 36). The instrument is especially well adapted for measuring the pulse sum during exercise and recovery.

2. By use of an ordinate recorder (Fig. 37), the pulse times (i.e., the duration of the pulse period) may be recorded. The recording, in the form of time expressed as the ordinate, is interrupted in this instrument by each pulse. Immediately thereafter, starting at the 0 line, the next pulse-time ordinate is drawn.

As a matter of fact, the instrument does not draw ordinates, but graphic representations of the slow phase of specific oscillations occurring at constant but regulable frequency and amplitude. The speed of the oscillating point (as nearly weightless as possible) must be directly proportional to the elapsed time. The slow, linear-time phase of the oscillation follows upon a very quick (practically negligible) return to the starting position. With a very great time difference between the deviation speed of the oscillation and the speed of the recording paper, vertical straight lines (ordinates) are drawn, whose angle to the base line is, however, never precisely 90°.

A device that makes possible mechanical recording of the pulse time was first mentioned by Fleisch (Fig. 37). An instrument that draws time ordinates electrically with points of ultra-violet light was constructed by the firm of Hartmann & Braun from plans worked up by Lillies and Stolzmann (of Böhm Co. in Berlin).

A cardiotachogram produced with the aid of an ordinate-writer (Fig. 38) affords a precise graphic representation and documentation of the behavior of HR during exercise and rest. By means of the jagged calibrations and a

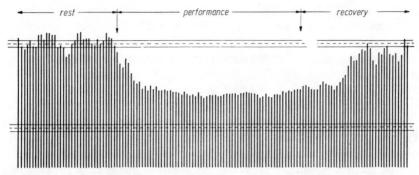

Fig. 38. Copy of an original cardiotachogram. Ordinates are drawn directly from the duration of each pulse period as recorded photoelectrically in the earlobe. (Performance: 2 watts per kg on a bicycle ergometer, trained male subject.)

known paper speed, the cardiotachogram makes it possible to determine the precise HR at every single phase of the performance. Regular, wave-like variations in HR and regulatory interferences leading to variations in heart time in the course of performance and their dispersion can be readily grasped through this method.

The performance HR can also be recorded by electrocardiogram. To eliminate excessive waste of paper, it is worthwhile to employ low paper speeds (5 to 10 mm per second). In commercially available instruments, a speed reducer will have to be added for this purpose. The electrocardiographic recording of the HR is less desirable, however, since the wire leads tend to interfere with free movement on the part of the subject and the recording comes solely from the subject's torso. This applies particularly in the case of cranking exercise while standing, less so with the subject seated or reclining.

Various manufacturers now produce instruments that operate on photoelectric and electrocardiologic principles for measurement, indication and recording of HR and pulse rate.

1.1 Sources of Error and Critique of Methodology

In measuring HR with a stopwatch, an inevitable error of $\pm 1/20$ second must be taken into consideration if the time is read in precise tenths of a second. In recalculating the time into frequencies per minute, the purely methodological error varies in various ranges of frequency as a result of the factor of hyperbole. This amounts to ± 0.5 at a frequency of 60 per minute, to ± 1 at 100 per minute, to ± 2 at 140 per minute, and ± 3 at 180 per minute. Over and above this comes the subjective error produced by the pressing of the stop button of the watch at somewhat different phases of the heart action. With practice, the methodological error can be reduced to about half, so that the greatest total error in a calculated frequency of 180 per minute is ±5 beats, which is ±2.8%. In auditory reading of the HR per minute over a period of six seconds, there arises a certain error in counting, which, with a maximal possible deviation of ±5 beats amounts to ±4.2% at a rate of 120 per minute and 2.8% at a rate of 180 per minute.

The error in HR measurement is greater, however, when measuring the rate during a recovery pause lasting six seconds. Approximately 10% of the O_2 consumed in the course of these six seconds may be used afterward. In counting pauses of six seconds per minute, therefore, a maximal endurance can be reached which is $\approx$10% above the actual steady-state performance (after recovery-breathing of an oxygen debt of $\approx$10% of the maximal O_2 consumption in each minute). The results obtained by the counting methods indicated, therefore, are $\approx$10% higher than the actual maximal steady-state values. This error can be approximately corrected for by deducting 10% from the borderline value obtained.

It is, moreover, to be borne in mind that the HRs measured in the initial seconds of the recovery period are not the same as the HRs at the end of the performance but are more or less lower.

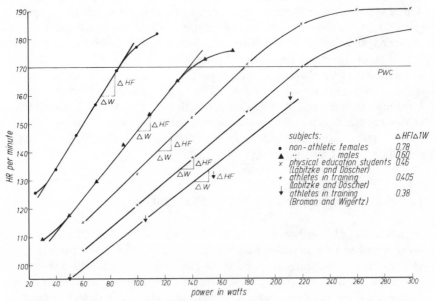

Fig. 39. Averages of the s-shaped static characteristic lines for the load frequency from four experiments on female and twelve on male non-athletes compared with data on physical education students and trained athletes. The comparison in steepness is based on the quotient of HR to stress ($\Delta HR/\Delta W$), after *Tiedt et al.*).

In minor to average ergometric performances, the HR can be affected by psychic influences, tending to increase the readings. In the case of less emotionally stable subjects, psychologically caused alterations in exercising HR are more pronounced (Antel and Cumming). In high ergometric performances, psychic factors have only a slight effect on the performance HR. Psychic effects on the heart rate in ergometric studies should be eliminated insofar as possible, as is provided for in the performance metabolism stipulations (Chapter III, 2).

2. Physiological Basis

Performance HR, physical performance and maximal cardiac and body power bear a regular relationship to one another. A linear relationship of HR and ergometric performance exists in the frequency range of ≈ 100–170 per minute in persons of average age. In the case of performances with a HR of >170 per minute, the power increases less steeply and approaches a

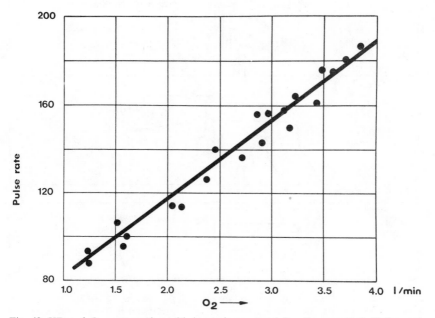

Fig. 40. HR and O_2 consumption with increasing power (after *Berggren* and *Christensen*).

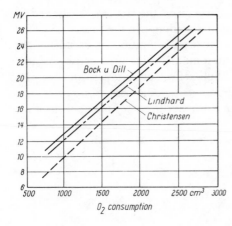

Fig. 41. O_2 consumption and cardiac output (after *Landen*) are in a linear relationship as power increases.

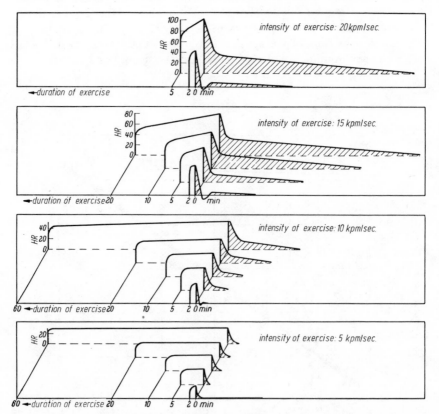

Fig. 42. Behavior of the HR during and after ergometric exercise of varying duration and intensity. The cross-hatched area represents the sum of the heart beats during recuperation (after *Karrasch* and *E. A. Müller*).

maximal value (Fig. 39, after Tiedt et al.). The steady-state HR increases with increased performance levels in almost linear proportion to the O_2 consumption (Fig. 40) and the cardiac output (Fig. 41), depending on the level of the arteriovenous O_2 difference. It is therefore of great practical importance to measure the HR, a simple, reliable matter requiring very little in the way of apparatus, and it is actually the basic method in ergometric studies.

The regulative setting of the HR during performance is controlled by a complex system of cortical, vegetative, reflex and hormonal interplay. HR increases immediately after the start of exercise (even the second beat period is already shorter!) in a definite and regular manner, depending on the intensity of the performance and on endogenous and exogenous factors. In power production of 10 to 50 watts, with a HR of 100 per minute, the HR increase does not take place linearly but increases in a steady curve (Grunert et al.). In strenuous performances following a state of rest of a few seconds, the sudden, brief bursts of maximal exertion increase the HR to 170 to 200 per minute easily.

HR levels off only in the lower endurance power levels, below the so-called pulse endurance performance limit (E. A. Müller). In the case of strenuous endurance power levels, there occurs a further, steady increase in HR depending on the degree of exertion, the performance state of the organism and the ambient temperature (Figs. 42 and 43). The greater the exercise intensity per unit of time, the more the HR increases. The greater the performance capacity of the vascular system and the better-trained it is, the less is the increase in HR for the same level of ergometric power (Fig. 44).

Maximal HR of $\approx$200 to 220 can be maintained for only very brief periods. These are attained in exhausting endurance power levels after a final spurt and maximal O_2 debt, especially by teenagers.

The maximal endurance limit of the heart for brief to average endurance exercise—in which the circulation is able to maintain its cardiac output for at least six minutes—is attained, according to recent studies and experience,

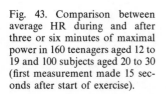

Fig. 43. Comparison between average HR during and after three or six minutes of maximal power in 160 teenagers aged 12 to 19 and 100 subjects aged 20 to 30 (first measurement made 15 seconds after start of exercise).

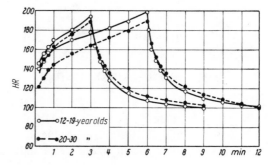

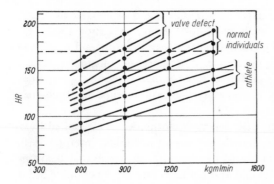

Fig. 44. Linear rise in HR with increasing exertion in trained athletes, normal individuals and cases of vascular insufficiency for work (VOC = valve defect) (after Sjöstrand).

at an average maximal HR of ≈160 to 200 in the case of individuals of average age, either sex, and various degrees of training (after Wahlund; Sjöstrand; Düntsch; Mellerowicz and Lerche; Dransfeld and Mellerowicz; etc.).

In the case of prolonged maximal endurance exercises of more than one hour duration, we must expect maximal steady-state HRs of less than ≈160. The acceptable HRs for an eight-hour day's work run 30 to 40 beats above the HR while resting, i.e., about 100 to 120 beats per minute (according to E. A. Müller and Karrasch).

A few seconds after the exercise, there occurs a steep, then a more gradual drop in HR. In a given individual, the time lapse until return to the resting HR and the total recovery pulse sum are approximately proportional to the amount and duration of the exercise. They are almost inversely proportional to the degree of training and performance of the cardiovascular system. The recovery period may last from a few seconds to a matter of hours after extreme exercise. The resumption of the normal HR usually takes place irregularly and may show great variations (as in cases of irregularly initiated "vagotonic braking"). The recovery period for the HR depends on numerous endogenous and exogenous factors.

3. Physiological Range of Variation in Performance HR in Standard Ergometric Performances

In order to evaluate the performance HR and cardiac performance capacity in ergometric studies, it is indispensable to know the range of physiological variation in HRs in healthy male and female members of the population at various ages in particular standard performances. The standard figures should, insofar as possible, be arrived at from observation of a representative cross-section of the total population. Exercise amounting to 1 and 2 watts per kg of body weight sets suitable standards. The graphic charts in Figures 48 and 49 demonstrate the relationship for the performance HR (at relatively equal powers of 1 or 2 watts/kg of body weight) in the case of healthy, untrained, teenagers aged 10–20 and men aged 20–30. The graphic chart in Figure 50 demonstrates the range of physiological variation in the recovery HR after a performance of 1 watt per kg of body weight for one minute in men aged 20 to 30.

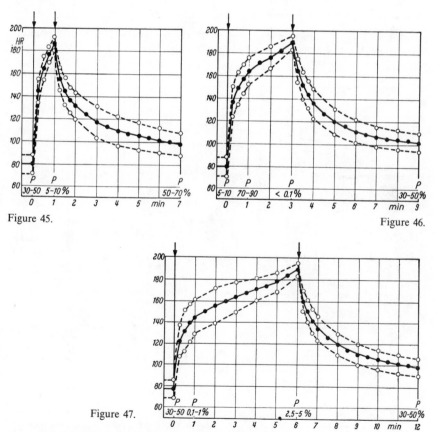

Figure 45.

Figure 46.

Figure 47.

Figs. 45, 46, and 47. HR and its standard deviations during and after maximal power 1, 3, and 6 minutes on the hand-crank ergometer in 100 untrained male subjects aged 20–30 (after *Dransfeld* and *Mellerowicz*).

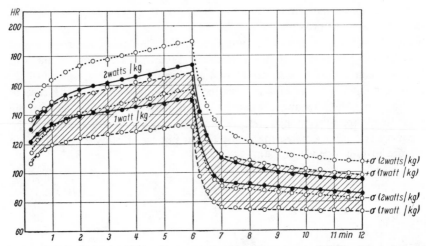

Fig. 48. HR during performance and recovery in 220 male teenagers aged 10 to 20 at relatively equal powers of 1 to 2 watts per kg of body weight (after *Mellerowicz* and *Lerche*).

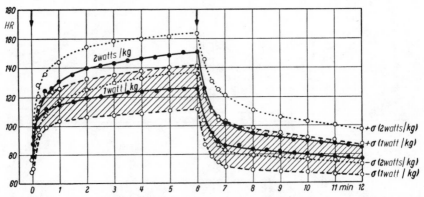

Fig. 49. HR during performance and recovery in 100 men aged 20 to 30 at relatively equal powers of 1 to 2 watts per kg of body weight (after *Dransfeld* and *Mellerowicz*).

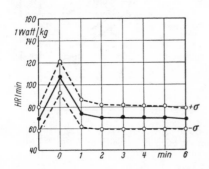

Fig. 50. HR in 100 healthy, untrained male students aged 20 to 30 after a performance of 1 watt per kg of body weight for one minute (after *Mellerowicz*, *Schmutzler* and *Maidorn*).

The relationship of HR to ergometric power in watts per kg of body weight in healthy male subjects aged 20 to 30 and 10 to 20 is shown schematically in Figures 48 and 49. The behavior of HR and its standard deviation with intensities of performance increasing from 30 to 230 watts in healthy men aged 20 to 30 are shown in Figure 51.

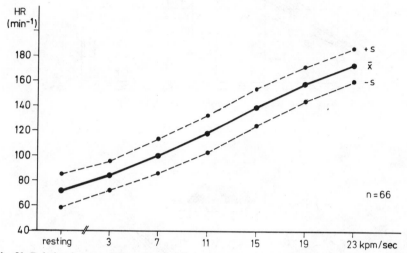

Fig. 51. Relation between HR and power in healthy male individuals aged 20 to 30 using the bicycle ergometer (after *Hollmann et al.*).

4. Endogenous and Exogenous Controlling Factors in Performance HR

4.1 The Relationships Between Performance HR and Age and Sex.

The graphic presentations in Figures 48 and 49 reveal, even at relatively equal performances, higher performance HRs in male teenagers than in (untrained) men aged 20 to 30. The differences are, however, slight and not significantly greater than those for HRs while at rest. The same is true of recovery HRs, which, after maximal exertion lasting three and six minutes, show a somewhat steeper drop and quicker reversion to normal in the teenagers (Fig. 43). This behavior indicates a capability for performance and recovery on the part of teenagers in brief endurance works that is relatively

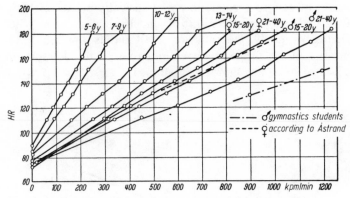

Fig. 52. Performance HR in various age groups (after *Bengtsson*).

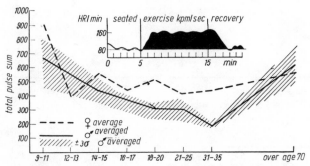

Fig. 53. Total pulse sum in healthy subjects in uniform ten-minute exercise on the bicycle ergometer (5 kpm/s); average values for 225 subjects (after *Nöcker* and *Böhlau*).

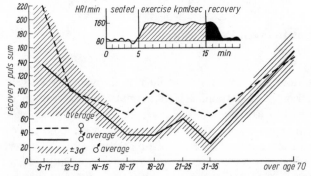

Fig. 54. Recovery pulse sum in healthy subjects after ten-minute uniform work on the bicycle ergometer (5 kpm/s); average values for 225 subjects (after *Nöcker* and *Böhlau*).

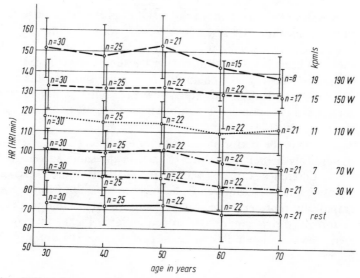

Fig. 55. Behavior of HR at given stages of stress in healthy male individuals aged 20 to 70 (after *Hollmann et al.*).

at least equal. On the other hand, at absolutely equal power levels the teen-agers performance HRs are distinctly and noticeably higher than those of adults, and the recovery time is considerably longer (Figs. 52, 53 and 54).

The behavior of performance HR in males aged 20 to 70 is shown in Figure 55. A tendency to a moderate drop in HR in absolutely equal exercise levels with advancing years is recognizable. In submaximal exercise levels based on body weight, however, Hertle et al. found no decline in HR in older subjects. The lower HR of older individuals with absolutely equal

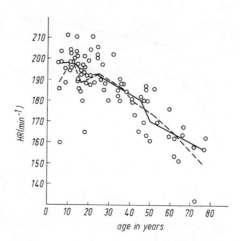

Fig. 56. The behavior of the maximal HR as presented by *Robinson*.

exercise levels is however not the result of greater cardiac performance capability, since the HR reserves decrease with advancing age.

Maximal HR declines at a regular rate with advancing biological age by about 10 heart beats per minute per decade of age (Fig. 56). According to studies by Nöcker and Böhlau, the total pulse sum and the recovery pulse sum decline with absolutely equal power (5 kpm/s of bicycle exercise lasting ten minutes) in various age groups up until age 30, and then rise again after about age 35 (Figs. 53 and 54).

In women, the performance HRs for absolutely equal exercise levels are significantly higher than those of men of the same age (Figs. 53 and 54). Lesser differences can be assumed for relatively equal exercise levels. The precise quantitative differences have yet to be defined for a series of demographically representative studies using irreproachable methodology. The performance pulse index is also considerably higher for women than for men. The sex-related differences in performance HR are probably smallest before the onset of puberty.

4.2   Performance HR and Degree of Training

Endurance training, depending on the nature and amount of training, leads to a reduction in resting HR amounting to as much as 50% of the figure observed before training was instituted. Resting HRs below 40 are no rarity among fully trained individuals. Those with the highest degree of training generally show the lowest HR.

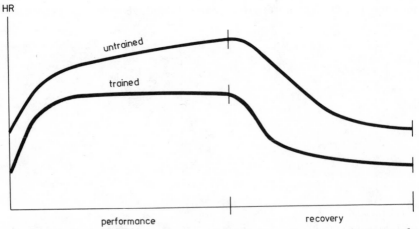

Fig. 57. Comparative schematic presentation of HR during performance and recovery after equal exercises in trained and untrained subjects.

In trained individuals, the performance HR increases more rapidly at the start of comparable exercise levels (Kössling). Depending on the state of training and performance, it reaches a considerably lower maximum. A constant HR sets in with trained individuals at higher performance rates than with the untrained. After equal power, the resting values are more rapidly reestablished by the trained individuals (Fig. 57). Through exaggerated vagotonic braking, the HR frequently drops in the trained individual, after brief but strenuous exercise, to a point lower than the resting level and then gradually returns to the resting value. The better-trained an individual is, the smaller is the total and the recovery pulse sum for comparable exercises.

In trained endurance athletes with greater cardiac volume, the maximal HRs are lower than in the untrained. They show a negative correlation to heart size (Israel).

4.3 Effect of Ambient Temperature, Atmospheric Pressure, Humidity and Time of Day on Performance HR

With equal physical and biological power performance, the HR reaches higher levels at higher ambient temperatures (see Fig. 18). Humidity above the comfort level gives rise to additional heat-regulation measures, resulting in further increase in performance HR. Therefore, in evaluating the performance HR and other data, the ambient temperature and humidity must always be recorded and taken into consideration. Insofar as possible, ergometric studies should be carried out at temperatures between 18° and 22°C and at humidities between 30% and 60%. More precise quantitative studies on the effects of temperature and humidity on performance HR, carried out on sufficiently large representative populations, have not been published.

It is certain that performance HR increases regularly in proportion to altitude above sea level, as barometric pressure decreases along with O_2 pressure in the air. The relatively slight variations in barometric pressure resulting from weather conditions, however, can be ignored in ergometric labs until more precise knowledge about quantitative relationships has been acquired.

As in the case of resting HR, it must also be assumed that performance HR is affected by time of day, and this must be taken into consideration. However, the more precise circadian rhythms of performance HR for various groups, defined by age, sex and constitution, are yet to be studied. To be comparable, ergometric studies must always be scheduled at the same time of day.

5.   Performance HR in Pathologic Conditions

When myocardial and valvular damage exists or there are congenital defects, performance HR at relatively equal levels of exertion will be higher than that of healthy subjects of average cardiac performance capacity, as cardiac output and O_2 pulse (at approximately equal arteriovenous O_2 difference) are reduced (Fig. 58). This is true for both pressure-stressed and volume-stressed hearts. But with full compensation for damage, the performance HR may lie within the $\pm 1\sigma$ range or even below that.

The latter effects are particularly noticeable when the damaged heart has been relieved of stress through increased O_2 difference and vascular economy as a result of (prescribed) training measures and its performance capacity with full compensation has not been increased beyond the $\pm 1\sigma$ range of norm. Not infrequently we encounter a relatively great or even above-average performance capacity in the case of damaged hearts presenting bradycardia.

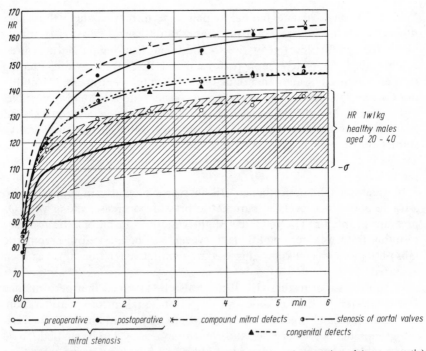

o—·— preoperative   ●—— postoperative   ×— — — compound mitral defects   ⊙— ··— stenosis of aortal valves
▲- - - - congenital defects

mitral stenosis

Fig. 58. Performance HR in the presence of mitral defects, aortic stenosis and (non-cyanotic) congenital defects (after *Schmutzler* and *Mellerowicz*).

As a rule, in the presence of myocardial or valvular damage with reduced volume performance and steeper increase in performance HR, the cardiac performance capacity is very likely to be further limited by reduction in the maximal HR. This is especially true in all more pronouncedly hypertrophic, pressure-stressed hearts, which more readily develop hypoxia in the presence of higher HR, and also in all hearts with reduced coronary O_2 reserve, regardless of etiology.

In the presence of damage to the heart and vascular system, especially in coronary insufficiency, there are many cases in which ergometric testing to the maximal effort should be avoided. Ergometric studies at submaximal power (e.g., 1 watt per kg of body weight) or in increasing submaximal power levels afford sufficiently accurate and reliable conclusions as to cardiac performance capacity.

In the presence of disturbed stimulations or conduction defects, it must be decided from case to case whether performance testing is indicated. In the presence of multifocal extrasystoles caution is advisable even during rest, but if they decrease during or after the exercise, the performance HR can be evaluated according to the usual guidelines. Should numerous extrasystoles develop upon exertion, it is advisable to interrupt ergometric study at an early stage. The ergometric performance in question can then be regarded as lying beyond the performance limit for the time being.

In the presence of hypertonic regulatory dystonia, performance HR are usually increased depending on the degree of disturbance and other endogenously controlled factors. Also, in the case of hypotonic regulatory dystonia, increases in performance HR are common. Hypotonic regulatory conditions are, however, a sign of an economical circulation with great performance reserves. They also occur as a rule in a trained and robust vascular system in connection with low performance HR. Orthostatic regulatory disturbances are very frequently found combined with a regulatory instability, inferior circulatory performance and high performance HR.

In the presence of all forms of anemia accompanied by a reduction in O_2 transport capacity, performance HR increases depending on the severity of the condition and other contributory factors.

In the case of all pulmonary diseases leading to greater stress on the right heart and cor pulmonale, HRs are usually increased. This is especially true in the case of all pulmonary defects involving disturbances of O_2 diffusion and O_2 saturation deficiency. In these instances, cardiac output is increased for equal exertion. Since the performance reserves of the respiratory system are usually greater than those of the vascular system, however, even widespread reduction in respiratory surface area and vital capacity may have little practical effect on performance HR and power.

In cases of vegetative regulatory dystonia, especially in ergotropic forms, high performance HRs are found as a rule. Considerable increases in per-

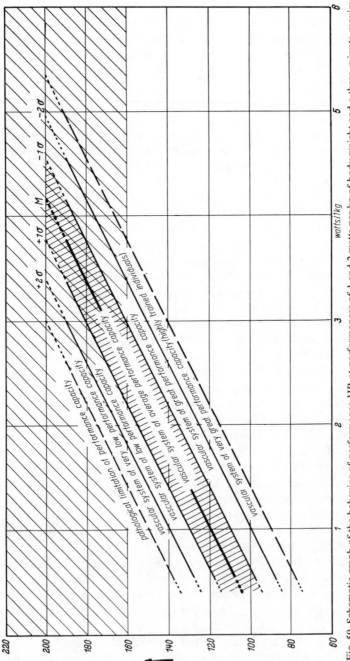

Fig. 59. Schematic graph of the behavior of performance HR at performances of 1 and 2 watts per kg of body weight and a three-minute maximal performance in 100 untrained men aged 20–30 on the hand-crank ergometer (after *Dransfeld* and *Mellerowicz*).

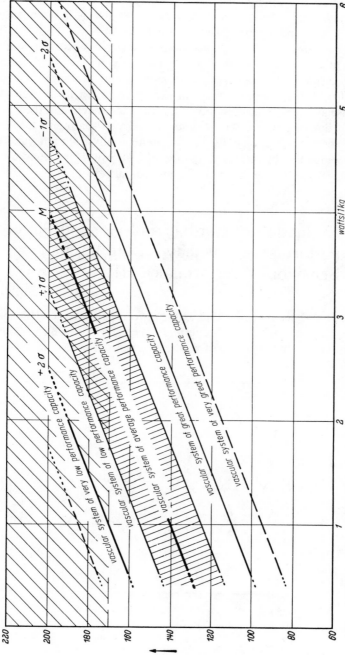

Fig. 60. Schematic graph of the behavior of performance HR at performances of 1 and 2 watts per kg of body weight and a three-minute maximal performance in 160 untrained male subjects aged 10–19 on the hand-crank ergometer (after *Mellerowicz* and *Lerche*).

formance HR also occur in cases of hyperthyroidism. The same is true for all other endocrine diseases leading to vascular changes and reduction of cardiac and bodily performance capacity, especially as is often observed in hypophyseal and suprarenal malfunction.

In the course of convalescence from all infectious diseases, performance HR is also increased, depending on the severity, nature and duration of the diseased state and duration of confinement to bed. Prolonged bed rest alone can also lead to sharp increases in performance HR as a result of loss of exercise and metabolic economy of the vascular system and the whole organism. Lack of physical activity and exaggerated sparing of the body may bring about a reduction in cardiac and general physical performance capacity accompanied by increased performance HR more pronounced than that found in cases of serious cardiovascular damage!

6.   Evaluation of Cardiac and General Physical Performance Capacity on the Basis of Behavior of Performance HR

The intimate relationships that exist between performance HR and degree of exertion and cardiovascular performance make it possible to evaluate and determine cardiovascular performance capacity. For this, it is necessary to

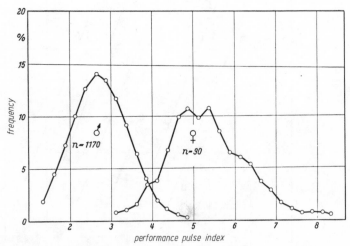

Fig. 61. Frequency distribution of the performance pulse index after *E. A. Müller*. Increase in pulse rate with a change in performance of 10 watts per minute on the bicycle ergometer at 60 rpm in male policemen aged 30 to 50 and women aged 20 to 30.

know the performance HR and its frequency distribution in certain relatively or absolutely equal exercise levels for particular age and sex groups, which should be as representative as possible. In making such evaluations, the ambient temperature, humidity, time of day, crank height, crank length, revolutions per minute and type of cranking exercise must all be taken into consideration. The graphic presentations in Figures 48 and 49 make possible a statistically based evaluation of cardiovascular performance capacity of teenagers and men aged 20–30 in tests at 1 or 2 watts per kg of body weight. In older men and women the age- and sex-dependency of performance HR must be considered.

Data lying within the ±1σ range indicate average (relative) cardiovascular (endurance) performance capacity. Performance HR above the ±1σ range (≈15% of healthy individuals) indicate a reltively low circulatory performance.

Five distinct levels of cardiocorporeal performance capacity can be established, corresponding to the physiological ±2σ range:

$$>+2\sigma$$
very poor circulatory performance capacity (slight, average or extensive pathological limitation)
$$+2\sigma$$

low circulatory performance capacity (≈15%)
$$+1\sigma$$

average   average circulatory performance capacity (≈67%)
$$-1\sigma$$

good circulatory performance capacity (≈15%)
$$-2\sigma$$

excellent circulatory performance capability (cases of excellent training and extreme constitutional excellence)
$$<-2\sigma$$

In the same way, the regulatory behavior of HR after a standard exercise of 1 watt per kg of body weight for one minute can be evaluated on the basis of the normal values for 100 healthy males aged 20–30, as seen in Figure 50.

If performance HR is determined using increasing wattage stages, the graphic representations of Figures 51, 59, and 60 provide a basis for evaluation. The resting HR, the increase in HR during the exercise and the maximal HR, are to be taken into consideration.

The behavior of the performance pulse index can be evaluated using the graphic presentation in Figure 61 on the basis of the frequency distribution among men and women of average age.

For the graphs in Figures 59 and 60, the average HR attained after each three minutes and its standard deviations were used. The measurement of the HR in one, two or three different power increments affords a comparative evaluation (corresponding to the statistical distribution) when using the

HR value measured after three minutes. With power increments of 10 watts for one minute, 25 watts for two minutes, and 50 watts for six minutes, no significant differences exist, according to Franz and Chintanaseri. (For a comparison of the HR in foot pedaling while seated and reclining and in hand cranking while standing, see Figs. 8 and 9.)

The behavior of the performance pulse index can be evaluated on the basis of the frequency distribution in men and women of average age according to the diagram in Figure 61.

References

Antel, J. and G. R. Cumming: The Research Quarterly Vol. 40 (1969) 2.

Åstrand, P. O.: Experimental studies of physical working capacity in relation to sex and age. Kopenhagen: Munksgaard, 1952.

Bengtsson, E.: Acta med. Scand. II, (1956) 91.

Chintanaseri, Diss. F. U. Berlin (1973).

Dransfeld, B. and H. Mellerowicz: Internat. Zschr. angew. Physiol. einschl. Arbeitsphysiol. 17, (1958) 207; 16, (1957) 464.

Düntsch, G.: Diss. Berlin (1960).

Ekelund, L.-G.: Rapid determination of work load at a heart rate of 170 beats/min with a heart-rate controlled ergometer. In: 3. Internationales Seminar für Ergometrie. Berlin: Ergon-Verlag, 1973.

Franz, J.: Diss. F. U. Berlin (1973).

Grunert, J. P., V. Hünerberg and H. Stoboy: Acta Card. 8/9, (1974) 111.

Hertle, F. H., H. Abel and H. Heidl: Int. Zschrf. angew. Physiol. 24, (1967) 320.

Hollmann, W. et al.: in Sportmedizin–Arbeits- und Trainingsgrundlagen. Stuttgart-New York: F. V. Shattauer Verlag, 1976.

Hollmann, W., W. Barg, G. Weyer and H. Heck: Med. Welt 21, (1970) 1288.

Hollman, W. and Th. Hettinger: Sportmedizin–Arbeits- und Trainingsgrundlagen. Stuttgart-New York: Schattauer, 1976.

Israel, S., H. Kuppardt, K. Gottschalk, G. Neumann and H. Böhme: Med. and Sport XIV, (1974) 297.

Karrasch, K.: Zbl. Arbeitswiss. soz. Betriebspraxis 10, (1952) 145.

Kössling, F.: Med. Welt 31, (1960) 1567.

Landen, H. C.: Die funktionelle Beurteilung der Lungen- und Herzkranken. Darmstadt: Steinkopff, 1955.

Mellerowicz, H. and D. Lerche: Zschr. Kinderhk. 81, (1958) 36; Internat. Zschr. angew. Physiol. einschl. Arbeitsphysiol. 17, (1959) 459.

Mellerowicz, H., H. Schmutzler and K. Maidorn: Zschr. Kreisl.forsch. 47, (1958) 792.

Müller, E. A.: Arbeitsphysiologie 14, (1950) 271.

Müller, E. A.: in Funktionsdiagnostik des Herzens. 5. Freiburger Symposium 1957.

Müller, E. A. and K. Karrasch: Zbl. Arbeitsmed. 2, (1953) 37.

Nicolai, G.: Physiologie des Menschen I. Braunschweig: Vieweg und Sohn, 1909.

Nöcker, J. and V. Böhlau: Theorie and Praxis d. Körperkultur 5, (1957) 29.

Robinson, S.: Arbeitsphysiol. 10, (1938) 251.

Rutenfranz, J., R. Mocellin: Untersuchungen über Beziehungen zwischen verschiedenen Paramtern der körperlichen Entwicklung und der Leistungsfähigkeit bei Kindern und Jugendlichen. In: Ergebnisse der Ergometrie. Berlin: Ergon-Verlag, 1974.

Schmidt, F. L.: Herzschlagfrequenz und Leistung. S. Karger Verlag, Basel 1973.

Schmidt, F. L.: Ergometrie bei Herzkranken. Basel: S. Karger Verlag, 1977.

Schmutzler, H., H. Mellerowicz and E. Carl: Zschr. Kreisl. forsch. 49, (1960) 445.

Sjöstrand, T.: Svenska läkartidn. 7, (1950) 349.

Stegemann, J.: Leistungsphysiologie—Physiologische Grundlagen der Arbeit und des

Sports. 2. ed. Stuttgart: Georg Thieme Verlag, 1977.

Tiedt, N., B. Wohlgemuth and P. Wohlgemuth: Med. und Sport XIII, (1973) 87.

Ulmer, H. V.: Zur Methodik, Standardisierung und Auswertung von Tests für die Prüfung der körperlichen Leistungsfähigkeit. Deutscher Ärzte-Verlag GmbH, Köln 1975.

Usami, M.: Erfahrungen mit einer ergometrischen Standardleistung von 1 Watt/kg Körpergewicht in Japan. In: 3. Internationales Seminar für Ergometrie. Berlin: Ergon-Verlag, 1973.

Valentin, H. and K. P. Holzhauser: Funktionsprüfungen von Herz und Kreislauf. FT 17, Deutscher Ärzte-Verlag GmbH, Köln 1976.

Wahlund, H.: Acta med. Scand. 215 (1948).

Wezler, K. R. and K. Thauer: Zeitschrift experimentelle Medizin 107, (1940) 751.

VI. Stroke Volume and Cardiac Output in Ergometric Performance

by Hans Stoboy

1. Methods of Measuring Stroke Volume and Cardiac Output

Direct measurement of the volume of blood moved by the human heart is frequently not possible in the course of ergometric examinations. Nevertheless, in well-equipped laboratories there are means available for measuring human cardiac output even under performance conditions.

The indirect or "physical" methods frequently used in clinics and industrial medicine in former times are inexact, frequently valid solely under certain conditions (e.g., with the body at rest), and therefore require only brief mention here.

1.1 Physical Methods

1.1.1 The product of amplitude and HR

Starting out from the consideration that amplitude of the blood pressure increases as the stroke volume (Q), Erlanger and Hooker stated the product of blood pressure amplitude times HR as a relative measure of the stroke volume (see Rushmer). A number of factors on which the pressure amplitude also depends are completely ignored in this procedure. From tables by Remington, the stroke volume is said to be obtainable with an error of around 25% as a function of pressure amplitude, body size and other factors. It is obvious that with such methodological variables, experimental distinctions can hardly be verified statistically.

1.1.2 Sphygmographic Methods

The basic ideas from which these methods are developed result from a number of complicated considerations concerning the hemodynamic circumstances of the cardiovascular system (see Wetterer and Kenner).

To calculate $\dot{Q}$ the following data must be recorded and determined*:

1. Synchronous recording of a central and a peripheral pulse curve (carotid artery or subclavian artery and the femoral artery)
2. Reading or recording of the systolic and diastolic blood pressure
3. Determination of the cross-section of the aorta.

If it is possible to record simultaneously also the EKG and heart sounds, further data can be obtained on the vascular system which will be useful in the functional diagnosis. From the data obtained can be found the values necessary for calculating Q:

1. Systolic blood pressure (P_S) in dynes per cm^{-2}
2. Diastolic blood pressure (P_D) in dynes per cm^{-2}
3. Systolic duration (S) in seconds
4. Duration of a cardiac period (T) in seconds
5. Diastolic duration (D) in seconds
6. Basic oscillatory duration of the arterial pulse (T_A) in seconds
7. Speed of the pulse wave (c) in cm per second
8. Density of the blood (σ) in g per ml
9. Cross-section of the aorta (Q) in cm^2.

The specific density of the blood runs about 1.055 to 1.062 g per ml in men and about 1.050 to 1.056 g per ml in women. The aortic cross-section can be obtained from tables as a function of age.

One of the formulae in which the data obtained can be used is (according to Broemser and Ranke):

$$Q = 0.48QT\frac{S}{D} \cdot \frac{(P_S - P_D)}{\sigma \cdot c}$$

Each method is based on considerable simplification of the hemodynamic situation and is therefore subject to corresponding degrees of error. Since in determination of the several key values (e.g., blood pressure), errors of $\pm 10\%$ are to be expected, the stroke volume obtained in the result will involve a factor of error of more than that figure. Comparative tests run with gas-analytical methods showed a variation of $\pm 20\%$.

---

*$\dot{Q}$ = Cardiac output (1/min); Q = stroke volume (ml); A-VO$_2\Delta$ = arteriovenous O$_2$ difference;

V_{O_2} = O$_2$ intake (ml/min); ESV = end-systolic volume; EDV = end-diastolic volume.

1.1.3   Determination of Stroke Volume by Means of Ballistocardiogram

In the ballistocardiogram (BKG) the recoil of the stroke volume or, in other words, the displacement of the center of gravity of the mass of the body and the ejected blood is recorded. If Q is driven in the direction of the head, the body experiences a displacement in the direction of the feet, which combines with the displacement of the blood toward the feet via the descending aorta and its concomitant placement of the body toward the head (Burger et al.).

In most procedures, the motions of the body are transmitted via its more-or-less elastic tissue to a movable table, the displacement of which is recorded either by means of a change in inductivity or photoelectrically. For the determination of Q only those procedures can be used, of course, in which the inherent frequency of the system itself diverges essentially from the frequencies of the process being measured, for otherwise resonance oscillations might arise and falsify the data (Haas and Klensch).

Objections to these procedures have to do with the oversimplified assumptions that:

1. Passage of the blood takes place in the small circulation without any displacement of the center of gravity in the long axis of the body
2. Venous backflow to the right side of the heart is temporally constant
3. At the end of systole, the blood stored in the entire chamber is distributed as in a static chamber
4. Movement of the heart within the thorax is negligible
5. Changes in the elastic factors are negligible.

Despite these objections, however, the values for stroke volume and cardiac output reported by Klensch and Eger, and Klensch and Hohnen, agree quite well with those obtained through other methods by other authors.

In the case of diseases of the heart, the form of the BKG may be very much altered. Thus, the choice of curve segments necessary for the calculation becomes more open to question (Nickerson et al.).

1.1.4   Impedance Plethysmography

In impedance plethysmography, the alteration in ohmic, capacitative and inductive resistance is measured. During systole there is more blood in a particular part of the body—for instance, in the legs—and this temporarily reduces impedance (Samek). The recorded variations in impedance are similar to a pulse curve. For the determination of stroke volume, the electrodes are applied to the neck and the abdomen and certain curve criteria are determined by various methods (Kubicek et al.), and from them stroke volume is calculated. In animal experiments a very high correlation was shown between flowmeter and impedance plethysmography measurements ($r = +0.98$) with regard to cardiac output (Baker et al.). Comparisons in man between these methods and the indicator method did not always afford a satisfactory agreement (Baker et al.; Pomerantz et al.; Siegal et al.).

1.2.1   Determination of the Cardiac Output According to Fick

The perfusion of an organ with blood can be determined by adding and removing a substance (indicator) while the blood is flowing through the organ. In the lungs, for instance, it is possible to determine the quantity of blood required to absorb a particular amount of O_2 and transport it to the periphery of the body. This amount of O_2 is ascertained by determining the difference between the O_2 content of the arterial and venous blood by volume in per cent (arteriovenous O_2 difference, or A-VO$_2$Δ). If, moreover, the volume of O_2 absorbed by the lungs in one minute ($\dot{V}_{O_2}$) is known, it becomes easy to calculate the quantity of blood which has transported the corresponding volume of O_2, that is, the cardiac output or $\dot{Q}$. If, for example, 100 ml of blood have transported five volume-per cent of O_2, and 250 ml of O_2 have been absorbed in one minute, then, by a simple calculation of proportion, the $\dot{Q}$ we are after must amount to 5000 ml. The corresponding formula is:

$$\dot{Q} \text{ (in ml/min)} = \frac{\dot{V}_{O_2} \text{ ml/min}}{\text{A-VO}_2\Delta/100 \text{ ml}}$$

$$\dot{Q} = \frac{\dot{V}_{O_2} \text{ (ml/min)} \cdot 100}{\text{A-VO}_2\Delta(\%)}$$

1.2.2   Determination of the Arteriovenous O_2 Difference (A-VO$_2$Δ)

The O_2 content of venous blood in different organs varies widely. While the venous blood in the kidneys has a relatively high O_2 content (19% by volume), the figure for coronary venous blood or venous blood in exercising muscles contains merely 5–10% by volume. The O_2 content of other organs varies between these extremes. To determine precisely the overall A-VO$_2$Δ, mixed venous blood must be used, to be representative of the O_2 consumption of the total organism. This is present in the pulmonary artery, since there we would find blood from all parts of the circulatory system thoroughly mixed together. Obtaining venous blood from the pulmonary artery is greatly facilitated by use of cardiac catheters (after Grandjean). The arterial blood sample may of course be taken at any point, e.g., the femoral artery.

1.2.3   Measurement of O_2 Consumption $(\dot{V}_{O_2})$

Oxygen consumption can most simply be measured with a spirometer; otherwise it is calculated in the open system from the respiratory volume $(\dot{V})$ and the difference between the O_2 concentration in exhaled air and that in the atmosphere.

Stroke volume can easily be ascertained by dividing $\dot{Q}$ by the HR. Accurate readings can of course be expected only if the HR remains approximately constant during the entire measuring procedure, that is, with the body fully at rest or during physical exercise with practically constant HR. Arrhythmias or considerable rise and fall of the HR can at best afford an average Q for the whole experiment. To assure accurate ascertainment of Q, the A-VO$_2\Delta$ should also remain constant. An obvious prerequisite for success of the determination is precise maintenance of the experimental conditions: precise measurement of the time consumed in the experiment and simultaneous and frequent or continuous drawing of both arterial and venous blood.

Average accuracy of the procedure is about $\pm 10\%$, though on occasion greater variations may occur (Rushmer).

Even if $\dot{Q}$ is ascertained carefully with strict observance of all conditions, it is questionable whether the readings obtained during "complete bodily rest" are actually correct. The catheterization procedure itself is a considerable ordeal for the subject or patient, often leading to disturbing factors at the outset and consequent elevated readings for $\dot{Q}$ which after all may not be representative of conditions of complete rest.

The disadvantages of this procedure lie in the performance of a catheterization of the pulmonary artery, in the possibility of slight error in timing the O_2 consumption, in the prerequisite of a steady state, and in the amount of work involved in analysis of blood gases (Blümchen). The margin of error involved in this procedure lies within the range of ± 5 to 15%.

1.3   Indicator-Dilution Methods (Hamilton)

The volume of a liquid in a container can be determined by adding a known amount of an indicator (a dye or a radioactive substance) and measuring its concentration after thorough mixing. Considering the vascular system as a closed container, the procedure is as follows: An indicator whose concentration in blood samples can easily be determined and which does not leave the system during the duration of the experiment is injected in known quantity and in a quick spurt into a vein. At the same time its concentration in an artery is either measured in blood samples taken in rapid succession or recorded continuously over a definite period of time. The indicators used

include old standbys like Evans blue and cardio-green, and newer substances such as radioactively tagged albumin and cool saline solutions
(thermodilution). In the latter method, a definite amount of the solution at
room temperature is injected and the dilution of this amount of chill (point
of reference being core-central temperature) is read by means of a quick-
registering thermistor in the aorta.

Thermodilution can be performed practically as often as desired, which is
not possible with Evans blue or radioactive tracers because the indicators
accumulate in the blood. Figure 62 presents an example of a curve obtained
in such an indicator-dilution procedure. Regardless of which indicator is
used, the shape of the curve obtained from the characteristics of the flow of
indicator from the point of injection to the point of registry is, to all intents
and purposes, the same. After the short transport time of the indicator between these two points, the concentration increases, and after some seconds
reaches a peak. The curve falls more slowly than it rises, and in an open

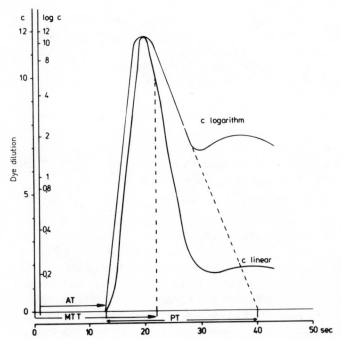

Fig. 62. Dye-dilution curve in arterial blood after injection of a known quantity of dye into the
vein at time zero.
AT = appearance time. The passage time (PT) can be ascertained by extrapolation of the
descending leg of the logarithmically presented concentration curve.
MTT = mean transit time (after *Gauer*).

system would necessarily drop to zero after all traces of the indicator had been washed away. In the closed vascular system, the transport of the indicator is so rapid that a second peak appears after a short time. This recirculation can lead to additional, ever smaller increases in concentration, which however are of no significance in the measurement of volume. The recirculation waves do interfere with an accurate calculation of volume, however, and for this reason the concentration of dye is frequently indicated logarithmically on the ordinate so as to allow linear extrapolation for time from the falling leg of the curve. Then the curve intersects the abscissa at the point of time at which, if there had been no recirculation, the indicator would have passed out of the system and its concentration thus would have been zero. In this way, the passage time, PT, in seconds, of the indicator at the point of measurement is determined. The data necessary for calculation of the dilution volume (cardiac output) by the following formula can be obtained from such a curve (Gauer):

$$\dot{Q} \text{ in ml per min} = \frac{\text{mg of indicator}}{\text{average concentration}} \cdot \frac{60}{\text{PT}}.$$

Upon the injection of 200 mg of a dye, the average concentration amounts to 10 mg per 100 ml of blood. Then 200 mg would have to be transported in the same time by 2000 ml of blood. If the passage time is 20 seconds, a cardiac output of 6 liters per minute is determined.

From a single indicator-dilution curve, the following circulatory data can in principle be calculated or measured:

1. Circulation time
2. Cardiac output
3. Volume between points of injection and reading
4. Plasma or blood volume
5. Presence and degree of valvular insufficiency
6. Presence and degree of shunts.

Depending on which of the above are to be studied, the choice of indicator and of points of injection and reading will vary.

In the circulatory system there are numerous parallel routes which differ in length and through which the blood travels at different speeds. The volume of such a route can be determined by multiplying the flow time-volume $\dot{Q}$, in ml/t, by the mean transit time, MTT. That can be determined from the linear indicator-dilution curve and is the average time required by an indicator to move from the point of injection to that of reading. It can be read at the point where the ordinate parallel intersects the lowest part of the linear indicator-dilution curve (Gauer).

The most important partial volume for further consideration is the intrathoracic volume, since on it depends, among other things, the extent of stroke volume. If, for example, a cardiac output of 6 liters per minute has been calculated and the MTT was 20 seconds, then according to the formula $Q = \dot{Q} \cdot MTT$ an intrathoracic blood volume of 2 liters is indicated.

2. Physiology of the Stroke Volume and Cardiac Output

It is the heart's job to transport a volume of blood suitable for the conditions prevailing at any given moment. The cardiac output $\dot{Q}$ must therefore, among other things, be adapted to any given requirement within the possible limits of the broad range between complete rest and maximal physical labor. The earliest observations of variation in the size of the $\dot{Q}$ were derived from animal experiments, performed on isolated hearts and heart-lung preparations. Because there was a lack of knowledge about what took place in a normal, intact cardiovascular system, it is understandable that at first the findings from such experiments were also applied to man and had great influence on the clinics for diseases of the heart and cardiovascular system.

2.1 Changes in Stroke Volume and Cardiac Output in the Classical Animal Experiment

In 1895, Frank applied knowledge of the function of skeletal muscles, namely the interconnection between length of fibers or tension and contractile power, to the isolated heart as well. He set up relationships between filling pressure and isometric contraction. From his pressure-volume diagrams, it appeared that with increased filling of the heart, the Q as well as the chamber pressure increased to a maximum and then decreased.

Straub, Wiggers, Starling and others succeeded in confirming these findings in the heart-lung preparation and extended them. An increase in peripheral resistance leads to temporary decrease in the Q and therewith to an increase in the end-systolic volume, ESV, and end-diastolic volume, EDV, until sufficient incipient fiber tension is reached and the initial Q can be transported with increased pressure. An increase in the venous inflow leads to an increase in the diastolic pressure in the atrium, the end-diastolic size of the ventricle and the Q. The increased initial filling was seen as the cause of these changes. Starling arrived at the opinion that the mechanical energy of the heart is ultimately dependent on the initial length of the muscle fibers. Considering an in situ heart, therefore, a relatively small heart would have at its disposal sufficient possibilities for increasing the Q because its fiber length is able to increase in proportion to the increase in the amount of venous blood introduced, while a large heart in end-diastolic position would have a low reserve.

A vast number of authors basically agreed with these findings as time went on.

2.2 Problems with the Classical Findings

2.2.1 Experimentally Based Objections

The results of studies mentioned up to this point depend on the situation of the isolated heart or heart-lung preparation. After careful and rapid preparation the isometric maxima occur considerably more steeply than in the further course of the experiment. The evaluation of the available findings is of course rendered difficult by the following points:

1. Usually the filling of the right side of the heart was altered, but volume changes in the left ventricle were also observed. In studies of the pressure-to-volume relationship in the adjacent parts of the heart considerable divergences arose (Sarnoff and Berglund; Berglund).
2. In general, the studies were carried out on hearts without a pericardium. The pericardium, however, sets a limit to the filling of the heart, so the results of the experiments also depend on whether the heart is suspended in air or in a liquid medium and what filling pressures are being used (Rushmer).
3. In earlier experiments, the blood supply to the coronary vessels was often insufficient (Gebhardt).

According to findings by Rushmer, anesthesia limits central regulatory influences or even cancels them out. An increase in the introduction of venous blood was for instance imitated by means of a rapid infusion of blood-substitute solutions. With increased filling pressure, then, increased Q can result. However, even under these conditions, increases in the central venous pressure without any change in the Q were observed (Fowler et al.).

Also, upon the opening of a thorax, heart volume and Q decrease, while the HR increases (Rushmer). The reduction in size of the heart can still be demonstrated about 24 hours after the thorax has been closed again.

2.2.2 Clinically Based Objections

Were we to assume that the heart behaves in situ the way it is expected to from the classical findings based on animal experiments, then we would necessarily observe at the start of a physical exercise an increase in the end-diastolic heart size. As early as 1926, Dietlen succeeded in determining in x-ray studies that end-diastolic heart size is actually reduced; this finding was confirmed by a number of authors. Almost without exception, the heart was found to remain the same size or shrink in size at systole, while the apical pulsations increased (Roskamm and Reindell). The end-diastolic pressure does not increase during physical exertion but shows rather a tendency to decrease (Roskamm and Reindell; Ekelund and Holmgren).

Roskamm and Reindell concluded from these findings that an increase in the supply of venous blood during adaptation of the heart to physical exercise is of no importance. Instead, the heart, at least at the start of the adaptive process, has to eject a residual volume increased by a greater degree of contraction and thus increase the stroke volume.

2.2.3   The End-Systolic Volume (ESV) and the End-Diastolic Volume (EDV)

Rushmer measured changes in the diameter of the ventricles in non-anesthetized dogs, practically free to move, during cardiac contraction. The difference between the end-systolic and end-diastolic diameter of the ventricles was relatively small, so that it must be assumed that there was an in-

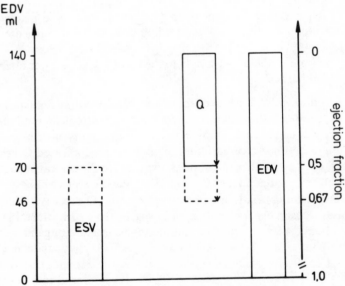

Fig. 63. Relationship between end-diastolic volume (EDV), stroke volume (Q) and end-systolic volume (ESV) of absolute values (left ordinate, ml) and as fraction (right ordinate). The areas marked with — — — lines demonstrate the variations quoted in the literature. The differences in the values of ESV and Q are due to methodology of testing. Ejection fraction angiographically established is 0.67; and established with dye methods is 0.5.

creased ESV in the heart. Clinical observations also indicated a larger ESV in the normal heart, and especially in the hearts of athletes. In animal experiments correlations of about 1:1 were verified. Even in an isolated frog heart, it was possible to eject (with the aid of electrical stimulation) ESVs that were about equal to Q (Stoboy and Nüssgen). According to Roskamm and Reindell, 67% of the EDV is ejected, on the average, as Q during the ejection period (Dodge and Baxley). The relationship between Q and EDV is also designated as the "ejection fraction." According to Lüthy and Kreuzer, the ejection fraction is given as about 50%; i.e., 33% to 50% of the EDV can be regarded as ESV under resting conditions (Figure 63). There is, therefore, doubtless a certain reserve amount of blood contained in the heart which the heart can fall back upon instantly if need arises.

In the transition from a reclining to a vertical posture, the EDV becomes smaller (Roskamm and Reindell). In the course of a physical exercise in erect position, there occurs a gradual increase in the size of the heart as a result of increased filling. The optimal filling while reclining is not exceeded, however. According to Guyton et al., this behavior is traceable to an increased venous backflow caused by the action of the venous muscular pump.

According to Lüthy et al., Kreuzer et al. and Krayenbühl, the EDV of the left ventricle under rest conditions while reclining is between 107 and 130 ml per square meter of body surface. Rapaport et al. give the EDV of the left ventricle while reclining as 98 ml per square meter of body surface and as 82 ml per square meter after passive placement in a 60° inclined posture on a tilt-table.

2.2.4 Changes in Stroke Volume with Constant Venous Supply

In animal experiments, it was possible to see findings showing considerable changes in the end-systolic volume with constant venous supply. Spontaneous or electrically induced HR changes had considerable effect on the ESV in an isolated frog heart while the peripheral resistance and venous supply remained constant (Stoboy and Nüssgen). With an increase in HR (a reduction in the duration of the cardiac period), Q was greater during several cardiac periods than the respective filling volume. The end-systolic volume was therefore reduced. Inversely, in a transition from high to low HR (a lengthening of the cardiac period's duration), there was a filling exceeding Q, and thus an increase in the end-systolic volume. The systolic reduction in the size of the heart observed at the start of a physical exercise, that is, the increase in Q by drawing on the stored-up ESV, can be traced to a positive inotropic effect such as might be found also after an accelerative stimulus or adrenal secretion in the hearts of both warm-blooded and cold-blooded creatures without increase in the diastolic volume (Bauereisen and Reichel; Ullrich et al.; Wezler).

Even after administration of beta-receptor blockers, there remains a slight HR-connected increase in contractility of the ventricular musculature (Sonnenblick et al.).

The first really definable indication of an adaptation to a physical exercise is an instantaneous increase in the HR (Rushmer; Mellerowicz; Stoboy and Nüssgen), which can be traced without doubt to an increased sympathetic innervation. There occurs thereupon a decrease in the duration of the cardiac period, and with that a lessening of the end-systolic volume before the increase in venous supply, as a result of, for example, a contraction of the skeletal musculature (Gauer) and the related reduction of the volume of the large blood vessels.

The conclusion therefore seems warranted that without any change in the venous supply, arterial pressure or end-diastolic pressure, Q can increase (Wezler); that is, that the normal in situ heart does not follow the Straub-Starling mechanism during physical exertion (Wezler; Hamilton; Richards; Monroe et al.).

2.2.5 Evaluation of the Phenomena of Adaptation of the Heart During Physical Exertion

When the HR in a healthy heart is subjected to an isolated increase to 150 per minute through electrical stimulation, Q increases only slightly, in contrast to its increase during physical exertion. Q is significantly lower than at the same HR during exercise (Rutishauser et al.; Braunwald et al.; Sonnenblick et al.). According to Guyton et al., a maximal stimulation of the sympathetic nervous system in animal experiments leads to an increase in the contractile force amounting to 60–70%, while stimulation of the parasympathetic reduces it by only 5–10% compared to the norm.

After total denervation of a dog heart, Q may increase to three or four times its former value while the HR rises to only 50% of its maximal value. The increase in Q in this situation is traceable chiefly to an increase in Q (Donald and Shephard). If denervated greyhounds are in addition treated with adrenergic blockers, they either give up a race, have to reduce their speed during the last third of the race or collapse just after reaching the finish line.

Nevertheless, after denervation and inhibition of the catecholamines, Q is said still to be able to increase to double or triple through the Straub-Starling mechanism (Guyton et al.).

When the increase in HR is limited, as for example in cases of total heart block, the stroke volume plays a greater role during physical exertion (Vatner and Pagani). These authors are of the opinion that the role of the stroke volume is reduced, and too great a Q is being measured during physical exertion. Under conditions of exertion, the diastolic heart size is said to be limited by the high HR because the filling time is shortened by it.

According to Roskamm and Reindell, the increase in $\dot{Q}$ during physical exertion does not ultimately depend on an increase in contractility, which may increase to five times the resting value. The increase in ejection speed is considerably reduced by beta-receptor blockade (Sonnenblick et al.) A decrease in EDV during physical exertion can no longer be detected under these conditions.

Also in experiments by Roskamm and Reindell, after administration of beta-receptor blockers, the increase in contractility occurring during exertion is largely suspended. At an exercise level of 200 watts, HR increased less and $\dot{Q}$ was reduced by about 15%. Maximal O_2 consumption was, however, only 10% less than in the control experiment, since Q was slightly greater— that is, at practically equal stroke volume. Ninety per cent of the maximal $\dot{V}_{O_2}$ was achieved. Without beta-receptor blockade, the end-diastolic pressure of the left ventricle drops during physical exertion. After such blockade, it increases considerably and is responsible for the constancy or slight increase in Q.

On the basis of the above findings, the participation of the Straub-Starling mechanism during adaptation of the normal heart to physical exertion is not to be entirely ruled out. Vatner and Pagani also report that in the course of an exercise in erect posture, the EDV may increase, but does not become greater than the EDV in the resting state while reclining. On the other hand, during an exercise while reclining, no further increase in the end-diastolic pressure is detectable (Roskamm and Reindell). According to Braunwald et al., the Starling mechanism is indeed at work, but is overshadowed by the positive inotropy. It becomes detectable only with the aid of a beta-receptor blockade. According to Roskamm and Reindell, the Straub-Starling mechanism makes its appearance as a replacement through nullification of the increase in contractility during a beta-receptor blockade.

3. The Magnitude of the Stroke Volume and Cardiac Output During Physical Performance

According to data supplied by Bühlmann and Lichtlen, and Åstrand and Rodahl, Q amounts to about 4–6 liters per minute in adults at rest, and in the event of maximal exertion, depending on the state of training, can reach values of 20 or even 40 liters per minute (see Tables 8 and 9). This increase can theoretically be effected by an increase in either HR or Q. In fact, the increase in $\dot{Q}$ is traceable almost exclusively to the increase in HR; at the

Table 8. The magnitude of Q̇, heart index, Q, stroke volume index and A-VO$_2$Δ in trained adult subjects during rest and exertion.

Authors	Q̇ in L per min	Heart index in L/min·m²	Q in ml	Stroke volume index in ml·m²	A-VO$_2$Δ in ml/100 ml	Commentary
Ekblom and *Hermansen*	28.4	14.8	149	77	16.1	endurance trainee: X̄ with V̇$_{O_2}$ max. 4.58 liters/min
	36.0	18.0	189	95	15.6	high-endurance trainee: X̄ with V̇$_{O_2}$ max. 5.57 L/min
	42.3	19.6	205	95	14.8	endurance trainee: performance with highest Q V̇$_{O_2}$ max. 6.24 L/min
Malarecki	13.6		115		11.1	♂ perf.: 600 kpm/min
	17.3		123		12.5	♂ perf.: 900 kpm/min
	22.5		139		13.8	♂ perf.: 1200 kpm/min } highly trained
	25.8		140		15.5	♂ perf.: maximal
	13.2		109		10.4	♂ perf.: 600 kpm/min
	16.4		114		11.3	♂ perf.: 900 kpm/min
	22.7		138		11.9	♂ perf.: 1200 kpm/min } poorly trained
	25.9		119		13.4	♂ perf.: maximal
Kindermann et al.	3.7		91		6.6	3000 m hurdler, resting (reclining)
	14.8		168		10.6	3000 m hurdler, perf.: 100 watts
	10.0		204		3.1	400 m runner, rest (reclining)
	15.5		158		8.9	400 m runner, perf.: 100 watts
	24.7		145		14.1	400 m runner, perf.: 300 watts
	10.5		205		3.1	oarsman, rest (reclining) } regulatory
	19.8		210		7.3	oarsman, perf.: 100 watts } disturbance
	30.4		177		12.6	oarsman, perf.: 300 watts
	10.1		205		3.3	middle rest (reclining)
	18.3		203		7.9	distance perf.: 100 watts
	29.4		173		12.7	runner perf.: 300 watts

same time, a distinct increase in stroke volume can be detected. This contradiction arises mainly because the measurements made at rest were performed under differing starting conditions. In the first case, the examination was made with the subject reclining while in the second he was standing. Stroke volume varies in magnitude during rest depending on the posture of the body. In the transition from standing to reclining, the hydrostatic pressure is eliminated, which while standing leads to considerable enlargement of the large blood vessels, especially in the lower extremities, and thus increases the volume of blood contained in them. This blood is stored in the intrathoracic section of the vascular system while the subject is reclining (about 400 ml). Through the greater end-diastolic filling which this involves, the stroke volume may rise to its maximum (about 120 ml) immediately in an untrained individual (Strandell). On the other hand the intrathoracic volume decreases correspondingly when the body is erect (Gauer). This reduces the filling volume and consequently stroke volume also (about 70 ml). In the transition from reclining to sitting, Q decreases by 5–20% and in that from reclining to standing by 20–30% (Guyton et al.). Consequently, Q may climb very much more during physical exertion while in an erect posture, in conjunction with the muscular pump, than while reclining—at least in the untrained individual (Fig. 64). While reclining, $\dot{Q}$ is about two liters greater than while standing, since the per cent increase in the stroke volume is greater than the per cent decrease in the HR (Fig. 64). Since the metabolism is definitely greater while standing than while reclining, a fur-

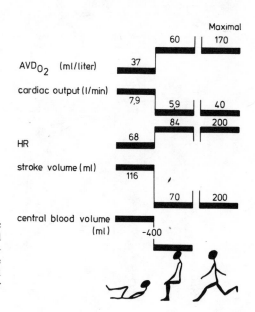

Fig. 64. The behavior of certain cardiac parameters (A-VO$_2\Delta$, HR, Q and central blood volume) in various postures (reclining and erect). At the right are the maximal values in endurance-trained subjects at maximal physical power (modified from *Gauer*).

Table 9. The magnitude of Q̇, heart index, Q, stroke volume index and A-VO₂Δ in untrained adult subjects during rest and exertion.

Authors	Q̇ in L per min	Heart index in L/min·m²	Q in ml	Stroke volume index in ml·m²	A-VO₂Δ in ml/100 ml	Commentary
Buhlmann	6.0	3.3	100		4.1	at rest, reclining
	5.0	3.0	72		5.2	at rest, seated
	18.0	10.0	110		14.0	performance: 175 watts, seated
Roskamm and *Reindell*	6.5	3.5 (2.5–4.5)	90	50 (45–55)	5.0	at rest, reclining
Grimby, Nilsson and *Sanne*	6.9		100		4.5	♂ 22–39 yrs., rest, reclining, untrained
	6.0		76			♂ 22–39 yrs., rest, seated, untrained
	14.6		108		10.6	♂ 22–39 yrs., perf., seated, untrained: 600 kpm/min, V_{O_2} 1.55 L/min
	17.0		109		13.0	♂ 22–39 yrs., perf., seated, untrained: 900 kpm/min, V_{O_2} 2.21 L/min
Jernérus, Lundin and *Thomson*	4.6		83			♂ 17–40 yrs., rest, reclining, untrained
	11.9		125			♂ 17–40 yrs., perf.: 300 kpm/min
	17.1		146			♂ 17–40 yrs., perf.: 600 kpm/min
	19.8		141			♂ 17–40 yrs., perf.: 900 kpm/min
	23.2		140			♂ 17–40 yrs., perf.: 1000 kpm/min
Strandell	≈7.5		≈120			young subjects
			≈70			at rest, reclining
	≈14.0		≈120			at rest, seated
	≈5.0		≈80			reclining, perf.: V_{O_2} 1.5 L/min or HR 150/min
			≈65			65–83 yrs., at rest, reclining
	≈12.5		≈105			65–83 yrs., at rest, seated
						65–83 yrs., perf., reclining: V_{O_2} 1.5/min or HR 125/min

ther factor must be present for a satisfactory O_2 supply. This can occur only through an increased O_2 use by the blood; that is, the A-$VO_2\Delta$ increases by about 23 ml per liter. With a $\dot{Q}$ of 8 liters per minute, then, about 180 ml more O_2 per minute would be available.

With increasing exertion, A-$VO_2\Delta$ increases. During maximal exertion, it amounts to about 14 ml per 100 ml in untrained individuals and about 17 in endurance athletes (Roskamm and Reindell).

Rowell gives the following reasons for the increase in A-$VO_2\Delta$ in connection with exertion:

1. A greater fraction of the $\dot{Q}$ is fed to the active muscles.
2. A greater amount of O_2 is extracted from the capillaries by the active muscles. During exertion, the number of the blood-filled capillaries increases. The affinity of the hemoglobin for O_2 is reduced and the increased metabolism in the active muscles lowers the intramuscular O_2 pressure.

The A-$VO_2\Delta$ plays a particular role especially in high ranges of exertion (those above 70% of the maximal $\dot{V}_{O_2}$). Therefore there is no positive linear relationship between the O_2 consumption under exertion conditions, and $\dot{Q}$ in the whole range between rest and maximal performance (Ekelund and Holmgren). From about 70% of the maximal $\dot{V}_{O_2}$ on, the regression curve is flatter as exertion increases; that is, in this range of performance, an increase in A-$VO_2\Delta$ is of greater importance than an increase in the cardiac output (Figs. 64 and 65). Reindell et al. in particular have pointed out the importance of this factor for the adaptation to physical exertion.

In the untrained individual, as already mentioned, Q may increase by about 30–60% during physical exertion while in an upright posture. This increase in Q does not, however, occur in a continuous linear fashion with the increase in exertion and/or HR and/or O_2 consumption. Maximal Q is reached at only about 40–50% of the maximal O_2 consumption (Åstrand and Rodahl; Rowell).

Starting from this relative performance, an increase in $\dot{Q}$ is achieved almost exclusively through an increase in HR (Fig. 65).

According to Roskamm and Reindell, a slight increase in A-$VO_2\Delta$ occurs as a result of endurance training, a slight increase in Q during an exercise with constant heart size because of an increase in the ejection fraction and finally an increase in Q through an increase in the EDV and accordingly in the heart volume.

Starting from a $\dot{Q}$ of 20 liters per minute in an untrained individual, the stroke volume would have to amount to about 110 ml at a maximal heart rate of 180 per minute (see Table 8). In athletes highly trained for great endurance, a $\dot{Q}$ as high as 40 liters per minute has been measured. At a maximal HR of 200 per minute, Q must then amount to 200 ml (see

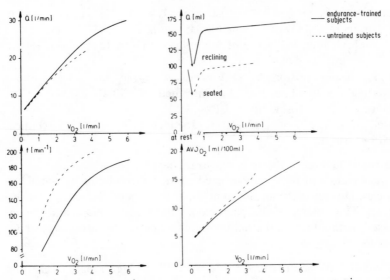

Fig. 65. The dependency of $\dot{Q}$, Q, HR and A-VO$_2\Delta$ on the magnitude of the $\dot{V}_{O_2}$ (— — — — — — = untrained subjects and ————— = endurance-trained subjects) (after *Rowell*).

Table 9). The $\dot{V}_{O_2}$ is calculated from the $\dot{Q}$ times the A-VO$_2\Delta$ in liters per liter of blood (Cumming). If in an untrained young man during maximal exertion $\dot{Q}$ is 20 liters and the A-VO$_2\Delta$ is 0.16 liters per liter, a maximal $\dot{V}_{O_2}$ of 3.2 liters per minute is observed. In a highly trained endurance athlete at a maximal $\dot{Q}$ of 40 liters per minute and an A-VO$_2\Delta$ of 0.17 liters per liter, the maximal $\dot{V}_{O_2}$ would be 6.8 liters per minute (see Table 9). In highly trained endurance athletes, Q may exceed 200 ml (Bevegard et al.; Ekblom and Hermansen; Reindell et al.).

Kindermann et al. report that in a highly trained endurance athlete at a maximal $\dot{Q}$ of 40 liters per minute maximal Q may exceed 200 ml. In endurance-trained individuals whose maximal HR corresponds approximately to that of healthy but untrained individuals of about the same age, the magnitude of $\dot{Q}$ is determined predominantly by the magnitude of the Q (Roskamm).

Even in trained individuals, Q increases only linearly during exercise while reclining, but steeply during exertion while in an upright posture (Roskamm and Reindell) (Fig. 65).

According to Ekelund and Holmgren, there is a close linear relationship between $\dot{Q}$ and $\dot{V}_{O_2}$ during conditions of rest and exertion up to an O$_2$ consumption of about 3 liters per minute (Roskamm; Lüthy et al.; Kubicek) and up to about 70% of the maximal $\dot{V}_{O_2}$ (Rowell). With an increase in the

$\dot{V}_{O_2}$ by 1 liter per minute, $\dot{Q}$ increases in this range by 6 liters per minute (Kindermann et al.). In various positions of the body, the steepness of the regression curve between $\dot{Q}$ and $\dot{V}_{O_2}$ is constant, but in youthful subjects in an upright posture at an equal $\dot{V}_{O_2}$ the $\dot{Q}$ is about 2 liters per minute, while in older subjects it is about 1 liter per minute less. A correlation of r = 0.87 between maximal $\dot{Q}$ and maximal $\dot{V}_{O_2}$ during exercise on the bicycle ergometer has been shown by Ekelund and Holmgren.

For a clinical and diagnostic evaluation of $\dot{Q}$, it suffices to determine this value nomographically from the magnitude of the venous pressure of mixed venous blood and the $\dot{V}_{O_2}$ in liters per minute. The agreement with $\dot{Q}$ obtained according to Fick's method is considered very good.

Many authors report a good correlation between maximal Q and cardiac volume (Bevegard et al.; Åstrand; Musshoff and Reindell). Athletes with the greatest cardiac volumes (about 950–1100 ml) accordingly also have the greatest Q (about 150–200 ml) during maximal performance. According to Ekelund and Holmgren, there exists a tenuous but linear correlation between cardiac volumes of about 550–1100 ml and Q during rest while reclining and during exercise.

The relationship between cardiac volume and Q while at rest is also very close in youthful subjects, but becomes less so in adults to such a degree that no relationship can be detected any longer (Musshoff and Reindell). In the adult, there is a correlation between cardiac volume and Q only during exercise. In older subjects, about 40 and upward, even this relationship becomes less noticeable as Q declines while cardiac volume remains constant.

According to Sjöstrand, the total quantity of hemoglobin correlates best with the magnitude of cardiac volume. Through a course of endurance training, the cardiac volume and blood volume are said to increase in about equal degrees. According to studies by Musshoff et al., there is a correlation of r = 0.725 between cardiac volume and total quantity of hemoglobin in a mixed population of young untrained male subjects, untrained females and trained males, while this relationship is less in each of the several subgroups, with r lying between 0.46 and 0.56.

3.1 Physiological Average Values and Range of Variation in Stroke Volume and Cardiac Output

In evaluating the magnitude of $\dot{Q}$ during the average exercise, it should be noted that according to Levy et al. the average coefficient of variation is 11.3% (3.5 to 20.7%). Grimby et al. report an average variability of 6.2% (3.2 to 14.7%). The difference between these two sets of figures is possibly of methodological origin. Ekelund and Holmgren arrive at about the same results.

During a workout in an upright posture, Q increases by about 30–50% (see Table 8). The highest value is attained five to seven minutes after the start of the exercise (Grimby et al.). With maximal physical exertion on the part of untrained individuals while reclining, there is found on the average an increase in Q of only 13-15% (Ekelund and Holmgren) or 18% (Saltin et al.). The maximal value for Q is reached at a HR of 110 per minute (Åstrand and Rodahl). Other authors give border values of 120-140 per minute for the HR up to which the Q is capable of increasing (Guyton et al.).

The rise in $\dot{Q}$ with increasing exertion depends on the posture of the body. The steepness of the regression curve for O_2 consumption does not of course change but is noticeably shifted downward, but parallel, while standing, so that for equal O_2 consumption $\dot{Q}$ is about 2 liters per minute less in younger persons and about 1 liter less in older persons (Ekelund and Holmgren).

Jernérus et al. used for their measurements a CO_2 rebreathing method. According to their data, $\dot{Q}$ while reclining at rest is 4.6 liters per minute; less than the volumes obtained according to the Fick principle or the dye-dilution method. They trace this small $\dot{Q}$ to the fact that, in the other methods mentioned, the $\dot{Q}$ is already greater during "rest conditions" than the actual resting value due to the experimental procedures and the mental state engendered by them. Even when using Jernérus's method, the first of a series of determinations during rest was greater than those taken after the subject had become accustomed to the apparatus being used (e.g., 6.0 liters per minute instead of 4.6). The exercising metabolism was likewise higher in the case of the initial determinations.

Since $\dot{Q}$ is subject to great variations with differences in body size, some standardization seems advisable. Since the magnitude of $\dot{Q}$ also depends on the magnitude of the exercising metabolism, and since there is better correlation between a calm metabolism at rest and body-surface area than between this exercising metabolism and body weight, the scatter of the $\dot{Q}$ becomes smaller when the cardiac index is calculated, that is, when $\dot{Q}$ is referred to 1 square meter of body-surface area (Guyton et al.).

According to Roskamm and Reindell, the $\dot{Q}$ of older individuals is less for the same amount of exertion than that of the young. With the same O_2 consumption, this reduction is compensated for by an increase in the A-$VO_2\Delta$. Based on a constant O_2 consumption, Q is also somewhat lower with advancing age (Lüthy et al.). According to Guyton et al., the maximal cardiac index declines by about 25 ml per minute per square meter for each year from age 15 on.

Women have in general a greater $\dot{Q}$ than men at equal power (Lüthy et al.), since A-$VO_2\Delta$ is smaller because of a lower hemoglobin count (Kindermann et al.).

The age-related decrease in $\dot{Q}$ and Q under identical conditions can be clearly seen in the data supplied by Strandell (Table 9). The orthostatically caused difference between Q while reclining and sitting, both at rest, is distinctly less in older subjects. However, Q is said to be capable of an increase of 25% during exercise while reclining. Strandell reports that end-diastolic pressure in the right ventricle is significantly increased during physical power in older persons, but he does not trace it necessarily to any performance insufficiency but rather to a greater rigidity in the ventricular musculature, whose collagenous components increase with age.

The highest values for Q and Q̇ at maximal performance have been reported by, among others, Ekblom and Hermansen, in Table 9. The high Q̇ values are caused almost exclusively by the high Q, since the HR is practically constant at maximal power.

According to Ekblom and Hermansen, the magnitude of A-VO$_2\Delta$ depends on the hemoglobin concentration. Thus the magnitude of the V̇$_{O_2}$ max is a function of the maximal Q̇ and the maximal A-VO$_2\Delta$. A reduction in the hemoglobin concentration occurring during hard endurance training is compensated for by an increase in Q. This determination does not, however, justify the claim made by Ekblom and Hermansen: "Because of the low O$_2$ capacity of the arterial blood, the maximal A-VO$_2\Delta$ in the top athletes averaged only 165 ml per liter." As is well known, hard endurance training leads to an increase in blood volume, brought about chiefly by an increase in the volume of plasma but to a lesser extent also by an increase in erythrocyte count (Röcker). This naturally means that the erythrocyte concentration must be reduced in the face of a greater O$_2$-transport capacity, but the total number of erythrocytes is increased. The advantage of this change lies in the approach of the hematocrit to the optimal value of 40% (Guyton et al.), and an improvement in thermoregulatory possibilities (Röcker).

According to Guyton et al., Q̇ may increase six- to seven-fold (Table 9) in the most highly endurance-trained individuals, but in the untrained by 500% at most. Only 40 seconds after the start of the physical effort, Q̇ is said to be capable of reaching 24 liters per minute (Guyton et al.). According to the above calculation, that would mean that at this point Q would have to amount to about 170 ml if its increase were limited by a HR of 140 per minute. However, a Q of this magnitude with a Q̇ of 24 liters per minute is reported nowhere in the literature. An increase in HR exceeding this borderline value should lead again to a decrease in Q because of the decreased filling time and the consequently reduced diastolic filling (Guyton et al.). Hints of this situation, even if not based on a borderline rate, are to be found in Table 9.

In highly trained individuals, Q̇ and Q increase steadily as exertion increases (Malarecki) (Table 8). In those less well trained, Q decreases during maximal performance only. This decline in the Q, says Malarecki, is a performance-limiting factor.

Table 10. The magnitude of $\dot{Q}$, cardiac index, Q and A-VO$_2\Delta$ in untrained adults and in patients with an exercise insufficiency, both while at rest and under stress. It should be noted that $\dot{V}_{O_2}$ remains constant in both groups.

Authors	$\dot{Q}$ in liters per min	Cardiac index in liters per min per m²	Q in ml	A-VO$_2\Delta$ in ml per 100 ml	Commentary
Kindermann et al.	8.05 6.44	4.33 3.47	108.0 92.1	4.13 5.35	1. norm. adults, rest, reclining, $\bar{X}$ 3 readings 2. cardiac insufficiency under exercise, at rest, reclining, 3 readings calc. $\dot{V}_{O_2}$: 1) 0.346 lit/min 2) 0.344 lit/min
	9.35 6.39	5.09 3.51	102.2 68.1	6.79 9.73	1. norm. adults, perf.: 25 watts 2. card. insuff. under exercise, perf.: 25 watts calc. $\dot{V}_{O_2}$: 1) 0.634 lit/min 2) 0.622 lit/min
	12.4 9.37	6.63 4.28	103.6 75.8	9.82 13.02	1. norm. adults, perf.: 75 watts 2. card. insuff. under exercise, perf.: 75 watts calc. $\dot{V}_{O_2}$: 1) 1.21 lit/min 2) 1.22 lit/min

According to studies by Kindermann et al., on trained athletes while at rest and during submaximal effort, (Table 10), the need for O_2 is met in different ways under the various conditions. At a power of 100 watts with more or less uniform O_2 consumption ($\overline{X} = 1.45$ to 1.55 liters per minute), $\dot{Q}$ varies between 15 and 19 liters per minute (Table 9), the A-$VO_2\Delta$ behaving compensatorially in the inverse direction (10.5 to 7.3 ml per 100 ml). With a lower HR compared to untrained individuals, Q sometimes shows a considerable tendency to decrease (Table 9) during submaximal power, starting out from the resting value while reclining.

The compensatory function of the A-$VO_2\Delta$ becomes especially evident when comparing normal adult subjects with patients suffering from cardiac insufficiency under exercise, studied while at rest and during various work levels (Kindermann et al.; Table 10). While maintaining uniform O_2 consumption, the $\dot{Q}$, the cardiac index and the Q are all considerably lower in patients with exercise insufficiency than in normal subjects. In the submaximal performance range, a reduced heart function is entirely compensated for by an increased A-$VO_2\Delta$. In these cases, an exclusive reliance on and evaluation of spiroergometric values may lead to misinterpretation, and so an invasive diagnosis of function is indicated.

According to Bühlmann, $\dot{Q}$ and Q are distinctly lower in children than in adults, both groups at rest and reclining, while the cardiac index and the A-$VO_2\Delta$ are more or less comparable in both children and adults (Table 11).

As a result of training, Q increases in boys aged 11 to 13 while reclining at rest at about the same rate as the $\dot{Q}$ (Eriksson and Koch) (Table 11). During submaximal and maximal exertion, the rise in Q is more pronounced (19%) than in $\dot{Q}$ (16%), caused by the slightly lower HR following training. No significant change in the A-$VO_2\Delta$ could be detected since, according to the opinion of Eriksson and Koch, children are more active physically than adults anyway and therefore have greater relative performance capacity to start with. In addition, the boys had a somewhat low average hemoglobin concentration (13 g per 100 ml), which may be regarded as normal for this age group. For the reasons given above, the O_2 binding capacity should be lower, so that the maximal A-$VO_2\Delta$ might have reached its maximum. The increase in performance capacity by 83 kpm/min resulting from training is therefore caused chiefly by the increase in Q.

At submaximal performance, the A-$VO_2\Delta$ is greater than generally reported for adults. The authors attribute this to the fact that organs whose activity does not increase during exertion are less perfused with blood in children than in adults. Since $\dot{Q}$ was not affected during submaximal power (250 kpm/min) by training, remaining at 7.7 liters per minute, the Q increased from 65.3 ml to 72.8. Before training, Q remained about constant during submaximal and maximal power and after training increased slightly in this range, while it was greater after training at each power from

Table 11. The magnitude of $\dot{Q}$, cardiac index, Q, stroke-volume index and A-VO$_2\Delta$ in children and teenagers during rest and exertion.

Authors	$\dot{Q}$ in liters per min	Cardiac index in liters per min·m²	Q in ml	Stroke volume index in ml·m²	A-VO$_2\Delta$ in ml per 100 ml	Commentary
Bühlmann	4.1	3.4	50		4.0	children at rest, reclining
Eriksson and Koch	5.0		62.2		4.6	♂ aged 11–13, rest, reclining, before training
	5.1		72.4		4.7	♂ aged 11–13, rest, reclining, after training
	3.9		49.4			♂ aged 11–13, rest, seated, before training
	4.5		56.9			♂ aged 11–13, rest, seated, after training
	11.8		68.9		13.3	♂ aged 11–13, perf.: 750 kpm/min, before training
	13.7		82.5		12.7	♂ aged 11–13, perf.: 750 kpm/min, after training
	12.5		66.9		14.2	♂ aged 11–13, perf.: 856 kpm/min, before training
	14.6		79.9		14.7	♂ aged 11–13, perf.: 939 kpm/min, after training
Cumming		10.1		56		♂ 12 yrs., max. perf., reclining, untrained
		8.6		46		♀ 12 yrs., max. perf., reclining, untrained
		9.2		49		♂ 12 yrs., max. perf., standing, untrained
		10.3		57		♂ 12 yrs., max. perf., standing, trained
		11.4		56		♂ 14 yrs., max. perf., standing, trained
Rode, Bar-Or and Shephard	3.4	2.8	43		8.2	♂ aged 11–13, seated, at rest, Eskimos
	3.6	2.6	43		7.4	♀ aged 13–15, seated, at rest, Eskimos
	12.5	10.3	64	1.6	17.9	♂ aged 11–13, max. perf. $\dot{V}_{O_2}$ = 2.24 l/min, Eskimos
	12.3	8.8	63	1.3	18.2	♀ aged 13–15, max. perf. $\dot{V}_{O_2}$ = 2.24 l/min, Eskimos
	9.9	7.9	51	1.3	18.1	♂ aged 10–12, max. perf. $\dot{V}_{O_2}$ = 1.79 l/min, Toronto
	9.9	7.9	51	1.3	14.4	♀ aged 10–12, max. perf. $\dot{V}_{O_2}$ = 1.43 l/min, Toronto
	20.5	12.8	100	1.8	16.8	♂ aged 14–19, max. perf. $\dot{V}_{O_2}$ = 3.45 l/min, Toronto
	13.5	9.1	71	1.3	18.0	♀ aged 16–19, max. perf. $\dot{V}_{O_2}$ = 2.48 l/min, Eskimos

250 kpm/min up to maximal power. According to the present author's opinion, this finding supports the theory that an increase in Q at submaximal power is to be regarded as a primary effect of training.

Sex-related differences in boys and girls aged 12 are detectable during maximal exertion while reclining, according to Cumming (Table 11). The cardiac index as well as the stroke volume index are lower in girls (about 15% and 18%, respectively) than in boys. The values reported by Cumming for the cardiac index and stroke volume index agree to a great extent with those of other authors (Eriksson; Eriksson et al.; Ekblom et al.). Cumming also calls attention to the fact that resting values may be too high because of psychological factors, and a more correct control value can be read fifteen to twenty minutes after the end of the exercise.

Rode et al. performed comparative experiments with Eskimo children and children from Toronto, using a CO_2 rebreathing method (Table 11). Even allowing for methodological error, the resting values for Q are clearly lower in the Eskimo children than in the young Canadians (Jegier et al.). The A-VO$_2\Delta$ is correspondingly high in the Eskimos. During maximal exertion, the Q is considerably higher in Eskimo boys and girls than in the children from Toronto, this difference being caused by a greater Q. The A-VO$_2\Delta$ in Eskimo children and Toronto boys seems to be extremely high, but declines as they grow older. Only the Toronto girls, with lower aerobic capacity (38.7 ml per kg · min) have a considerably lower maximal A-VO$_2\Delta$. Even bearing in mind that the hemoglobin concentration (14 g per 100 ml) is higher than that reported by Eriksson and Koch, an A-VO$_2\Delta$ of about 18 ml per 100 ml in boys seems extremely high. Rode et al., like Eriksson and Koch, attribute this extremely high figure to very low perfusion of blood in the organs not involved in exertion. Compared with older subjects, the perfusion of the skin, necessary for heat radiation and caused by thinner skin folds, should be only slight. It is assumed, moreover, that the enzyme activity in the musculature is greater in children than in older subjects.

Strehler calculated Q during physical exertion in 1500 children and adults aged 5 to 65 (Table 12). Q was obtained by the following formula:

$$Q = \frac{L_A}{\Delta F \cdot \alpha \cdot 1.0}$$

Q   = stroke volume in ml
L_A = performance in kpm/min
ΔF = difference between exercise HR and basic HR
α = specific circulatory exercise capacity in kpm per ml of blood, being calculated as follows from the hemoglobin:

$$\alpha = \frac{Hb\ g\% \cdot 6.25}{1000}$$

Although the calculated Q need not necessarily agree with the observed Q and must involve a greater factor of error for methodological reasons, the data reported by Strehler are used, because of the large sampling and broad range of subject age, to show age-related tendencies.

The performance capacity of male and female subjects increases uniformly from age five and in males reaches a maximum at about age 24, in women between ages 17 and 19. After that, it decreases slowly but uniformly in both sexes. Q increases in male subjects to about age 18, in females to about 15. This change matches more or less the cessation of growth in stature. In male subjects, Q decreases during their 40s and 50s; in females it remains constant, more or less (Table 12). In men of each age group, it is greater than in women of the same age. The Q per kg of body weight in male subjects, up to about age 18, remains constant and then declines slightly. In female subjects, it climbs until about age 12, remains at a low figure until about age 24, and then declines slightly during the remainder of life. The high Q/kg in male subjects until age 18 is attributable to great physical activity in childhood and youth. Its decline at subsequent ages correlates with a reduction in motor activity. In women, the decrease with advancing age is thought to be caused by an increase in fatty tissue, since the weight increase in women aged 20 to 55 is on the average about 18% but only 5% in men of the same age group.

Table 12. Capacity for physical exertion, Q and Q per kg of body weight, as compared with age and sex.

Author		Age	n	Perf. in kpm per min	Q in ml	Q in ml per kg
Strehler	♂	5–7	56	494	41	1.7
	♂	8–10	76	657	54	1.7
	♂	11–13	87	852	69	1.7
	♂	14–16	108	1135	95	1.7
	♂	17–19	114	1307	111	1.7
	♂	X̄ 23.4	45	1357	109	1.5
	♂	X̄ 34.7	47	1301	112	1.5
	♂	X̄ 45.4	47	1215	112	1.4
	♂	X̄ 55.6	34	1087	107	1.4
	♂	X̄ 62.2	26	1016	103	1.4
	♀	5–7	63	402	32	1.4
	♀	8–10	77	525	44	1.5
	♀	11–13	79	741	67	1.6
	♀	14–16	131	863	75	1.4
	♀	17–19	130	891	77	1.4
	♀	X̄ 24	97	838	75	1.4
	♀	X̄ 34.9	69	820	76	1.3
	♀	X̄ 45.0	59	777	79	1.3
	♀	X̄ 54.7	41	742	30	1.2
	♀	X̄ 63.5	14	665	75	1.2

A Q measured at 104 while reclining will drop after three weeks' bedrest to 74 ml. Through a subsequent eight weeks' continuous training, it can climb well above the initial level to 120 ml (Saltin et al.).

Under conditions of heat, Q reaches its maximum with a relatively low $\dot{V}_{O_2}$ and remains practically constant as the performance level continues to climb. If the skin temperature climbs from 35.0 °C to 40.5 °C and the core-central temperature from 36.7 °C to 39.1 °C, the Q̇ increases from 6.4 liters per minute to 13.1, while the perfusion of the muscles with blood rises by only 0.2 liters per minute (Rowell). Under the effects of heat, the central blood volume first falls but then climbs again (+ 100 ml). Q̇ is reduced by only 0.2 to 0.4 liters per minute with slight exertion under the effects of heat (43.3 °C), and with great exertion by 1.1 to 1.2 liters per minute. $\dot{V}_{O_2}$ remains constant through compensatory increase in the A-VO$_2$Δ. Q may decline by about 20 ml during exertion in the heat (Rowell).

Since the perfusion of the skin must necessarily be greater during exertion in heat than in a cooler environment, a redistribution of the blood perfusion occurs. During these conditions, both a reduction of renal perfusion (Radigan and Robinson) and lowered hepatic perfusion (Rowell et al.) have been reported.

3.2 Regularity and Variability in the Adaptation Mechanisms

The basic mechanisms for adaptation to various body postures, physical exertions, certain environmental conditions (heat) and to endurance training have been described in sections 3 and 3.1.

There is no dispute about the fact that the HR increases linearly in youthful subjects with increases in exertion or $\dot{V}_{O_2}$, at least in the range between 100 and 170 per minute (Mellerowicz; Ekelund and Holmgren). Q likewise increases linearly between a $\dot{V}_{O_2}$ of about 0.4 liters per minute and 3.0 (Asmussen and Nielsen; Ekelund and Holmgren). However, it is reported that Q increases in an untrained adult only up to an HR of 110–140 per minute (Åstrand and Rodahl; Guyton et al.), or to a $\dot{V}_{O_2}$ of about 1.2 liters per minute (Rowell). Until maximal $\dot{V}_{O_2}$ is reached, it then remains practically constant (Rowell). From these values, the HR would have to climb more steeply with increasing exertion if the linearity of the relationship between Q̇ and exertion or $\dot{V}_{O_2}$ is to be maintained. Such a nonlinearity on the part of the HR in this range is not reported in the literature, however. According to Smith et al., at low ranges of exertion the increase in HR suffices to explain the increase in Q̇. In the range of maximal exertion, however, an increase in Q̇ is caused chiefly by an increase in Q. According to Ekelund and Holmgren, Q usually increases somewhat in the untrained with exertion while reclining, but in some subjects it also declines a bit. Even in athletes, Q reaches a constant value after a slight increase.

An increase in Q at maximal exertion has been reported by Chapman et al., but could not be confirmed by Åstrand et al. According to Ekblom and Holmgren, a linear relationship exists between $\dot{Q}$ and Q and the $\dot{V}_{O_2}$ in well-trained and topflight athletes at maximum performance. The increase in both functions is about equally steep. This relationship holds, however, only for a $\dot{V}_{O_2}$ greater than 4 liters per minute.

In the HR range of 130-170 per minute, the mechanisms causing the linearity in $\dot{Q}$ for this range seem not to have been sufficiently studied. According to Guyton et al., an exclusive increase in HR above 125 per minute is incapable of raising the pumping performance of the heart any further, but even leads to a decrease in the Q.

The differences between readings for $\dot{Q}$, Q and A-VO$_2\Delta$ under approximately equal conditions of rest and exertion in Tables 8-11, can, to a certain extent, be attributed to differences in method and methodological error.

The statement that in athletes the circulation tends to be hyperkinetic during rest and light exertion but hypokinetic during high performance (Ekelund and Holmgren) describes only the magnitude of $\dot{Q}$ as compared with the corresponding O$_2$ consumption.

According to Cumming and Jernérus et al., there is an ever-present danger of exaggeration in measuring $\dot{Q}$. The confrontation of the subject with the procedures of experimentation and unfamiliar apparatus, especially when employing the invasive methods, can in itself lead to a "hyperkinetic" circulatory situation. Under these conditions, the actual resting value is impossible to read. With a hyperdynamic interference with regulatory processes (König), $\dot{Q}$ is increased even with the subject still at rest or during performance, because of a considerable increase in either Q or HR. Thus, the A-VO$_2\Delta$ falls. The $\dot{V}_{O_2}$ for each stage of exercise level up to 200 watts matches the values for untrained and trained subjects under "normodynamic" conditions (Reindell). The athletes described by Kindermann et al. in Table 8, who have a $\dot{Q}$ of at least 10 liters per minute, would, according to Ekelund and Holmgren, have to be counted as hyperkinetic circulatory cases, although they can in no way be designated as clearly hypokinetic, with their $\dot{V}_{O_2}$ of over 3 liters per minute. According to König, these athletes would have to be classed as having hyperdynamic regulatory disturbances, although in no cases are elevated values reported for arterial blood pressure. Such regulatory disturbances are relatively frequent among youthful athletes (Kindermann et al.).

Besides the parameters described above in detail ($\dot{Q}$, Q and A-VO$_2\Delta$), other biological factors play a significant role in the attainment of a correspondingly high $\dot{V}_{O_2}$ at a particular level of exercise. In endurance-trained athletes, the quantity of erythrocytes and the plasma volume are also significantly greater (Röcker). Since the plasma volume increases more than the quantity of erythrocytes as a result of training, the erythrocyte concentration and that of hemoglobin must decrease. The A-VO$_2$Δ is said by Eriksson and Koch and by Rode et al. to depend on the concentration of hemoglobin. In the training-caused increase in blood volume described, the hematocrit value is lowered. This, according to Guyton et al., then approaches a reported optimal value of about 40%, which represents the most favorable compromise between the maximal O$_2$ transport capacity and the viscosity, which hampers the free flow of the blood.

Lastly there exists the possibility that the enzyme activity of the muscle fibers is of importance for the magnitude of the O$_2$ consumption by the muscle tissue. The assumption that genetic factors are of importance to muscular enzyme activity was greatly supported by studies on the part of Komi et al.

The range of possibilities for adaptation is so great for a given $\dot{V}_{O_2}$ that individual variations in the individual data are very probable, depending on the validity of one or several factors, and therefore loom larger than methodologically caused differences.

References

Asmussen, E. and M. Nielsen: Cardiac output in rest and work determined simultaneously by the acetylene and the dye injection methods. Acta Physiol. Scand. 27, 217 (1952).

Åstrand, P.-O., Cuddy, T. E., Saltin, B. and J. Stenberg: Cardiac output during submaximal and maximal work. J. Appl. Physiol. 19, 268 (1964).

Åstrand, P.-O. and K. Rodahl: Textbook of Work Physiology. McGraw-Hill Book Company. New York, London (1970).

Baker, L. E., Judy, W. V., Geddes, L. E., Langley, F. M. and D. W. Hill: The measurement of cardiac output by means of electrical impedance. Cardiovasc. Res. Ctr. Bull. 9, 135 (1971).

Bauereisen, E. and H. Reichel: Über die inotrope Wirkung der Herznerven. Klin. Wschr. 24/25, 785 (1947).

Berglund, E.: The function of the ventricles of the heart. Acta Physiol. Scand. 33, Suppl. 119, 1 (1955).

Bevegard, S., Holmgren, A. and B. Jonsson: Circulatory studies in well trained athletes at rest and during heavy exercise, with special reference to stroke volume and the influence of body position. Acta Physiol. Scand. 57, 26 (1963).

Blümchen, G.: Messung des Herzzeitvolumens und der Kreislaufzeiten. In: H. Reindell und H. Roskamm: Herzkrankheiten. Springer-Verlag. Berlin-Heidelberg-New York 1977.

Braunwald, E., Sonnenblick, E., Ross, J., Glick, G. and S. H. Epstein: An analysis of cardiac response to exercise. Circulation Res. 20, Suppl. 1, 44 (1967).

Braunwald, E., Ross, J. and E. H. Sonnenblick: Mechanisms of contractions of the normal and failing heart. London: Churchill 1968.

Broemser, P. and O. F. Ranke: Die physikalische Bestimmung des Schlagvolumens des Herzens. Z. Kreislaufforsch. 25, 11 (1933).

Bühlmann, A. A.: Herz und Kreislauf, physiologische Grundlagen. In: A. A. Bühlmann und E. R. Froesch: Pathophysiologie. Springer-Verlag. Berlin, Heidelberg, New York 1972.

Bühlmann, A. A. and P. Lichtlen: Herz und Kreislauf. In: A. A. Bühlmann und E. R. Froesch: Pathophysiologie. Springer-Verlag. Berlin, Heidelberg, New York 1972.

Burger, H. C., Noordergraaf, A. and A. M. W. Verhagen: Physical basis of the low-frequency ballistocardiograph. Amer. Heart J. 46, 71 (1953).

Chapman, C. B., Fischer, J. N. and B. J. Sproule: Behavior of stroke volume at rest and during exercise in human beings. J. Clin. Invest. 39, 1208 (1960).

Cumming, G. R.: Cardiac stroke volume of athletic training. J. Sports Med. 3, 18 (1975).

Cumming, G. R.: Hemodynamics of supine bicycle exercise in "normal" children. Amer. Heart J. 93, 617 (1977).

Dietlen, H.: Herzgröße, Herzmeßmethoden: Anpassung, Hypertrophie, Dilatation, Tonus des Herzens. Handbuch der normalen und pathologischen Physiologie. Bd. VII, 1, 306, Springer Vlg. Berlin 1926.

Dodge, H. T. and W. A. Baxley: Hemodynamic aspects of heart failure. Amer. J. Cardiol. 22, 24 (1968).

Donald, D. E. and J. T. Shepherd: Initial cardiovascular adjustment to exercise in dogs with chronic cardiac denervation. Amer. J. Physiol. 205, 393 (1963).

Donald, D. E. and J. T. Shepherd: Sustained capacity for exercise in dogs after complete cardiac denervation. Amer. J. Cardiol. 14, 835 (1964).

Ekblom, B., Åstrand, P. O., Saltin, B., Stenberg, J. and B. Wallstrom: Effect of training on circulatory response to exercise. J. Appl. Physiol. 24, 518 (1968).

Ekblom, B. and L. Hermansen: Cardiac output in athletes. J. Appl. Physiol. 25, 619 (1968).

Ekelund, L. G. and A. Holmgren: Circulatory and respiratory adaptation during long-term, non-steady state exercise in the sitting position. Acta Physiol. Scand. 62, 240 (1964).

Ekelund, L. G. and A. Holmgren: Central hemodynamics during exercise. Circulation Res. 20/21, Suppl. 1, 33 (1967).

Eriksson, B.: Physical training, oxygen supply and muscle metabolism in 11- to 13-year old boys. Acta Physiol. Scand. Suppl. 384, 1 (1972).

Eriksson, B., Grimby, G. and B. Saltin: Cardiac output and arterial blood gases during exercise in prepubertal boys. J. Appl. Physiol. 31, 348 (1971).

Eriksson, B. and G. Koch: Effect of physical training on hemodynamic response during submaximal and maximal exercise in 11- to 13-year old boys. Acta Physiol. Scand. 87, 27 (1973).

Fowler, N. O., Franck, R. H. and W. L. Bloom: Hemodynamic effects of anemia with and without plasma volume expansion. Circulation Res. 4, 319 (1956).

Frank, O.: Zur Dynamik des Herzmuskels. Z. Biol. 32, 370 (1895).

Gauer, O. H.: Kreislauf des Blutes. In: O. H. Gauer, K. Kramer und R. Jung: Physiologie des Menschen. Bd. 3: Herz und Kreislauf. Urban und Schwarzenberg. München-Berlin-Wien 1972.

Gebhardt, W.: Die Druck-Volumenbeziehungen des Warmblüterherzens. Arch. Kreislaufforsch. 34, 201 (1961).

Grandjean, T.: Une microtechnique du cathétérisme cardiaque droit practicable au lit du malade sans contrôle radioscopique. Cardiologie (Basel) 51, 184 (1967).

Grimby, G., Nilsson, N. J. and H. Sanne: Repeated serial determination of cardiac output during 30 min exercise. J. Appl. Physiol. 21, 1750 (1966).

Guyton, A. C., Jones, C. E. and Th. G. Coleman: Circulatory Physiology: Cardiac output and its regulation. W. B. Saunders Company, Philadelphia-London-Toronto 1973.

Haas, H. G. and H. Klensch: Kritik ballistokardiographischer Methoden. Pflügers Arch. Physiol. 262, 107 (1956).

Hamilton, W. F.: Role of the Starling concept in regulation of the normal circulation. Physiol. Res. 35, 161 (1955).

Jegier, W., Sekelj, P., Auld, P. A. M., Simpson, R. and M. McGregor: The relation between cardiac output and body size. Brit. Heart J. 25, 425 (1963).

Jernérus, R., Lundin, G. and D. Thomson: Cardiac output in healthy subjects determined with a CO_2 rebreathing method. Acta Physiol. Scand. 59, 390 (1963).

Kindermann, W., Reindell, H. and J. Keul: Hämodynamik bei Gesunden und Kranken unter körperlicher Belastung. Sportarzt u. Sportmedizin 28, 195 (1977).

Klensch, H. and W. Eger: Ein neues Verfahren der physikalischen Schlagvolumenbestimmung (Quantitative Ballistographie). Pflügers Arch. Physiol. 263, 459 (1956).

Klensch, H. and H. W. Hohnen: Bestimmung von Schlag- und Minutenvolumen nach Arbeitsleistung mit der ballistischen Methode. Pflügers Arch. Physiol. 265, 207 (1957).

Komi, P. V., Viitasalo, J. H. T., Havu, M. et al.: Skeletal muscle fibres and muscle enzyme activities in monozygous and dizygous twins of both sexes. Acta Physiol. Scand. 100, 385 (1977).

König, K.: Psychovegetativ bedingte Herz- und Kreislaufstörungen. In: H. Reindell a.

H. Roskamm: Herzkrankheiten. Springer-Verlag. Berlin, Heidelberg, New York 1977.

Krayenbühl, H. P.: Die Dynamik und Kontraktilität des linken Ventrikels. Bibl. cardiol. (Basel) 23, (1969).

Kreuzer, H.: Ventrikelvolumina und ihre Beziehungen zur Herzinsuffizienz. In: H. Reindell, J. Keul und E. Doll: Herzinsuffizienz. Stuttgart: Thieme-Verlag 1968.

Kreuzer, H., Bostroem, B. and F. Loogen: Das Enddiastolische und Endsystolische Volumen des rechten Ventrikels beim Menschen in Ruhe. Z. Kreislaufforsch. 39, 790 (1964).

Kubicek, W. G., Patterson, R. P. and D. A. Witsoe: Impedance cardiography as a non-invasive method of monitoring cardiac function and other parameters of the cardiovascular system. Amer. N. Y. Acad. Sci. 170, 724 (1970).

Kubicek, F.: Der Einsatz der Ergometrie in der Beurteilung der kardiovasculären Arbeitskapazität. Wien. klin. Wschr. 85, Suppl. 19, 1 (1973).

Levy, A. M., Tabakin, B. S. and J. S. Hanson: Cardiac output in normal men during steady-state exercise utilizing dye-dilution technique. Brit. Heart. J. 23, 425 (1961).

Lüthy, E.: Die Hämodynamik des suffizienten und insuffizienten rechten Herzens. Basel-New York: Karger 1962.

Lüthy, E., Wirz, P., Rutishauser, W., Krayenbühl, H. P. and H. Scheu: Herz. In: W. Siegenthaler: Klinische Pathophysiologie. Georg Thieme Verlag, Stuttgart 1970.

Malarecki, I.: Cardiac output in assessment of physical fitness. In: J. Kral and V. Novotny: Physical fitness and its laboratory assessment. Universitas Carolina Pragensis 1970.

Mellerowicz, H.: Die Herzschlagfrequenz bei ergometrischer Leistung. In: H. Mellerowicz: Ergometrie. Urban und Schwarzenberg. München-Berlin 1974.

Monroe, R. C., La Farge, C. G. Gamble, W. J., Rosenthal, A. and S. Honda: Left ventricular pressure-volume relations and performance as affected by sudden increases in developed pressure. Circulation Res. 22, 233 (1968).

Musshoff, K., Schmidt, H. E. A., Reindell, H., König, K., Bilger, D., Held, E. and J. Keul: Beziehungen zwischen Herzvolumen, Körpergewicht, körperlicher Leistungsfähigkeit und Blutvolumen bei gesunden Männern und Frauen unterschiedlicher Leistungsfähigkeit. Acta Radiol. 57, 377 (1962).

Musshoff, K. and H. Reindell: Zur Rönt-gendiagnostik des Herzens. In: H. Reindell und H. Roskamm: Herzkrankheiten. Springer-Verlag. Berlin, Heidelberg, New York 1977.

Nickerson, J. V., Warren, J. V. and E. S. Brannon: Cardiac output in man: studies with low frequency, critically damped ballistocardiograph and method of right atrial catheterization. J. Clin. Invest. 26, 1 (1957).

Pomerantz, M., Delgado, F. and B. Eiseman: Unsuspected depressed cardiac output following blunt thoracic or abdominal trauma. Surgery 70, 865 (1971).

Radigan, L. and S. Robinson: Effect of environmental heat stress and exercise on renal blood flow and filtration fraction. J. Appl. Physiol. 2, 185 (1949).

Rapaport, E., Wong, M., Ferguson, R. E., Bernstein, P. and B. D. Wiegand: Right ventricular volumes in patients with and without heart failure. Circulation 31, 531 (1965).

Rapaport, E., Wong, M., Escobar, E. E. and G. Martinez: The effect of upright posture on right ventricular volumes in patients with and without heart failure. Amer. Heart J. 71, 146 (1966).

Reindell, H.: Beitrag der Klinik zur Dynamik des Herzens. Verh. dtsch. Ges. Inn. Med. 70, 100 (1964).

Reindell, H., Klepzig, H., Steim, H., Musshoff, K., Roskamm, H. and E. Schildge: Herz, kreislauferkrankungen und Sport, Johann Ambrosius Barth Verlag. München 1960.

Reindell, H., Gebhardt, W. and H. Steim: Ein Beitrag der Klinik zur Dynamik des gesunden und kranken Herzens. Arch. Kreislaufforsch. 34, 145 (1961).

Remington, J. W.: Volume quantitation of the aortic pressure pulse. Fed. Proc. 11, 750 (1952).

Richards, D. W.: Discussion of Starling's law of the heart. Physiol. Rev. 35, 156 (1955).

Rode, A., Bar-Or, O. and R. J. Shephard: Cardiac output and oxygen conductance. A comparison of Canadian eskimo and city dwellers. Pediatric work physiology proceedings of the fourth international symposium. Edt. O. Bar-Or. Wingate Institute, Israel 1972.

Röcker, L.: Der Einfluß körperlicher Aktivität auf das Blut. In: W. Hollman: Zentrale Themen der Sportmedizin. Springer-Verlag. Berlin,. Heidelberg, New York 1977.

Roskamm, H.: Funktionsprüfung von Herz und Kreislauf. In: H. Reindell und H. Roskamm: Herzkrankheiten. Springer-Verlag. Berlin, Heidelberg, New York 1977.

Roskamm, H. and H. Reindell: Die Arbeitsweise des gesunden Herzens. In: H. Reindell und H. Roskamm: Herzkrankheiten. Springer-Verlag. Berlin, Heidelberg, New York 1977.

Rowell, L. B.: Circulation. Med. Sci. sp. 1, 15 (1969).

Rowell, L. B.: Human cardiovascular adjustments to exercise and thermal stress. Physiol. Rev. 54, 75 (1974).

Rowell, L. B., Bringleman, G. L., Blackman, J. R., Twiss, D. and F. Kusumi: Splanchnic blood flow and metabolism in heat stressed man. J. Appl. Physiol. 24, 474 (1968).

Rushmer, R. F.: Cardiac diagnosis. A physiologic approach. W. B. Saunders. Philadelphia-London 1955.

Rushmer, R. F.: Cardiovascular dynamics W. B. Saunders. Philadelphia-London 1961.

Rutishauser, W., Wirz, P., Gauder, M. and G. Noseda: Vergleich der Herzdynamik bei Frequenzsteigerung unter Arbeitsbelastung und elektrischer Stimulation. In: E. Wollheim und K. W. Schneider: Herzinsuffizienz. Thieme-Verlag. Stuttgart 1968.

Rutishauser, W., Noseda, G., Wirz, P. and M. Gauder: Left ventricular performance at rest, during exercise and electrical pacing in conscious man before and after beta-blockade. Z. Kreislaufforsch. 29, 1037 (1970).

Saltin, B., Blomquist, G., Mitchell, J. H. et al.: Response to submaximal and maximal exercise after bedrest and training. Circulation 38, Suppl. 7, 1 (1968).

Samek, L.: Impedanzplethysmographie. In: H. Reindell und H. Roskamm: Herzkrankheiten. Springer-Verlag. Berlin, Heidelberg, New York 1977.

Sarnoff, St. J. and E. Berglund: Vertricular function: I. Starling's law of the heart studied by means of right and left ventricular function curves in the dog. Circulation 9, 706 (1954).

Siegel, J. H., Fabian, M., Lankau, Ch., Levine, M., Cole, A. and M. Nahmad: Clinical and experimental use of thoracic impedance plethysmography in quantifying myocardia contractility. Surgery 67, 907 (1970).

Sjöstrand, T.: Volume and distribution of blood and their significance in regulation of the circulation. Physiol. Rev. 33, 302 (1953).

Smith, W. M., Damato, A. N. and J. G. Galante: Response of the heart to exercise. Clin. Res. 12, 81 (1964).

Sonnenblick, E. H., Braunwald, E., Williams, J. F. Jr. and G. Glick: Effects of exercise on myocardial forcevelocity relations in intact unanesthetized man: relative roles of changes in heart rate sympathic activity, and ventricular dimensions. J. clin. Invest. 44, 1051 (1965).

Starling, E. H.: The Linacre Lecture of the law of the heart. Cambridge 1915. Longmans, Green & Co., London and New York 1918.

Stoboy, H. and W. Nüssgen: Anpassungserscheinungen am isolierten Froschherzen. Z. Kreislaufforsch. 45, 820 (1957).

Strandell, T.: Circulation during exercise in healthy old men. In: E. Jokl and E. Simon: International Research in Sport and Physical Education. Charles C. Thomas. Springfield 1964.

Straub, H.: Die Dynamik des Herzens. Die Arbeitsweise des Herzens in ihrer Abhängigkeit von Spannung und Länge unter verschiedenen Arbeitsbedingungen. Handbuch der normalen und pathologischen Physiologie. 7/I, 237. Hrsg.: A. Bethe und G. v. Bergmann. Springer-Verlag. Berlin 1926.

Strehler, E. H.: Ergometrische Bestimmung des Herzschlagvolumens bei 1500 schweizerischen Kindern und Erwachsenen beiderlei Geschlechts im Alter von 5-65 Jahren (1. Teil). Z. Kardiol. 65, 270 (1976).

Strehler, E. H.: Ergometrische Bestimmung des Herzschlagvolumens bei 1500 schweizerischen Kindern und Erwachsenen beiderlei Geschlechts im Alter von 5-65 Jahren (2. Teil). Z. Kardiol. 65, 283 (1976).

Ullrich, K., Rieker, G. and K. Kramer: Das Druckvolumendiagramm des Warmblüterherzens. Isometrische Gleichgewichtskurven. Pflüg. Arch. Physiol. 259, 481 (1954).

Vatner, St. F. and M. Pagani: Cardiovascular adjustments to exercise: Hemodynamics and mechanisms. Progress in cardiovascular diseases. 19, 91 (1976).

Wetterer, E. and Th. Kenner: Grundlagen der Dynamik des Arterienpulses. Springer-Verlag. Berlin-Heidelberg-New York 1968.

Wezler, K.: Wesen, Rangwert und Zusammenwirken der physikalischen und regulativen Kräfte der Herzdynamik. In: H. Reindell und H. Roskamm: Herzkrankheiten. Springer-Verlag. Berlin, Heidelberg, New York 1977.

Wiggers, C. J.: Circulatory Dynamics. Grune and Stratton. New York 1952.

Wood, E. H.: Symposium on use of indica-tor-dilution technics in the study of circulation. Circulation Res. 10, 377 (1962).

Wyndham, C. H. and N. B. Strydom: Körperliche Arbeit bei hoher Temperatur. In: W. Hollmann: Zentrale Themen der Sportmedizin. Springer-Verlag. Berlin, Heidelberg, New York 1977.

VII. The O_2 Pulse in Ergometric Performance

1. Significance, Calculation and Evaluation of the O_2 Pulse

The O_2 pulse is the quantity of O_2 which is absorbed during one cardiac period (systole plus diastole). As a rule, the O_2 consumption per minute is divided by the HR to get the average O_2 consumption in the course of a heartbeat of average duration. The O_2 pulse depends on the stroke volume and the A-$VO_2\Delta$ of the blood (Fig. 66). Regular relationships exist between the O_2 pulse while at rest and during exertion, and between the resting O_2 pulse and the performance capacity of the vascular system (Åstrand; Reindell; Mellerowicz and Petermann). The determination of the O_2 pulse in a given period of time during exertion—

$$\frac{O_2 \text{ Consumption (SPTD)}}{HR}$$

affords conclusions as to the cardiac, pulmonary and overall bodily power. Even at lower exercise levels results can be obtained which are useful in evaluation without resorting to powers of the level of the *vita maxima*.

As early as 1948, the concept of "oxygen pulse" was coined by Åstrand. He even established regular relationships among pulse rate, O_2 consumption and physical exertion. Later, Wahlund and Sjöstrand confirmed linear relationships between HR and physical exertion and also between O_2 consumption and physical exertion in both patients and healthy individuals. Not until recently have Knipping, Reindell, Nöcker, Mellerowicz and their associates turned to determining O_2 pulse as a functional test in performance diagnosis, thus enriching the process of functional diagnosis of the cardiovascular system.

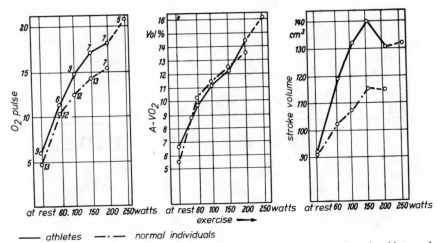

— athletes   —·— normal individuals

Fig. 66a. Average values of O$_2$ pulse, arteriovenous difference and stroke volume in athletes and normal individuals while at rest and during ergometric pedaling performance while reclining. The difference in the steepness of the curve for O$_2$ pulse is chiefly the result of a difference in the stroke volume (after *Roskamm, Reindell, Musshoff,* and *König*).

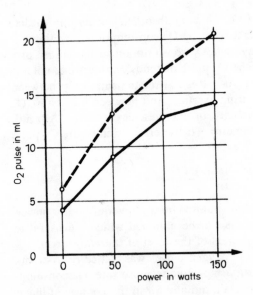

Fig. 66b. O$_2$ pulse in ergometric power of 50, 100, and 150 watts in untrained and trained subjects (after *Pickenhain*).

However, without detailed knowledge of the average physiological values and standard deviations, power evaluation studies on patients lack a basis for comparison. Tests of relatively equal power involving a comparison with body weight are especially well adapted for comparative physical performance studies. In healthy individuals, too, the O$_2$ pulse stands in close correlation with body weight (Brody, 1947). A power of one watt per kg of body weight has been shown to be a practical unit in comparative ergometry. It is a small submaximal power well adapted for use even with patients suffering from heart disease and circulatory disorders resulting in slight or moderate limitation of performance capacity.

With equal submaximal ergometric power, the cardiac and general bodily performance capacity can be assumed in general to be generally proportional to the O_2 pulse and the stroke volume (when the A-$VO_2\Delta$ is approximately the same) and inversely proportional to the HR.

Since the reading for the O_2 pulse at approximately equal O_2 consumptions is determined almost exclusively by the HR, it may be concluded that the reading for HR, at relatively equal power, can be taken alone as an expression of the performance capacity of the heart and vascular systems. Not even the changes from psychic causes in the resting HR refute this. These have relatively slight influence during physical exertion compared with the far-overriding performance regulation. Under similar experimental conditions, they are practically insignificant. Constitutional and psychic differences in the regulatory behavior mechanism affect the cardiac and general bodily performance capacity.

The kind of ergometric exercise being performed leads to no significant differences in the O_2 pulse rate, either at equal submaximal power (Figs. 67 and 68) or at maximal power (Galle and Mellerowicz). O_2 consumption and HR are affected to equal degrees by different kinds of ergometric exercise.

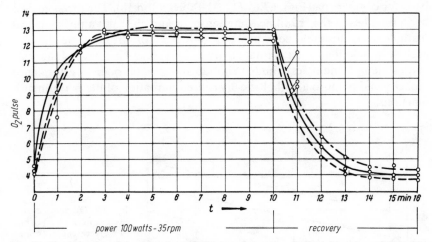

Fig. 67. The behavior of the O_2 pulse (STPD) in comparative studies of hand cranking while standing and pedaling while seated or reclining at equal power (100 watts) during a ten-minute exercise and six-minute recovery in 36 untrained male subjects aged from 20 to 40 years (after *Mellerowicz* and *Nowacki*).

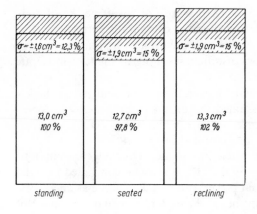

$\sigma = \pm 1.6 \, cm^3 = 12.3\,\%$

$\sigma = \pm 1.9 \, cm^3 = 15\,\%$

$\sigma = \pm 1.9 \, cm^3 = 15\,\%$

13,0 cm³
100 %

12,7 cm³
97,8 %

13,3 cm³
102 %

standing   seated   reclining

Fig. 68. Average O_2 pulse (STPD) in the steady state in hand cranking while standing and pedaling while seated.

2. Physiological Average Values and Range of Variation in the O_2 Pulse in Ergometric Performance

In evaluating the performance O_2 pulse, the physiological average values and standard deviations at different exercise levels can be drawn upon as a basis for comparison (Figs. 67 to 73 and Tables 13 to 18). The physiological borderline lies at the $\pm 2\sigma$ line. Between $\pm 2\sigma$ and $\pm 3\sigma$ lies a physiological (pathological) threshold zone in which only 2.5% of all the values lie in a healthy population with a normal distribution. Values lying beyond the $\pm 2\sigma$ borderline indicate a very limited cardiac and general bodily performance capacity and point to a pathologically caused limitation of the performance functions.

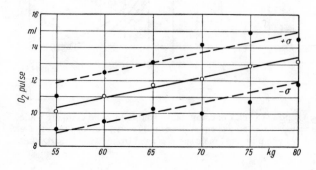

Fig. 69. O_2 pulse during exercise of one watt per kg of body weight in 100 men aged 20 to 30; hand cranking, standard conditions (after *Dransfeld* and *Mellerowicz*).

Table 13. The O_2 pulse in the steady state at a power level of 1 watt per kg of body weight in children and teenagers, arranged by age and weight groups (after *Dressler* and *Mellerowicz*).

Weight groups	Boys				Girls		
kg	n	M_y	$\pm\sigma_y$	$\pm\nu_y$	n	M_y	$\pm\sigma_y$	$\pm\nu_y$
17.5 to 22.4	2	3.66						
22.5 to 27.4	11	5.03	0.269	5.34	9	4.62	0.387	8.37
27.5 to 32.4	31	5.77	0.726	12.59	20	4.46	0.687	15.40
32.5 to 37.4	18	6.32	0.835	13.20	20	5.32	1.021	19.20
37.5 to 42.4	24	7.00	1.247	17.82	9	5.94	1.150	19.37
42.5 to 47.4	15	7.63	1.545	20.25	5	6.29	0.974	15.49
47.5 to 52.4	20	8.70	1.434	16.48				
52.5 to 57.4	17	8.70	1.508	17.33				
57.5 to 62.4	10	10.84	1.267	11.69				
62.5 to 67.4	8	11.81	1.139	9.69				
67.5 to 72.4	4	12.43	1.126	9.06				
Age groups in years								
6	1	3.52						
7	4	5.72	1.406	24.58				
8	14	5.49	0.739	13.45				
9	19	5.45	0.581	10.66	20	4.91	1.055	21.48
10	16	5.91	1.038	17.56	24	4.90	0.995	20.31
11	16	6.22	0.777	12.49	16	5.79	0.978	16.90
12	8	6.83	1.142	16.73	3	7.31		
13	22	8.31	1.445	17.25				
14	29	8.94	1.722	19.26				
15	14	9.31	2.336	25.09				
16	7	10.28	1.710	16.63				
17	8	10.74	1.681	15.65				
18	3	12.53						

Explanation of symbols: n = number of subjects
M_y = average
σ_y = average quadratic deviation from average
ν_y = coefficient of variation

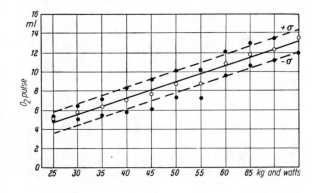

Fig. 70. The O_2 pulse in the steady state in relation to body weight with a power level of 1 watt per kg of body weight (hand crank exercise) in 167 boys aged 7 to 18 (after *Dressler* and *Mellerowicz*).

Table 14. The relationship between cardiac volume and O$_2$ pulse at an ergometric pedaling power (while reclining) of 100 and 200 watts and at maximal steady-state power in normal 20- to 30-year olds of both sexes as well as of 20- to 30-year old athletes of both sexes (after *Roskamm, Musshoff* and *König*).

	Number	Cardiac vol. in cm³	O$_2$ pulse at 100 watts							Significance
	n	x̄	x̄	εx̄	δ	V%	r	εr	t	
Normal individuals aged 20 to 30	50	797.2	12.35	0.15	1.08	8.75	+0.3820	0.122	2.87	**
Male athletes	103	904.2	13.85	0.19	1.98	13.68	+0.5739	0.067	7.04	***
Professional cyclists	19	1083.4	14.33	0.41	1.77	12.36	+0.7700	0.096	4.97	***
Normal females aged 20–30	45	586.1	9.68	0.14	0.94	9.71	+0.2648	0.142	1.80	not
Female athletes	32	680.2	10.83	0.19	1.06	9.80	+0.3200	0.161	1.88	not

The relationships between cardiac volume and O$_2$ pulse at 200 watts.

	Number	Cardiac vol. in cm³								Significance
	n	x̄	x̄	εx̄	δ	V%	r	εr	t	
Normal individuals aged 20 to 30	18	797.2	16.93	0.41	1.74	10.50	+0.3260	0.217	1.46	not
Male athletes	89	929.2	18.62	0.12	2.05	11.00	+0.6612	0.060	8.23	***
Professional cyclists	19	1083.4	19.36	0.47	2.05	10.60	+0.7439	0.105	4.58	***

The relationships between cardiac volume and maximal O$_2$ pulse attainable in the steady-state.

	Number	Cardiac vol. in cm³								Significance
	n	x̄	x̄	εx̄	δ	V%	r	εr	t	
Normal individuals aged 20 to 30	45	792.20	14.69	0.37	2.48	16.90	+0.3690	0.130	2.60	**
Total male athletes	89	912.6	19.72	0.36	3.40	17.24	+0.8100	0.037	12.89	***
Professional cyclists	20	1085.0	22.74	0.67	3.00	13.20	+0.7606	0.097	4.98	***
Normal females aged 20 to 30	43	586.6	10.13	0.21	1.39	13.70	+0.3800	0.132	2.86	**
Female athletes	34	674.7	11.36	0.31	1.80	15.20	+0.5200	0.127	3.45	**

Explanation of symbols: x̄ = the average value. εx̄ = the average error in the average value. δ = the average quadratic deviation. V% = the coefficient of variation which represents the relationship and thus a measure of percent distribution. r = the coefficient of correlation. ** = 1–0.1% probability of excess of significant values. *** = less than 0.1% probability of excess of significant values.

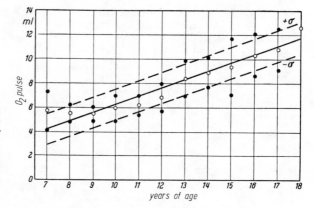

Fig. 71. The O_2 pulse in the steady state at a power level of 1 watt per kg of body weight (hand cranking) in 157 boys and male teenagers in relation to age in years (after *Dressler* and *Mellerowicz*).

The behavior of the O_2 pulse in male youths aged 7 to 18 is shown in Figure 71. If the O_2 pulse in children is taken in relation to body weight, then there are no significant differences in comparison with the values for healthy, untrained men aged 20 to 30 (Fig. 69), in overlapping weight groups. A surprisingly exact agreement is to be seen in the results obtained by different observers working with distinct subject populations. Åstrand found, even with maximal physical exertion, no differences in the O_2 consumption in youngsters and adults calculated on the basis of body weight (Fig. 118). On the other hand, it is not surprising that children and teenagers, with their smaller hearts and greater HRs, have a smaller O_2 pulse at equal O_2 consumption (Fig. 72).

Table 15. Average values for maximal O_2 pulse in normal individuals from childhood to old age and in athletes of all ages in all sports (after *Hollmann*).

Age classes normal individuals	Number	O_2 pulse	$\pm 3\sigma$
12 and 13	55	9.1	± 2.4
14 and 15	51	12.4	± 3.8
16 and 17	38	14.6	± 3.2
18 and 19	43	17.1	± 3.5
20 to 40	80	16.8	± 3.3
41 to 50	36	15.6	± 2.9
51 to 60	42	13.0	± 3.8
61 to 70	18	11.1	± 2.0
71 to 80	11	11.0	± 3.1
Athletes in all sports 20 to 40	127	21.6	3.4

Table 16. Relationships between cardiac volume and O$_2$ pulse while at rest, during ergometric foot pedaling while reclining at maximal steady state and under *vita-maxima* conditions in normal individuals aged 20 to 60. Absolute values, quotients and correlations. (After *König, Reindell, Musshoff,* and *Kessler*).

Group	Power	Number n	Cardiac volume in cm³	O$_2$ pulse O$_2$ consumption per pulse	Cardiac volume O$_2$ pulse	Correlation of cardiac volume to O$_2$ pulse	Certainty of the correlation
			$\bar{x}$	$\bar{x}$ / $\varepsilon\bar{x}$ / δ / Variation	$\bar{x}$ / $\varepsilon\bar{x}$ / δ / Variation	r / εr / B	P
Age in years							
I 20–29	at rest	50	797	4.6 / 0.12 / 0.83 / 2.8–6.2	179.4 / 5.08 / 35.92 / 122–269	0.295 / 0.129 / 0.09	*
	50 watts	50		9.3 / 0.14 / 1.00 / 7.8–12.0	86.0 / 1.59 / 11.00 / 61.2–108	0.438 / 0.113 / 0.19	**
	100 watts	50		12.4 / 0.15 / 1.08 / 10.4–14.4	64.8 / 1.21 / 8.54 / 47.2–85.1	0.382 / 0.121 / 0.15	**
	maximal steady state	45		14.7 / 0.37 / 2.48 / 10.5–21.0	55.2 / 1.46 / 9.79 / 40.0–83.6	0.369 / 0.122 / 0.14	**
	Vita maxima	41		17.0 / 0.31 / 1.99 / 12.6–21.2	46.7 / 0.97 / 6.20 / 37.5–69.3	0.504 / 0.114 / 0.26	*** / ***
II 30–39	at rest	50	762	4.3 / 0.14 / 1.00 / 2.1–8.1	183.1 / 6.85 / 48.45 / 94–352	0.400 / 0.119 / 0.16	**
	50 watts	50		9.4 / 0.16 / 1.14 / 77.–11.7	81.6 / 1.89 / 13.37 / 55.6–127	0.454 / 0.112 / 0.21	***
	100 watts	50		12.3 / 0.19 / 1.34 / 9.9–15.5	62.4 / 1.51 / 10.66 / 41.2–93.7	0.460 / 0.111 / 0.21	***
	maximal steady state	39		13.5 / 0.30 / 1.88 / 9.9–18.1	56.5 / 1.29 / 8.04 / 41.3–69.8	0.631 / 0.085 / 0.40	***
	Vita maxima	30		15.8 / 0.46 / 2.52 / 11.8–21.0	49.8 / 1.21 / 6.61 / 32.9–62.6	0.654 / 0.101 / 0.43	***

Table 16, continued.

Group	Power	Number n	Cardiac volume in cm³	O_2 pulse O_2 consumption per pulse	Cardiac volume O_2 pulse	Correlation of cardiac volume to O_2 pulse	Certainty of the correlation
Age in years			$\bar{x}$	$\bar{x}$ $\varepsilon\bar{x}$ δ Variation	$\bar{x}$ $\varepsilon\bar{x}$ δ Variation	r εr B	P
III 40–49	at rest	30	796	4.8	169.5	0.315	∅
				0.13	5.71	0.163	
				0.75	31.30	0.11	
				3.7–6.8	130–240		
	50 watts	30		9.6	83.8	0.461	**
				0.21	3.35	0.144	
				1.14	11.26	0.21	
				7.7–12.7	61.8–108		
	100 watts	27		12.5	63.4	0.728	***
				0.28	1.22	0.086	
				1.45	6.34	0.53	
				9.9–15.1	47.7–77.3		
	maximal steady state	23		13.5	57.9	0.736	***
				0.46	1.36	0.095	
				2.20	6.52	0.54	
				9.9–17.3	46.2–69.8		
	Vita maxima	17		14.8	49.1	0.335	∅
				0.68	2.46	0.215	
				2.82	10.15	0.11	
				11.2–21.6	40.2–69.5		
V 50–60	at rest	29	800	4.6	176.5	0.556	***
				0.13	4.53	0.122	
				0.72	24.41	0.32	
				3.0–6.0	144–240		
	50 watts	29		9.9	82.6	0.522	**
				0.25	2.06	0.131	
				1.38	11.27	0.27	
				7.8–13.2	69.2–116		
	100 watts	28		13.2	61.4	0.573	***
				0.32	1.39	0.121	
				1.71	7.33	0.33	
				10.6–16.2	49.7–78.7		
	maximal steady state	27		13.8	59.7	0.462	*
				0.37	1.53	0.151	
				1.93	7.94	0.21	
				10.8–17.1	47.7–78.7		
	Vita maxima	20		16.0	51.6	0.296	∅
				0.53	1.77	0.204	
				2.35	7.89	0.09	
				12.3–21.2	40.7–65		

Explanation of symbols: $\bar{x}$ = the average value. $\varepsilon\bar{x}$ = the average error in the average value. δ = the average quadratic deviation. V% = the coefficient of variation which represents the relationship and thus a measure of percent distribution. r = the coefficient of correlation. ** = 1–0.1% probability of excess of significant values. *** = less than 0.1% probability of excess of significant values.

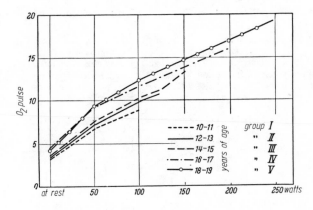

Fig. 72. Averages of the O₂ pulse in the individual age groups (ages 10 to 19) while at rest and under exercise (steady state) (after *König, Reindell, Keul,* and *Roskamm*).

With increasing age the maximal O_2 pulse steadily declines, as shown in Tables 14, 16 and 17. However, the behavior of the O_2 pulse at powers of 50 and 100 watts shows no significant differences among men aged 20 through 60 (Table 16).

Exercise O_2 pulse in women is less than in men at approximately the same O_2 consumption and higher HR with absolutely equal power levels (Table 15) and also to some extent with relatively equal power levels.

Table 17. Cardiac volume, maximal O_2 consumption, maximal O_2 pulse and quotient of cardiac volume divided by maximal O_2 pulse in normal individuals aged 10 to 60 and athletes (after *Reindell, König, Roskamm* and *Keul*).

Age groups (yrs.)	Number	Kg	Cardiac volume in cm³		Cardiac volume in body wt		Maximal O₂ pulse		Maximal O₂ consumption		Cardiac volume max. O₂ pulse
	n	σ	X̄	σ	X̄	σ	X̄	σ	X̄	σ	
10 to 11	42	35.4	411.5	63.5	11.6	1.3	7.2	1.2	1125.5	206	57.1
12 to 13	41	44.6	508.6	80.8	11.4	1.5	9.0	1.3	1430.8	233	56.5
14 to 15	42	52.2	610.8	114.7	11.7	1.2	10.8	2.1	1669.9	368	56.5
16 to 17	49	62.0	717.7	100.2	11.4	1.3	13.5	1.9	2181.7	342	53.1
18 to 19	51	67.5	769.5	112.8	11.4	1.4	16.1	2.0	2668.7	298	47.7
20 to 29	50	68.1	797.2	107.4	11.7	1.2	14.7	2.5	2373.0	459	54.2
30 t 39	50	70.5	762.2	132.8	10.8	1.0	13.5	1.9	2008.0 ≈85%	268	56.4
40 to 49	31	75.0	795.8	120.6	10.6	1.2	13.5	2.2	1847.8 ≈78%	231	58.9
50 to 59	30	75.5	808.1	102.0	10.7	1.1	13.8	1.9	1642.6 ≈69%	289	58.5
Athletes	108	61.2	906.2	111.1	14.8	2.0	19.8	2.8	3202.6	680	45.7
Athletes over 30	10	66.0	945.0	64.1	14.3	1.4	20.3	3.2	3288.5	510	46.5

Explanation of Symbols: n = number of cases studied. X̄ = average value. σ = standard deviation.

3. The Relation Between Maximal O_2 Pulse and Cardiac Volume

The maximal O_2 pulse stands in regular relationship to the cardiac volume, as was successfully demonstrated by Reindell and associates. It increases in approximately linear proportion to the cardiac volume, depending on age (Figs. 73 and 74). From the results of studies on 207 healthy male subjects aged 20 to 75, the average values and the $\pm 2\sigma$ range of the quotients of cardiac volume over maximum O_2 pulse were calculated (Table 19). They provide a physiological basis for comparison for the evaluation of the relation of maximal O_2 pulse (as an expression of the performance of the cardiovascular system, provided the respiratory system is functioning physiologically) to cardiac volume. If through x-ray measurement a cardiac volume has been detected that is enlarged compared to normal values (Table 17), the determination of the maximal O_2 pulse affords a very useful indicator of whether the physiological relation between cardiac size and performance is altered.

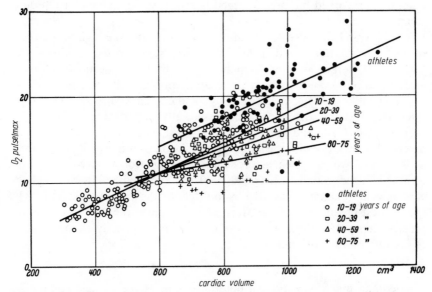

Fig. 73. Relationships between cardiac volume and maximum O_2 pulse in normal male individuals aged 10 to 70 (n = 389) and athletes (n = 89); in addition, the regression lines are given for the individual groups (after H. Reindell: Verh. Dtsch. Ges. inn. Med. 1961). Composite presentation from the following individual articles: Mushoff, Reindell, et al.: Arch. Kreisl. forschg. 35 (1961) 12; König, Reindell, et al.: Arch. Kreisl. forschg. 35 (1961) 37; König, Reindell, et al.: Arch. Kreisl. forschg. 39 (1962) 143; Roskamm, Reindell, et al.: Arch. Kreisl. forschg. 35 (1961) 67.

Table 18. The quotient of cardiac volume and maximal O_2 pulse in male and female normal individuals and athletes (average values and average quadratic deviation, average error in average value and coefficient of variation) (after *Roskamm, Reindell, Musshoff* and *König*).

	n	x̄	σ	εx̄	V%
Normal males, 20–30 yrs.	41	55.2	9.8	1.46	17.70
Total male athletes	89	46.6	4.6	0.48	10.51
Professional cyclists	20	47.9	4.4	0.99	9.19
Normal females	43	59.2	8.7	1.33	14.70
Female athletes	34	57.8	8.3	1.43	14.43

Explanation of symbols: n = number of cases studied. x̄ = the average value. εx̄ = the average error in the average value. σ = the average quadratic deviation. V% = the coefficient of variation which represents the relationship and thus a measure of percent distribution. r = the coefficient of correlation.
** = 1–0.1% probability of excess of significant values.
*** = less than 0.1% probability of excess of significant values.

If the calculated quotient lies within the $\pm 2\sigma$ range (Tables 18 and 19), it points to a physiological enlargement of the heart with correspondingly increased performance. If, however, it lies beyond the $\pm 2\sigma$ limit, it is to be regarded as indicative of a pathological cardiac enlargement with relatively deficient performance (Fig. 77). The relationship may also be altered in cases of overworked but non-enlarged hearts or those damaged from other causes.

The maximal O_2 pulse is determined by finding out the highest quotients of O_2 consumption divided by HR using standardized methods (see Chapter III) at increasing performance levels. In this connection it is apparently of no importance whether the examination is made by means of foot pedaling while reclining or sitting or by hand cranking while standing, since the maximal O_2 pulse does not differ essentially among these three forms of performance (Galle and Mellerowicz) (Fig. 75). The cardiac volume can be determined by x-ray with the subject prone, two exposures being made from a distance of two meters each, one sagittal and one frontal. According to the formulae introduced by Rohrer and Kahlstorf and modified by Reindell, the cardiac volume can be calculated by multiplying the maximum length (1) by the greatest breadth (b) of the Moritz quadrangle in the A.P. exposure, the greatest depth (t) in the frontal exposure and an empirically obtained factor of 0.4 (after Musshoff and Reindell):

$$\text{cardiac volume} = 1 \cdot b \cdot t \cdot 0.4.$$

Friedman made *post mortem* determinations of the cardiac volume according to the Rohrer-Kahlstorf formulas as modified by Liljestrand, Lysholm, Nylin and Zachrisson and by Jonsell, and compared the result with the volume as measured by flooding a specially prepared heart with water. The x-rayed and water-flooded volume findings differed by not more than 5%.

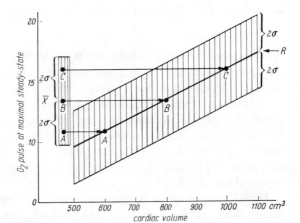

Fig. 74. O$_2$ pulse at "maximal steady-state" in relation to cardiac volume. Physiological median line and ±2σ range (after *Reindell et al.*) A = cardiac volume 600 cm^3, B = cardiac volume 800 cm^3, C = cardiac volume 1000 cm^3.

Table 19. Averages of quotient of cardiac volume over maximal O$_2$ pulse in 207 healthy males aged 20 to 75 years (after *Reindell et al.*).

Age in years	Number	Average quotients of cardiac volume over maximal O₂ pulse (cardiac performance quotient)	Distribution ±2σ
20–40	100	55–56	16–20
40–60	59	57–59	13–15
60–75	48	67	23

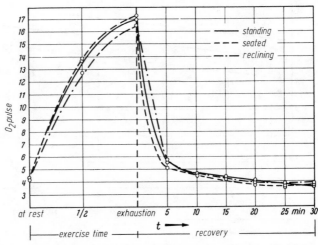

Fig. 75. O$_2$ pulse with increasing power levels (stages of 50 watts per two minutes until exhaustion) in hand cranking while standing and pedaling while sitting and reclining in ten untrained subjects aged 20 to 40, standard conditions (after *Galle* and *Mellerowicz*).

4.   The O_2 Pulse Under Pathological Conditions

The O_2 pulse is very strikingly lower in patients with congenital (noncyanotic) and subsequently acquired cardiac defects as well as in cases of weak, damaged myocardium, even during performances far below their endurance limit, than in healthy untrained individuals (Fig. 76). This characteristic behavior is probably caused by a reduction in the cardiac volume performance and not a reduction in the peripheral O_2 extraction of the blood. The determination of O_2 pulse therefore makes it possible to evaluate the cardiac and general physical performance capacity even at relatively small submaximal exercise levels.

The O_2 consumption at physically and biologically equal submaximal steady-state performance is approximately the same in healthy individuals as in cardiac patients. Therefore the magnitude of the O_2 pulse is determined overwhelmingly by the behavior of the exercising heart rate. The greater the latter is, the less is the O_2 pulse and the less are in general the cardiac and general bodily endurance reserves. Exceptions to this rule are highly hypertrophic, hypertensive hearts, those with coronary insufficiency, and those of the very old. The measurement of the HR at physically and

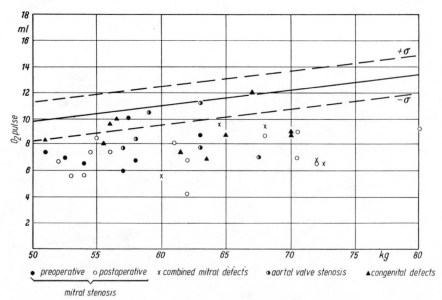

Fig. 76. O_2 pulse at a power level of 1 watt per kg of body weight in acquired and congenital (noncyanotic) defects in comparison with the normal values of Dransfeld and Mellerowicz (after *Schmutzler, Mellerowicz* and *Carl*).

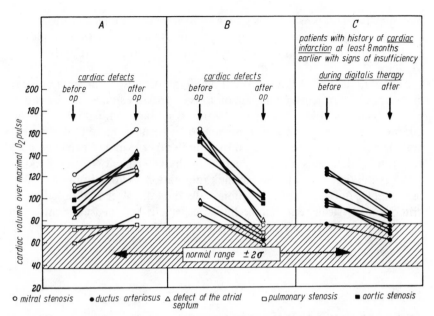

Fig. 77. The quotient of cardiac volume over maximal O_2 pulse in cases of heart damage before and after operations and in patients after cardiac infarction during digitalis therapy (after *Reindell et al.*).

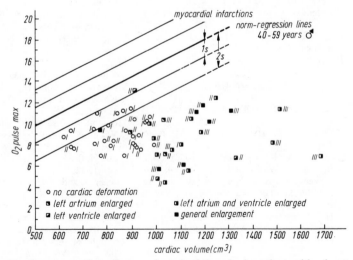

Fig. 78. Relationships between cardiac volume and maximal O_2 pulse in patients with a heart condition after healed cardiac infarction with and without pathological alterations in the shape of the heart, based on the range of correlation of norms in healthy individuals of the same age (after *Reindell, König,* and *Roskamm*).

biologically equal power levels under equivalent conditions and subsequent comparison with norms for the same age groups therefore permit simple and fairly reliable evaluation of the cardiac and general physical performance capacity.

According to Reindell a too-small maximal O$_2$ pulse or an enlarged cardiac-capacity quotient in comparison to the cardiac volume may be caused by a reduction of the cardiac performance resulting from pathological conditions (Figs. 77 and 78). It is, however, to be borne in mind that the maximal O$_2$ pulse may also be reduced by a limited performance capacity in the respiratory apparatus and a reduction of the O$_2$ capacity of the blood.

An evaluation as to whether, in the examination and determination of the maximal O$_2$ pulse, maximal exertion really did take place is afforded by the criteria of physical performance limits, especially the measurement of the HR (see Chapter III, 5.1 and Chapters V and XIV).

References

Åstrand, P. O.: Experimental studies of physical working capacity in relation to sex and age. Kopenhagen: Munksgaard, 1952.

Brody: after Sjöstrand: Verh. Dtsch. Ges. Kreisl.forschg. 22 (1956).

Christensen, E. H.: Arbeitsphysiol. 4, (1931) 470.

Dransfeld, B. and H. Mellerowicz: Zschr. Kreisl.forschg. 48, (1959) 901.

Dressler, F. and H. Mellerowicz: Zschr. Kinderhk. 85 (1961) 31.

Friedman, C. E.: Amer. Heart J. 39, (1950) 397.

Galle, L. and H. Mellerowicz: Sportarzt 10 (1962) 332.

Hollmann, W.: Habilitations-Schrift. Köln 1961.

Kahlstorf, A.: Klin. Wschr. 17, (1938) 223.

Knipping, H. W., W. Bolt, H. Valentin and H. Venrath: Untersuchung und Beurteilung des Herzkranken, Stuttgart: Enke, 1955.

König, K., H. Reindell, J. Keul. and H. Roskamm: Internat. Zschr. angew. Physiol. einschl. Arbeitsphysiologie 18, (1961) 393.

König, K., H. Reindell, H. Roskamm, K. Musshoff and M. Kessler: Arch. Kreisl. forschg. 35 (1961) 12 and 37; 39 (1962) 143.

König, K., H. Reindell: Über die Bedeutung der korrelativen Betrachtung bei der ergo-metrischen Funktionsdiagnostik. In: 2. Internationales Seminar für Ergometrie. Berlin: Ergon-Verlag 1967.

Mellerowicz, H.: Arch. Kreisl.forschg. 24, (1956) 70.

Mellerowicz, H. and P. Nowacki: Zschr. Kreisl.forsch. 50, (1961) 1002.

Mellerowicz, H. and A. Petermann: Arzt u. Sport 4/2, (1956) 9.

Mellerowicz, H. and D. Lerche: Zschr. Kinderhk. 81, (1958) 36.

Mellerowicz, H., H., Schmutzler and K. Maidorn: Zschr. Kreisl.forschg. 47, (1958) 792.

Musshoff, K. and H. Reindell: Dtsch. med. Wschr. 81, (1956) 1001.

Musshoff, K., H. Reindell, K. König, J. Keul and H. Roskamm: Arch. Kreisl.forschg. 35, (1961) 12.

Nöcker, J. and V. Böhlau: Verh. Dtsch. Ges. Kreisl.forschg. 24 (1958).

Pickenhain, L.: In: Findeisen, Linke, Pickenhain: Grundlagen der Sportmedizin, Leipzig: Barth 1976.

Reindell, H. et al.: Herz und körperliche Belastung. Vortr. 67. Tagg. d. Dtsch. Ges. inn. Med. Wiesbaden 1961.

Reindell, H. and H. W. Kirchhoff: Verh. Dtsch. Ges. Kreisl.forschg. 22 (1956); Dtsch. med. Wschr. 17, (1957) 613.

Reindell, H., K. König, H. Roskamm and J. Keul: Mkurse ärztl. Fortbild. 4 (1959).

Reindell, H., K. König, and H. Roskamm: Funktionsdiagnostik des gesunden und kranken Herzens. G. Thieme, Stuttgart (1967).

Rohrer, F.: Fortschr. Röntgenstr. 24, (1961/17) 285.

Roskamm, H., H. Reindell, K. Musshoff and K. König: Arch. Kreisl.forschg. 35, (1961) 67.

Schmutzler, H., H. Mellerowicz and E. Carl: Zeitschrift f. Kreislaufforschung 49, (1960) 445.

Schwalb, H.: Zur Beurteilung des Sauerstoffpulses bei Übergewichtigen. In: Ergebnisse der Ergometrie. Köln: Wissenschafts-Verlag, 1974.

Schwalb, H., J. Eberl: Das kymographisch bestimmte Herzvolumen und seine Beziehung zum Sauerstoffpuls. In: Ergebnisse der Ergometrie. Berlin, Ergon-Verlag, 1974.

Sjöstrand, T.: Verh. Dtsch. Ges. Kreisl.forschg. 22 (1956).

Wahlund, H.: Acta med. Scand. 215 (1948).

VIII. Arterial Pressure in Ergometric Performance

by Kurt Maidorn

1. Methodology of Measurement and Registration of Arterial Pressure During and After Ergometric Performance

The arterial blood pressure can be measured directly and indirectly during ergometric performance in pedaling while seated or reclining and after hand cranking while standing. In practice the indirect measurement is common and indispensible despite its limited precision. The method of determination is simple, quick, repeatable as often as desired and involves no elaborate apparatus. As in measurement while at rest, it follows the principle of Riva-Rocci and Korotkoff. It must be borne in mind that under the influence of physiological, pathophysiological and clinical methodological studies new modifications of the measuring techniques are again and again recommended and new points of view are discussed as to evaluation of the findings. These efforts lead mainly in the direction of better comparability of results in the medical and scientific spheres.

In the present state of our knowledge, the indirect measurement of the blood pressure while at rest is best performed according to the recommendations of the German Society for Cardiovascular Research, which follow closely those of the American Heart Association. It is in fact expected that the indirect measurement of blood pressure will be employed as recommended during ergometric performance. Practical experience in the ergometric field points in the same direction. In a memorandum entitled "Recommendations on the indirect measurement of blood pressure in man," published by a committee of the German Society for Cardiovascular Research, the following recommendations are outlined[1]:

---

[1] Since January 1, 1978, the new units are used in Germany when measuring the blood pressure (Table 20).

1.1   Instruments for Measurement

Mercury as well as membrane manometers may be used for indirect measurement of blood pressure. Each instrument must be calibrated and correspondingly characterized by its manufacturer. Recalibration at two-year intervals is required by law.

The fabric portion of the cuff for adult use shall be 13 to 14 cm wide and about 50 cm long. On the inner surface of its end, the cuff has a fabric pocket 25 to 30 cm long to receive an inflatable rubber portion. This rubber portion shall be 23 to 30 cm long and 12 to 13.5 cm wide. The fastening of the cuff must ensure that the rubber portion is uniformly covered for its entire length and breadth by the nonstretchable fabric portions of the cuff.

1.1.1   Application of the Cuff

When applying the deflated cuff, make sure that the inflatable rubber portion covers at least the total inner semi-circumference of the arm. The cuff must fit tightly without constriction and end about 2.5 cm above the elbow.

1.2   Measuring the Systolic and Diastolic Pressures

Regardless of the posture of the patient, the elbow and the forearm (bent slightly at the elbow), shall be located at the same level as the heart. In order to estimate the level of the systolic pressure without overlooking a possible

Table 20. New units of measurement of blood pressure (in effect as of January 1, 1978).

1. Scale of comparison							
2. Enlarged partial scale							
3. Comparative table for determining intermediate values							
torrs	millibars	torrs	millibars	torrs	millibars	torrs	millibars
0	0	50	66.7	120	160.0	190	253.3
1	1.3	60	80.0	130	173.3	200	266.6
5	6.7	70	93.3	140	186.7	210	280.0
10	13.3	80	106.7	150	200.0	220	293.3
20	26.7	90	120.0	160	213.3	230	306.6
30	40.0	100	133.3	170	226.6	240	320.0
40	53.3	110	146.7	180	240.0	250	333.3

4. Conversion factor: 1 torr = 1.33 millibars
                        1 millibar = 0.75 torrs

After *Pharmazeutische Zeitung* 122, 18 (1977)

"auditory gap," the pressure in the cuff is pumped up rapidly, while palpating the radial pulse, to a point about 30 mm of mercury beyond the manometric pressure, at which the radial pulse disappears. Then the pressure in the cuff is gradually reduced and at the same time the brachial artery in the pit of the elbow is auscultated. At the first "Korotkoff sounds" the systolic pressure is read on the manometer. The diastolic pressure is read when the Korotkoff sounds become distinctly softer (more damped) but not entirely silenced. Damping and silencing may occur simultaneously. The cuff pressure must drop not more than 2 to 3 mm of mercury per second within the measuring range of the systolic and diastolic pressures. An interval of at least 1 minute shall intervene between two successive pressure readings and during this time the cuff must be completely deflated in order to preclude a blockage of the vein.

The pressure readings, despite the well-known range of error inherent in this method, must not be rounded off upward or downward but be read precisely.

1.2.1 Details

Do not allow for the thickness of the soft parts of the arm by applying corrections to the pressure readings unless the upper arm is above 40 cm in circumference and a non-standard cuff is being used, since for one thing, the customary normal values have also been arrived at without consideration of the "soft-part factor of error." In children, narrower cuffs are employed (2.5 or 8 cm wide); select the size which covers approximately 2/3 of the upper arm. With upper arms above 40 cm in circumference, the frequently considerable factor of error can be reduced by use of a wider cuff, but can not be entirely compensated for in each individual instance. In such cases, use a fabric cuff 15 to 20 cm wide and 60 to 80 cm long with a comparably sized rubber portion, the kind used when taking the readings from the thigh.

Bear in mind, however, that during and after physical performance differences between direct and indirect readings have been proven to occur which are sometimes greater than in readings taken with the patient at rest. Thus Anschütz has determined in comparative studies that the systolic values are read 5 to 10 mm of mercury too high by auscultation during exercise levels above 1000 kpm per minute as compared with readings obtained by the direct method. The differences are smaller in the case of lesser exercise levels. A relationship to the speed of blood flow is obvious. However, the indirect determination of the systolic pressure during exercise is indispensible. It must surely be assumed that the reading errors within the range of physiological variation are smaller than the elevations of blood pressure in cases of pathological change.

The latter leads at first to nonphysiological elevations of the exercise blood pressure before this development shows up in the readings while the patient is at rest. The knowledge of the behavior of the systolic blood pressure during physical performance is thus of diagnostic value and is of considerable importance in determining therapeutic measures.

The value of the indirectly obtained diastolic pressure during exercise is dubious. The differences between direct and indirect readings are relatively great, even with the subject at rest. The criterion of determination is inexact and there is constant discussion as to whether the cuff pressure should be read at the damping phase (phase IV) or not until total disappearance of the sounds (phase V) in determining the diastolic pressure. Meanwhile the predominant feeling is, as described, to read the diastolic pressure at the first distinct damping of the Korotkoff phenomena, that is, in phase IV.

Under physical exercise this criterion becomes more and more imprecise (Anschütz; Henschel et al.; Kleinhanss et al.; Schellong and Lüderitz; Krestownikow; Metzner; Parade and Ohr). Such great differences are possible between direct and indirect reading methods, and the statement and evaluation of the readings are no longer acceptable. This is true, at any rate, if neither the damping nor the disappearance of the Korotkoff phenomena is audible until the cuff pressure reaches 0 mm of mercury. The heightened blood-flow speed is probably responsible. Even at low or nonexistent cuff pressures, turbulences arise, so that the Korotkoff phenomena of phase III[1] remain unaltered and the pressure must be read as zero. Under these circumstances, the indirect measurement of the diastolic pressure is impossible.

If, however, the damping of the Korotkoff phenomena becomes more audible by auscultation, or if it even coincides with their disappearance, this value can be of practical significance. This occurs especially with an elevation of the diastolic pressure obtained by auscultation, since under this circumstance an actual elevation is to be expected.

There is in addition a practical significance to the zero phenomenon. According to Krestownikow, Parade and Ohr, and also Valentin and Holzhauser, the Korotkoff sounds can be heard even during the exercise, but more frequently at the beginning of the rest period, down to 0 mm of mercury, if individually high performances are achieved or if the subjects are to be regarded as untrained (Fig. 79).

It would be desirable to measure the blood pressure during exercise not only by the given method but also by registering it continuously and obtaining it both systolically and diastolically at the same pulse beat. Various more or less reliable apparatus have been developed for this purpose, but they have no importance in practice.

---

[1] In phase III, the acoustic phenomenon takes on a loud, noisy character like a rhythmic hissing.

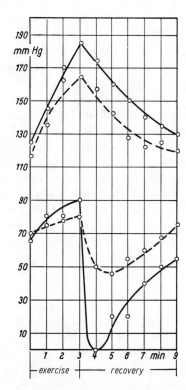

Fig. 79. The behavior of the blood pressure, determined by Korotkoff's auscultation method during and after an ergometric performance of 2 watts per kg of body weight in two highly trained and six untrained students (average).

However, fully automatic recording blood-pressure and pulse-rate apparatus now on the market are of practical value. They operate completely by the Riva-Rocci-Korotkoff method and are well-adapted for bloodless measurement of blood pressure with the subject at rest and very useful in series or monitoring studies. But for ergometry, they can be recommended for the most part only with caution and reservations. If, during physical stress, mechanical noises occur under the sound pick-up device (these apparatus usually involve body-sound microphones built into the cuff), inaccurate readings can occur. The noises can occur when the arm muscles are actively involved, through direct transmission of bumping and friction noises through the body or from contact with the inflated cuff. Most such apparatus are fitted with a constant pressure drop. The speed of pressure drop is often too rapid and therefore does not conform to the usual recommendations. In the reading ranges of the systolic and diastolic pressures, therefore, the systolic readings tend to be too low and the diastolic too high. At high blood pressure readings, such as are to be expected during physical exertion, a noncontinuous pressure drop would be more suitable. The drop must run about 2 to 3 mm of mercury per second in the range of the systolic and diastolic pressures in order to conform to the usual recommendations. Beyond this range it should be as rapid as possible. It is important that the individual reading not take too long, for methodological reasons.

Moreover, no venous blockage must be allowed to occur. With standardization of the release speed, these considerations should be borne in mind. With manual regulation, the conditions can be relatively easily maintained after a little practice.

Moreover, most microphones do not register the damping of the Korotkoff sounds when determining the diastolic pressure, but only their disappearance. The former, as indicated above, agree better with the invasively obtained readings. Bearing in mind these sources of error, the available apparatus is adaptable to ergometric use only under certain conditions. At all events, only such fully automatic blood-pressure apparatus as is equipped with a high-grade static eliminator, and is thus capable of accurate readings, can be recommended for ergometric studies in the submaximal range. For reliable readings under vita maxima conditions no apparatus as yet produced fulfills the necessary requirements.

For methodological reasons, the determination of blood pressure is carried out most reliably when the patient is pedaling while reclining. It is more difficult with pedaling while seated and impossible with hand cranking while standing. However, after hand-cranking work, the determination of blood pressure during the recovery period is possible even with the subject standing. If the cuff is put in place before the exercise, just tight enough that it will not fall off, then immediately after the exercise the arterial pressure can be read with the subject standing or reclining and its further progress followed at equal intervals of one minute. It is useful to determine the heart rate for six seconds first before reading the blood pressure. These are just the

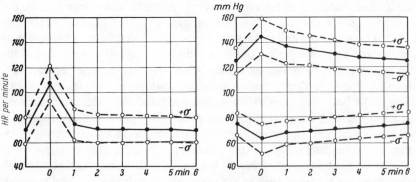

Fig. 80. HR and arterial pressures in 100 healthy, untrained students aged 20 to 30 after performance of 1 watt per kg of body weight per minute (after *Mellerowicz, Schmützler* and *Maidorn*).

data which permit conclusions to be drawn as to the regulation and capacity of the vascular system (Fig. 80).

In the indirect measurement of blood pressure by auscultation using the Riva-Rocci-Korotkoff method, reading errors may arise before, during and after physical exercise:

1. Through incorrect handling of the equipment in taking the reading; e.g., too-slow or too-rapid release of the cuff pressure, too-tight or too-loose application of the cuff and too-firm or incomplete emplacement of the stethoscope
2. Through false readings of the Korotkoff sounds and their coordination with cuff pressure
3. Through displacement of the diastolic criterion toward 0 mm of mercury after physical exertion
4. Through too-great or too-small upper arm circumference without proper selection of cuff width
5. Through the effect of psychic, reflex and mechanical events on blood pressure

2. On the Physiology of the Arterial Pressure in Ergometric Performance

In the study of the physiological background of the blood pressure during exertion, we are still only on the threshold. Still, some relationships between blood pressure and physical performance are already known. Results of studies using ergometric methods obtained to date show that the systolic pressure rapidly increases with the HR at the start of the exercise, and remains in close coordination as the exercise proceeds, as Figure 81 shows. The amount of the increase as well as the increase in amplitude (Fig. 82) stand in close relationship (almost linear in the submaximal ranges) with the degree of performance for the same individual (after Bock et al.; Hollmann; Mellerowicz; Rutenfranz et al.).

With light and medium-heavy exercise levels, a blood pressure steady-state is reached after a few minutes; at heavy exercise levels, the systolic blood pressure climbs until the conclusion of the exercise (Hollmann). There are no available experimental data on the maximal systolic pressure, including amplitude of pressure and its physiological border values at maximal physical performance. In ranges of performance not attainable by the untrained individual, we have found systolic blood pressure values above 250 mm of mercury in professional athletes.

Pressure and volume performance of the heart stand in lawful relationship (see Fig. 83, after Ekelund and Holmgren). Measurable expression of

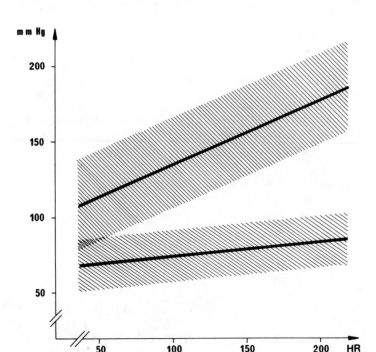

Fig. 81. Systolic and diastolic pressures in relation to HR during increasing ergometric performance (66 healthy male and female subjects aged 16 to 41) (after *Ekelund* and *Holmgren*).

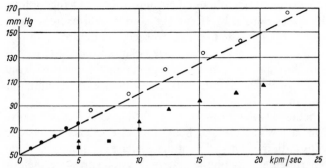

Fig. 82. Interdependence of the average blood pressure amplitude and the intensity of performance. With increasing exercise intensity, the blood pressure amplitude increases linearly. In our
studies (●), it followed on the average an equation having the formula "y = 50.75 + 5.0 x"
between 1 and 5 mkp per second. The blood pressure amplitudes at higher work obtained by
Hollmann, marked with ○, correspond with sufficient precision to a projection of this regression
line, while the values obtained by Kirchhoff, Reindell and Hauswaldt (■ and ▲) on children of
maturity-level "K" and teenagers of maturity-level "PR" deviate sharply from this regression
line (after *Rutenfranz, Hellbrügge and Keilhacker*).

the cardiac pressure performance is afforded by the performance pressure reserves. They correspond to the difference between systolic pressure at maximal ergometric performance and the systolic pressure while at rest. The greater the cardiac performance capacity is, the greater are the systolic performance pressure reserves. They are:

In trained athletes with high-performance hearts	100–150 mm Hg
In healthy nontrained of average age	75–100 mm Hg
In cardiac low-performers and those with performance insufficiency	75 mm Hg

The systolic pressure reserves are also more or less reduced in the case of hypotonic subjects. Measuring those reserves makes possible a reliable evaluation of the cardiac performance capacity by simple, bloodless methods. The contraindications for such measurement in coronary patients, high-level hypertension in elderly arteriosclerotics, etc., must not be lost sight of (after Mellerowicz).

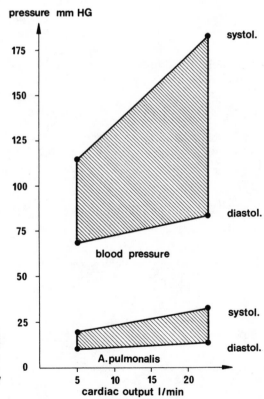

Fig. 83. The relations of the arterial blood pressure in the major and minor circulatory systems to the cardiac output at increasing physical exercise level (after *Ekelund* and *Holmgren*).

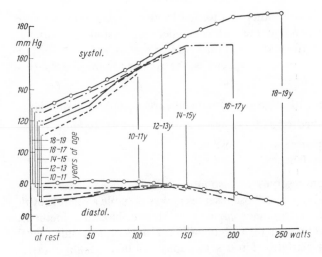

Fig. 84. Average readings of the systolic and diastolic pressures in the various age groups (10–19 years) while at rest and during exercise levels (steady-state), pedaling while reclining (after *König, Reindell, Keul* and *Roskamm*).

Immediately after the conclusion of the exercise, there occurs a steep drop in the systolic pressure, which then continues on with decreasing steepness. Under certain conditions of regulation, training vagotonia, hypertonic regulation, etc., the systolic pressure readings may fall to below the resting levels.

In view of the above statements about the determination and evaluation of diastolic blood pressure, it must be noted that under physiological conditions during a workout it shows a small increase of varying amount (Emery;

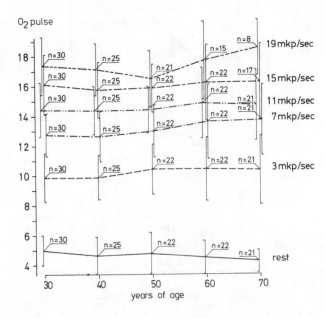

Fig. 85. Averages of the systolic pressure in males in their third to seventh decades of life at equal power levels during bicycle-ergometer exercise (Standard Test Method) (after *Hollmann et al.*).

Reindell et al.). According to Hollmann, however, a drop may also occur up to a maximum of 30 mm Hg. In the higher decades of life, he found a significant rise at a similar exercise level.

In the recovery phase, the diastolic pressure usually falls very sharply (Emery; Fraser and Chapman; Henschel et al.; Korner; Mellerowicz; Reindell et al.). The magnitude of the drop depends on the degree of exertion and the regulatory conditions of the vascular system. The return to resting value then takes place in different ways. Toward the end of the recovery period, systolic and diastolic pressures approach the starting levels more and more slowly but as a rule almost simultaneously. The recovery period is again in lawful relationships to the magnitude and duration of the exercise as well as to the performance capacity of the vascular system and the organism as a whole. It can take minutes or hours.

3. Physiological Variation Capacity of the Arterial Pressure in Ergometric Performance

In order to be able to evaluate the performance capacity of the vascular system on the basis of the performance and recovery blood pressures, a knowledge of the physiological variation capacity of these vascular values is essential (see Figs. 79, 81, 84, 85, 86, and 87). As for other performance functions, 1 watt per kg of body weight and 2 watts per kg of body weight are suitable as standard power levels alongside the absolute performances. The graphic representation (Fig. 80) shows the physiological range of variation of the blood pressure during recovery after a standard power level of 1 watt per kg of body weight for one minute in men aged 20 to 30 (see also Figs. 84 and 85).

4. Endogenous and Exogenous Conditioning Factors of the Arterial Pressure in Ergometric Exercise

4.1 Age and Sex

Comparative studies on the behavior of the blood pressure under exercise in teenagers and adults of various age groups are shown in Figures 84 and 85. In ergometric studies on older people, Hollmann et al. found at the same exercise level a greater increase in the systolic pressure than in younger ones.

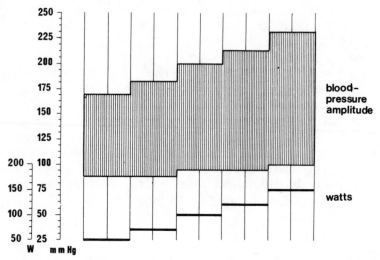

Fig. 86. Averages of the systolic and diastolic pressures during increasing ergometric power levels in stages of 25 watts per two minutes, 50 and 100 watts, pedaling while sitting (after *Halhuber*).

In the 30 seconds after the conclusion of the exercise, a further increase in the systolic pressure may occur in older persons, according to Fraser and Chapman, a phenomenon not observed in younger individuals. Contrary to expectation, there has to date been found no difference in behavior between men and women as to blood pressure during absolutely equal exercise, in contrast to the behavior of the HR (Fraser and Chapman; Brouha and Harrington; Hollmann). On the other hand, according to available data, the return of the systolic pressure to the resting level occurs more rapidly in the male than in the female subjects.

Verified age and sex differences in the diastolic pressure during exercise and recovery have not yet been proven. More detailed studies on age- and sex-related phenomena of the blood pressure during exercise seem to be necessary.

4.2   Arterial Pressure and State of Training

The behavior of the arterial pressure and amplitude while at rest for various age levels of the total population is compared to that for well-trained endurance athletes in Figures 88 and 89.

Depending on kind, magnitude and duration of the training, endurance athletes generally show lower systolic pressures. The diastolic pressure is usually somewhat elevated in these individuals and the amplitude while at rest thereby reduced. Teenagers, even those engaged in sports, turn up not infrequently above the scatter range for the norm with blood pressures as high as (or even higher than) 150 or 160 mm Hg.

Endurance athletes in good form reach the steady state of blood pressure earlier at slight total elevation (Fig. 90). However, a considerable amount of training, especially in endurance training, is necessary until its influence on the behavior of the arterial pressure under stress of exercise becomes defi-

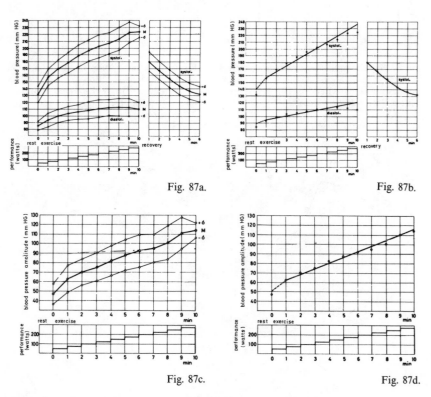

Fig. 87a.   Fig. 87b.

Fig. 87c.   Fig. 87d.

Fig. 87a. Behavior of the systolic and diastolic pressure at increasing performance load in 50 untrained, male subjects aged 20 to 30 (after *H. Al-Eshaiker* and *H. Mellerowicz*).

Fig. 87b. Behavior of the systolic and diastolic blood pressures during increasing ergometric exercise, represented by means of the regression lines.
y = 0.35x + 139.86 for systolic pressure and
Y = 0.11x + 89.37 for diastolic at increasing power (after *H. Al-Eshaiker* and *H. Mellerowicz*).

Fig. 87c. Behavior of the blood pressure amplitude at increasing ergometric power (after *H. Al-Eshaiker* and *H. Mellerowicz*).

Fig. 87d. Behavior of the blood pressure amplitude, represented by a regression line according to the equation y = 0.24x + 50.49 at increasing power (after *H. Al-Eshaiker* and *H. Mellerowicz*).

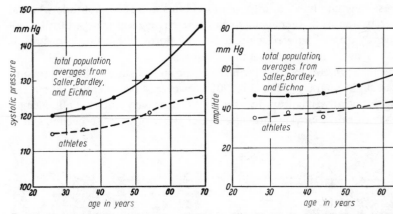

Fig. 88. Systolic pressure at various age levels in the total population (averages from Saller, Bordley and Eichna) and in 107 well-trained athletes (after *Mellerowicz*).

Fig. 89. The amplitude in the total population (after Saller, Bordley and Eichna) compared with 107 well-trained endurance athletes, with the body at rest (after *Mellerowicz*).

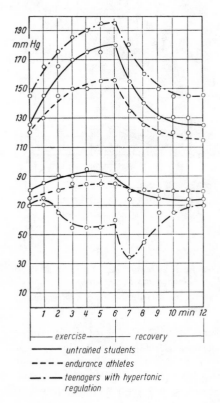

exercise ——— recovery ———
—————— untrained students
— — — — endurance athletes
—·—· teenagers with hypertonic regulation

Fig. 90. The behavior of the blood pressure, determined by auscultation. (Korotkoff's method) during and after an ergometric power of 100 watts in five highly trained endurance athletes, seven untrained students and five teenagers with hypertonic regulation.

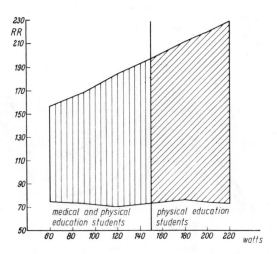

Fig. 91. The systolic and diastolic pressures in ten non-sports-participating medical students and ten students of physical education at the tenth minute of a constant exercise of, first 60, then 90, 120, etc., watts on the bicycle ergometer. Up to 150 watts no differences between the two groups appear. Exercise levels of over ten minutes beyond 150 watts were not possible with the medical students (after *Hollmann*).

nitely verifiable. Hollmann was unable to detect any differences in the level of the systolic pressure between medical students and students of physical education at equal power levels up to 150 watts (Fig. 91). Although students of physical education are generally very well trained physically, the effects on heart and vascular systems are irregularly less as a result of this training than of special endurance training. This explains the lack of differences in the blood pressure during exertion of equivalent magnitude between these two groups.

While normal individuals on the average perform maximally between 100 and 150 watts in the steady state (only a small percentage reach 200 watts), top trained athletes perform in the steady state up to 350 watts and attain systolic pressures up to 250 mm of mercury. Maximal values during athletic events go even higher.

The performance amplitude of the well-trained also shows a lower absolute total increase. The relative increase in such individuals is however greater (Figs. 92a and b). This may be caused by a relatively (compared to the stroke volume while at rest) increased stroke volume during exertion on the part of well-trained athletes.

4.3 Circadian and Seasonal Variations in the Arterial Pressure

The arterial blood pressure while at rest is subject to various physiological rhythmic and arrhythmic variations which are caused by various exogenous influences. The average circadian variations, which lead to a minimum in

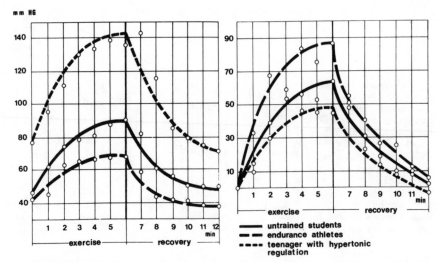

Fig. 92. Absolute (a) and relative (b) behavior of the blood pressure amplitudes in relation to the arterial amplitude with the body at rest, determined according to the infratone method of Boucke-Brecht, during and after exercise at 100 watts in five highly trained endurance athletes, seven untrained students and five teenagers with hypertonic regulation.

the first hours of sleep and a maximum in late afternoon, amount to between 10 and 20 mm of mercury, which includes the slight blood pressure elevations during ingestion of food (Hantschmann). Seasonal variations between winter, spring, summer and fall amount to about 8 mm of mercury (higher in summer), according to Kusui and Miyano.

5.   On the Pathological Physiology of the Arterial Pressure During Ergometric Performance

The physiological blood pressure is the important prerequisite for sufficient and economic blood supply to the organs, and depends mainly on stroke volume and peripheral and elastic resistance. It is kept nearly constant by a complex and finely tuned system of regulators. The neurovegetative and endocrine processes play a role in this. In the presence of pathological processes, sometimes a change in only one function is sufficient to produce upsets in the physiological blood pressure situation. Upsets of a repeated or continuous nature lead in time to either an elevation in the arterial pressure (hypertonia) or a lowering of it (hypotonia). This is not a matter of disease but a symptom whose pathogenesis may be very varied and often very difficult to explain. (Details on this are to be found in monographs on the subject by Hantschmann; Sack and Koll; Pierach and Heynemann.)

The exact distinction between hypertonia and normotonia is a difficult, mainly biological-statistical problem. During absolutely equivalent power levels of 100 watts per six minutes, there occurs in hypertonic subjects a greater absolute increase in systolic pressure and HR (Fig. 90). The increase also persists longer. The relative increase in the systolic pressure is smaller, however, in agreement with Mellerowicz. Even at average lower levels that have little effect on the heart and vascular system of normotonics, hypertonics and patients with mitral stenosis show elevated systolic pressures (Fig. 93). Ergometric studies up to the maximal power should therefore be particularly avoided in elderly hypertonics.

That the changes in the systolic pressure are measurable only during and after physical power levels, and not during rest periods, is clear from Figure 94.

In the recovery phase, the drop in pressure is often delayed in comparison with normotonics. Chiefly in teenage hypertonics (Weiss), and also in people

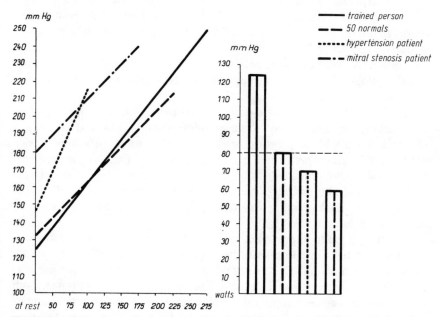

Fig. 93. Systolic pressure reserves in normals and typical cases of trained persons and cardiacs (after *Mellerowicz* and *Schmutzler*).

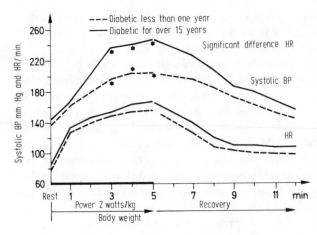

Fig. 94. Behavior of the systolic blood pressure and HR before, during and after an ergometric power level of 2 watts per kg of body weight for five minutes in diabetics, in relation to duration of the diabetic condition. Diabetes up to one year n = 11; diabetes above 15 years n = 7.

older than they whose hypertension is not yet manifest, the systolic pressure often drops during the recovery phase to a point below that of the resting phase before returning to its original level, which often takes hours.

The diastolic pressure during exercise behaves very differently in hypertonics. Sharper increases and, more commonly, sharper decreases are found. Often the "O phenomenon" occurs which can be observed by auscultation almost regularly at the beginning of the recovery phase after relatively low-grade exercise levels (Fig. 79).

Comparative studies on the behavior of the arterial pressure during exertion in etiologically and pathogenetically different forms of hypertension are yet to be undertaken.

Schleusing et al. studied two groups of patients with essential hypertension, seeking an explanation of the question whether adequate training is able to affect the blood pressure behavior in hypertonics in a similar way. While the one group performed prescribed amounts of training exercise for 8 months along with the medication therapy, those in the control group were assigned no exercise. Spiroergometric studies with determination of the behavior of the blood pressure served to objectivize the success of the treatment (Fig. 95).

The training led to improvement in the subjective sense of well-being and performance. In connection with the improvement in performance, an increase in the maximal O_2 consumption and the maximal O_2 pulse was detectable by spiroergometric means. The blood pressure was lower, both while at rest and at the comparable levels of exercise. The untrained patients on the other hand showed no improvement during the same period of time but rather a worsening in their readings.

The importance of training in sports in the alleviation of neurovegetative disturbances leading to hypertension is obvious from these studies.

In hypotonic disturbances of regulation, only slight elevations in blood pressure and limitation of the performance reserves in the vascular system are found, even during exercise with high HR. Symptomatic hypotension can occur as a result of acute and chronic infectious diseases, valvular defects, anemias, adrenal insufficiencies, hypophysis insufficiency and during convalescence. Low performance capacity at high HR during exercises and low arterial performance amplitude, caused by meager increase in systolic pressure, are the results. Many hypotonic individuals, however, can show very good performance under normotonic regulatory conditions during exertion. In the case of well-trained athletes, "hypotonic" arterial pressure readings are the rule while at rest, coupled with great performance capacity of both heart and vascular systems (Figs. 79, 92 a and b).

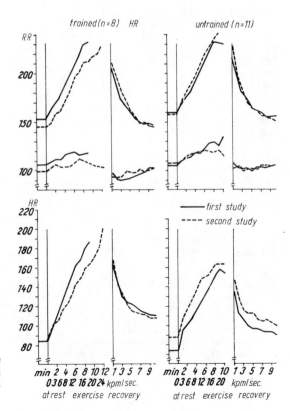

Fig. 95. Effect of training on the behavior of blood pressure and HR (averages). See text (from *Schleusing et al.*).

The German Federal Republic accepted the SI (Système International d'Unités) as a new law. The conversion tables from mm Hg to kPa and from mm Hg to mbar are presented. The unit, kPa, is recommended by WHO and

Conversion table of blood pressure from mm Hg to kPa and from mm Hg to mbar following the SI International Unit System.

mm Hg (= Torr) → kPa

	0	1	2	3	4	5	6	7	8	9
0	—	0.1	0.3	0.4	0.5	0.7	0.8	0.9	1.1	1.2
10	1.3	1.5	1.6	1.7	1.9	2.0	2.1	2.3	2.4	2.5
20	2.7	2.8	2.9	3.1	3.2	3.3	3.5	3.6	3.7	3.9
30	4.0	4.1	4.3	4.4	4.5	4.7	4.8	4.9	5.1	5.2
40	5.3	5.5	5.6	5.7	5.9	6.0	6.1	6.3	6.4	6.5
50	6.7	6.8	6.9	7.1	7.2	7.3	7.5	7.6	7.7	7.9
60	8.0	8.1	8.3	8.4	8.5	8.7	8.7	8.8	8.9	9.2
70	9.3	9.5	9.6	9.7	9.9	10.0	10.1	10.3	10.4	10.5
80	10.7	10.8	10.9	11.1	11.2	11.3	11.5	11.6	11.7	11.9
90	12.0	12.1	12.3	12.4	12.5	12.7	12.8	12.9	13.1	13.2
100	13.3	13.5	13.6	13.7	13.9	14.0	14.1	14.3	14.4	14.5
110	14.7	14.8	14.9	15.1	15.2	15.3	15.5	15.6	15.7	15.9
120	16.0	16.1	16.3	16.4	16.5	16.7	16.8	16.9	17.1	17.2
130	17.3	17.5	17.6	17.7	17.9	18.0	18.1	18.3	18.4	18.5
140	18.7	18.8	18.9	19.1	19.2	19.3	19.5	19.6	19.7	19.9
150	20.0	20.1	20.3	20.4	20.5	20.7	20.8	20.9	21.1	21.2
160	21.3	21.5	21.6	21.7	21.9	22.0	22.1	22.3	22.4	22.5
170	22.7	22.8	22.9	23.1	23.2	23.3	23.5	23.6	23.7	23.9
180	24.0	24.1	24.3	24.4	24.5	24.7	24.8	24.9	25.1	25.2
190	25.3	25.5	25.6	25.7	25.9	26.0	26.1	26.3	26.4	26.5
200	26.7	26.8	26.9	27.1	27.2	27.3	27.5	27.6	27.7	27.9
210	28.0	28.1	28.3	28.4	28.5	28.7	28.8	28.9	29.1	29.2
220	29.3	29.5	29.6	29.7	29.9	30.0	30.1	30.3	30.4	30.5
230	30.7	30.8	30.9	31.1	31.2	31.3	31.5	31.6	31.7	31.9
240	32.0	32.1	32.3	32.4	32.5	32.7	32.8	32.9	33.1	33.2
250	33.3	33.5	33.6	33.7	33.9	34.0	34.1	34.3	34.4	34.5
260	34.7	34.8	34.9	35.1	35.2	35.3	35.5	35.6	35.7	35.9
270	36.0	36.1	36.3	36.4	36.5	36.7	36.8	36.9	37.1	37.2
280	37.3	37.5	37.6	37.7	37.9	38.0	38.1	38.3	38.4	38.5
290	38.7	38.8	38.9	39.1	39.2	39.3	39.5	39.6	39.7	39.9
300	40.0	40.1	40.3	40.4	40.5	40.7	40.8	40.9	41.1	41.2
310	41.3	41.5	41.6	41.7	41.9	42.0	42.1	42.3	42.4	42.5
320	42.7	42.8	42.9	43.1	43.2	43.3	43.5	43.6	43.7	43.9
330	44.0	44.1	44.3	44.4	44.5	44.7	44.8	44.9	45.1	45.2

Conversion: (mm Hg) $\times$ 0.133 = (kPa); (kPa) $\times$ 7.501 = (mm Hg)
Example: 118 mm Hg = 118 Torr = 15.7 kPa
Name of new unit: Kilopascal (kPa)
Notice: mm Hg is practically identical with Torr. During the printing of this book, the discussion concerning the unit Millibar was in process.

recognized by Germany. There is still a discussion about the Millibar. It has been suggested that the first two units be used in the next five years—mm Hg and kPa, placing mm Hg in parenthesis (*Lippert*).

mm Hg (= Torr) → mbar

	0	1	2	3	4	5	6	7	8	9
0	—	1	3	4	5	7	8	9	11	12
10	13	15	16	17	19	20	21	23	24	25
20	27	28	29	31	32	33	35	36	37	39
30	40	41	43	44	45	47	48	49	51	52
40	53	55	56	57	59	60	61	63	64	65
50	67	68	69	71	72	73	75	76	77	79
60	80	81	83	84	85	87	88	89	91	92
70	93	95	96	97	99	100	101	103	104	105
80	107	108	109	111	112	113	115	116	117	119
90	120	121	123	124	125	127	128	129	131	132
100	133	135	136	137	139	140	141	143	144	145
110	147	148	149	151	152	153	155	156	157	159
120	160	161	163	164	165	167	168	169	171	172
130	173	175	176	177	179	180	181	183	184	185
140	187	188	189	191	192	193	195	196	197	199
150	200	201	203	204	205	207	208	209	211	212
160	213	215	216	217	219	220	221	223	224	225
170	227	228	229	231	232	233	235	236	237	239
180	240	241	243	244	245	247	248	249	251	252
190	253	255	256	257	259	260	261	263	264	265
200	267	268	269	271	272	273	275	276	277	279
210	280	281	283	284	285	287	288	289	291	292
220	293	295	296	297	299	300	301	303	304	305

	0	10	20	30	40	50	60	70	80	90
200	267	280	293	307	320	333	347	360	373	387
300	400	413	427	440	453	467	480	493	507	520
400	533	547	560	573	587	600	613	627	640	653
500	667	680	693	707	720	733	747	760	773	787
600	800	813	827	840	853	867	880	893	907	920
700	933	947	960	973	987	1000	1013	1027	1040	1053
800	1067	1080	1093	1107	1120	1133	1147	1160	1173	1187
900	1200	1213	1227	1240	1253	1267	1280	1293	1307	1320

Conversion: (mm Hg) × 1.333 = (mbar); (mbar) × 0.7501 = (mm Hg)
Example: 118 mm Hg = 157 mbar
Notice: The preferred unit to replace mm Hg or Torr is Kilopascal (see the previous table).

6. Evaluation of the Cardiac and Physical Performance Capacity on the Basis of the Behavior of the Arterial Pressure During Physical Performance

The performance capacity of the vascular system can be evaluated on the one hand by means of the relationship existing between the blood pressure during exertion and recovery and on the other by the magnitude of the power and the performance capacity. Extensive fundamental studies must still be carried out, however, in order to determine the blood pressure during exercise and recovery at certain relatively and absolutely equivalent performances and its distribution in certain age and sex categories, kept as representative as possible. Power levels of 1 to 2 watts per kg of body weight while reclining and seated seem well adapted for a standardization. On the basis of the statistical frequency distributions it will also be possible to evaluate by actual readings the performance capacity from the behavior of the arterial pressure during exercises.

On the basis of the normal readings taken from 100 healthy men aged 20 to 30 after a standard power level of 1 watt per kg of body weight, the regulatory behavior of the blood pressure during recovery can be evaluated (Fig. 80). For further evaluations see Figures 81, 84, 85, 86, 87, 88, 89, 90, 91, 93 and 94.

According to our present knowledge, it can be assumed that changes in arterial pressure ranging above or below the physiological and economic border values ($\pm 2\sigma$ thresholds) have the effect of reducing performance capacity.

References

Al-Eshaiker, M. H. and H. Mellerowicz: Untersuchungen des arteriellen Druckes bei ansteigender ergometrischer Leistung. In: 2. Internationales Seminar für Ergometrie, Ergon Verlag Berlin, 1967.

Anschütz, F.: Fortschr. Med. 88, 1931 (1970).

Anchütz, F. and H. Ch. Drube: Verh. Dtsch. Ges. Kreisl.forschg. 20. Tagg. 1954.

Bock, A. V., C. Vaucaulaert, D. B. Dill, A. Folling and L. M. Hurxthal: J. Physiol. 66, 136 (1928).

Brecht, K., G. Amann and H. Boucke: Münchner med. Wochenschrift 97, 112 (1955).

Brecht, K. and H. Boucke: Pflügers Arch. Physiol. 43, 256 (1952); Klin. Wschr. 31, 668 (1953).

Brouha, L. and M. E. Harrington: Lancet Vol. 77, 79 (1957).

Ekelund, L. G. and A. Holmgren: Circ. Research, Suppl. 1 Vol. XX and XXI, 1–33 (1967).

Emery, F. E.: Texas Rep. Biol. Med. 13, 23 (1955).

Fraser, F. F. and C. B. Chapman: Circulation 9, 193 (1954).

Frey, U.: Die sportärztliche Untersuchung. Sportmed. Schriftenreihe, H. 2.

Halhuber, M. J.: after Schmidt, F. L.: S. Karger Verlag Basel-München-Paris-London-New York-Sydney 1977.

Hantschmann, L.: Die krankhafte Blutdrucksteigerung. Stuttgart: Thieme, 1952.

Henschel, A., F. de la Vega and H. L. Taylor: J. Appl. Physiol. 6, 506 (1954).

Hollmann, W.: Der Arbeits- und Trainingseinfluß auf Kreislauf und Atmung. Kreislauf-Bücherei, Bd. 17. Darmstadt: Steinkopff, 1959.

Hollmann, W., W. Barg, G. Weyer and H. Heck: Die medizinische Welt 28, 2 (1970).

Hollmann, W. and H. Venrath: Med. Klin. 54, 1311 (1959).

König, K., H. Reindell, J. Keul and H. Roskamm: Internat. Zschr. angew. Physiol. einschl. Arbeitsphysiol. 18, 393 (1961).

Korner, P. J.: Austral. J. Exper. Biol. 30, 375 (1952).

Krestownikow, A. W.: Physiologie der Leibesübungen. Berlin: Volk und Gesundheit, 1953.

Krethlow, A.: Physikalisch-Technisches Praktikum für Mediziner, S. 221. Berlin: Springer, 1930.

Kusui, K. and Y. Miyano: Wakayama, med. Rep. 2, 97 (1955).

Lippert, H.: SI-Einheiten in der Medizin, 2. ed. Urban & Schwarzenberg, München-Wien-Baltimore 76, 77 (1978).

Maidorn, K. In: Jahnke, K., H. Mehnert, H. E. Reis: Muskelstoffwechsel, körperliche Leistungsfähigkeit und Diabetes mellitus. F. K. Schattauer Verlag, Stuttgart-New York, 1977.

Mellerowicz, H.: Arch. Kreisl.forschg. 24, 70 (1956); Herz- und Blutkreislauf beim

Sport. In: Lehrbuch der Sportmedizin, Hrsg. A. Arnold. Leipzig: Barth, 1956.

Mellerowicz, H. and H. Schmutzler: Malattie Cardiovascolari, Vol. Xn, 1–2, (1969).

Mellerowicz, H., H. Schmutzler and K. Maidorn: Zschr. Kreisl.forschg. 47, 792 (1958).

Metzner, A.: Untersuchung und Beurteilung des Kreislaufs. In: F. Heiss, Praktische Sportmedizin. Stuttgart: Enke, 1960.

Parade, G. W. and A. Ohr: Zschr. klin. Med. 143, 242 and 252 (1943).

Pierach and Heynemann: Der niedrige Blutdruck und die Hypotonie. Enke-Verlag, Stuttgart 1959.

Reindell, H., E. Schildge, H. Klepzig and H. W. Kirchhoff: Kreislaufregulationen. Stuttgart: Thieme, 1955.

Reindell, H., H. Klepzig and H. Steim: Die sportärztliche Herz- und Kreislaufberatung. Sportmed. Schriftenreihe, H. 3.

Rutenfranz, J., Th. Hellbrügge und E. Keilhacker: Zschr. Kinderhk. 85, 317 (1961).

Sack and Koll: Die Erkennung, Beurteilung und Behandlung des symptomatischen Hochdrucks. Enke-Verlag. Stuttgart 1959.

Schellong, F. and B. Lüderitz: Regulationsprüfung des Kreislaufs. Darmstadt: Steinkopff, 1954.

Schleusing, G. and H. Pissarek: Med. u. Sport 3, 79 (1963).

Schleusing, G., Th. Luther, F. Liebold and F. Kunadt: Med. u. Sport 9, 197 (1969).

Valentin, H. and K. P. Holzhauser: Funktionsprüfungen von Herz und Kreislauf, Deutscher Ärzte-Verlag GmbH, 1976.

Weiss, A.: Verh. Dtsch. Ges. Kreisl.forschg. 15. Tagg. 1949. Darmstadt-Steinkopff, 1949.

Wezler, K.: Verh. Dtsch. Ges. Kreisl.forschg. 15. Tagg. 1949. Darmstadt: Steinkopff, 1949.

Kommission der Deutschen Gesellschaft für Kreislaufforschung: Merkblatt, Empfehlungen zur indirekten Messung des Blutdrucks beim Menschen.

IX. O_2 Consumption in Ergometric Performance

1. Methods of Measurement

It is desirable to maintain basal metabolic conditions, of course, but this is not always psychologically or practically possible. The inclination to undergo physical exertion on an entirely empty stomach is generally very slight. This attitude can have more effect on the results of a study than a shift in experimental conditions. Besides, by subtracting the metabolism while at rest from the total metabolism, the actual metabolism (net performance metabolism) during a stress test can always be determined and evaluated. As suggested, the performance-metabolism conditions described in Chapter III should be observed.

1.1 O_2 measurement in open systems

In so-called open systems, atmospheric air (20.95% oxygen) is inspired and the O_2 concentration in the expired air is measured. Since in enclosed spaces we can not always count on the normal O_2 content of 20.95%, the difference between the O_2 in the inspired and expired air must be determined more precisely. A comprehensive survey of methods of measuring O_2, including sources of error, was reported in 1975 by H. V. Ulmer.

1.1.1 Total-Volume Methods

The expired air needed for O_2 analysis can be collected in 100- and 300-liter bags (Douglas bags). For protracted studies at high performance rates a number of bags are needed. By this method mixed air samples are obtained from long or short portions of the performance time. Rapid alterations in O_2 consumption can not be detected by this method, Douglas bags are rela-

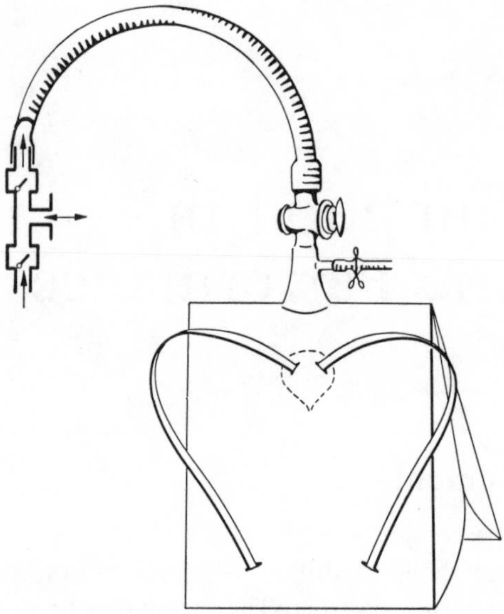

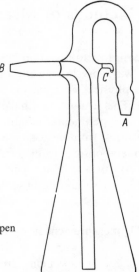

Fig. 96. The "bag method" for study of respiratory metabolism in man (Douglas). Through a mouthpiece fitted with valves the expired air is led in such a way that the total amount of the expiration is collected in a large bag, worn on the back of the subject during muscular exercise and the like and holding 100 to 200 liters. The time it takes to completely inflate the bag is accurately measured. Then the bag is removed and its contents measured via the gasometer. But previously an air sample has been removed via a small side tube for chemical analysis (after *Rein and Schneider*)

Fig. 97. Mixing flask for mixing the expired volume in open systems.
A = intake
B = outlet
C = outlet for removal of the volume for analysis.

tively clumsy to handle and the determination of their volume takes considerable time, using spirometers. However, the absence of any air resistance when they are being filled is a considerable advantage in the case of high- or maximal-performance tests. The material of the air bags must be as O_2- and CO_2-tight as possible. Most commercially available bags meet this requirement, but not completely. Therefore, the analysis must be done as quickly as possible after the experiment. Samples can be taken immediately from Douglas bags by means of (Scholander) pipettes or (completely gas-tight) glass hypodermic syringes. These can be inserted into a glass container whose bottom is covered 1 to 2 cm deep with mercury and can then be analyzed later. In order to test the gas-tightness of Douglas bags and determine the degree of error they lead to, several comparative analyses should be undertaken at intervals of three to thirty minutes after they are filled. This procedure should be repeated every three to six months in order to check up on the possibility of deterioration or damage to the bags (Fig. 96).

1.1.2   Sample-Volume Methods

In order to avoid the fuss with the Douglas bags, it is possible to take a sample directly from expired air. The following methods are suitable for this:

Expired air is led into a bottle, which affords satisfactory mixing (Fig. 97). For use with performances of some magnitude, the content of the bottle must correspond to at least a maximal-performance tidal volume of approximately 3 liters. From the mixing bottle one can either remove individual samples with a pipette or else draw out continuously a volume for analysis with the aid of a small electric pump.

A sample of air can also be obtained by means of a perforated tube. The perforated portion of the tube, about 30 centimeters long, is inserted into the expiration tube. It permits simultaneous removal of samples from various portions of the tidal volume. This method is less suited for the removal of individual samples but more so for continuous analysis by physical methods.

Zuntz was the first to use a gasometer equipped with a device for removing aliquot portions of the expired air. A gasometer developed by Kofranyi and Michaelis in 1941 uses a small piston pump to insert 1% of the expired air into a rubber balloon. The "integrating motor pneumotachograph" developed by Wolff[1] collects samples of the expired air on a continuous basis.

1.1.3   Chemical Analysis of Expired Air

For chemical analysis of the gases in the expired air (O_2 and CO_2), the Haldane procedure can be recommended. It makes use of the O_2-bonding properties of pyrogallol and determines the reduction in volume of the air sample (Fig. 98).

Scholander's gas analysis device (Fig. 99) makes it possible to measure O_2 and CO_2 even in amounts of air as small as 0.5 cm^3. In a measuring chamber CO_2 is absorbed by a solution containing potash lye and potassium bichro-

---

[1]Wolff, H. S., "IMP," manufactured in England under license from the National Research Development Corporation by J. Langham Thompson Ltd., Bushey Heath, (Herts.) England.

mate. A solution containing sodium dithionide (Na$_2$S$_2$O$_4$) and sodium anthrachinon sulfonate is used for O$_2$ absorption. The decrease in volume can be canceled out through an equalization chamber by altering the volume of the measuring chamber and be measured by means of a micrometer screw. The precision of measurement is relatively high in experienced, skilled hands ($>$0.1 volume %).

Scholander and Evans described an apparatus with which even quantities of air down to 0.07 mm^3 can be analyzed in six minutes for O$_2$ and CO$_2$ with an accuracy of $\pm$0.05 volume %.

The van Slyke apparatus has been modified by Shepard and Sperling for microanalysis of amounts down to 0.1 cm^3. CO$_2$ and O$_2$ can be determined in about ten minutes to $\pm$0.1 vol %.

0.2 cm^3 of gas are needed for Dirken and Heemstra's micro-gas-analysis apparatus. This amount can be analyzed for O$_2$ and CO$_2$ in ten minutes with a degree of precision as great as $\pm$0.05 volume %.

According to a method by Krogh, 1 to 7 cubic millimeters of air can be measured absorptively for O$_2$ and CO$_2$ in a calibrated thermometer capillary with a precision of $\pm$2 to $\pm$0.2 volume %.

Other chemical methods are presented summarily in the chapter "Gasanlyse" in E. Opitz's *Handbuch der physiologisch- und pathologisch-chemischen Analyse.*

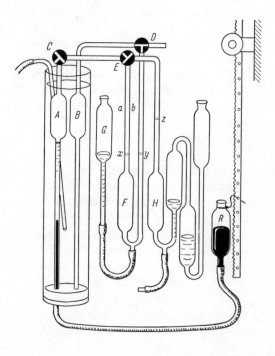

Fig. 98. Device for gas analysis after Haldane. A gas burette (10–20 cm^3) in water bath, filled with mercury to serve as "blocking liquid." With proper setting of the three-way cock C and lowering of the overflow vessel R, the mercury can run out of the bottom of the burette and the air to be analyzed can flow into it at the top. After C is reset, the gas is forced toward F via proper setting of cock E (by the raising of R), where CO$_2$ is bonded out of the gas by means of potash lye. Most of the lye escapes toward G in the course of this. After resetting cock E, the CO$_2$-free air is compressed into H. The pyrogallol solution in H bonds O$_2$. After sucking the gas remainder back into A until meniscus level z is restored, the decrease in volume that has just taken place (equal to the O$_2$ content) can be read. B, D, and y are an equalizing device for temperature errors. (after *Rein* and *Schneider*)

Fig. 99. Scholander micro-
gas-analysis device.

A = compensation chamber
B = reaction chamber
C = side-chamber for car-
bon-dioxide absorbtion
D = side-chamber for oxy-
gen absorbtion
E = shut-off cock
F = shut-off cock
G = vessel for cleansing
H = micrometer screw
J = pipette for transfer of
gas sample
K = pipette for cleansing
L = micrometer burette
M = mercury-level bulb
N = three-way cock
O = thermobarometer cock
P = ring mark

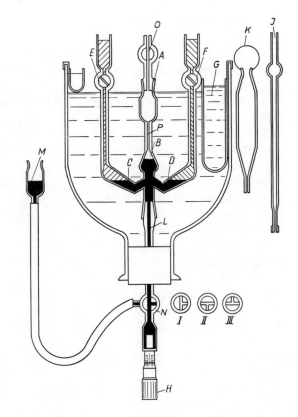

1.1.4 Physical Analysis of Expired Air

These are based on various physical properties of the gases of the atmosphere, such as variable heat conductivity, magnetic susceptibility, light dif-
fraction and differing mass. They take relatively little time and, unlike the
chemical methods, are useful for continuous monitoring.

Analysis according to the principle of heat conductivity: The O_2 content
of the expired air can be determined on the basis of the dependence of air's
heat conductivity on its composition and O_2 content. In a measuring chamber kept at constant temperature, a wire made of a precious metal and
having a uniform current passing through it takes on a particular temperature depending on the heat conductivity of the surrounding gas. This temperature is higher the more poorly the gas conducts heat. The electrical
resistance of the wire is determined by its temperature. This reading permits
a quantitative pronouncement as to the composition of a mixture of two to
three gases whose identity is known qualitatively. Breathed-air analyses
were first carried out by Hill, using this principle in an apparatus by Daynes.

Rein described his "metabolism recorder" in 1932, a sensitive and relatively fast-operating device, which is, however, cumbersome to operate.

Devices that measure by this principle are manufactured by various firms. The Diaferometer, designed by Noyons and manufactured by Kipp and Sons, of Delft, Netherlands, permits the running measurement of O_2 and CO_2, using two separate measuring systems. The setting delay in this device runs from ≈ 15 seconds to 2 minutes, and its precision can run as high as ± 0.1 volume %.

Analyses on the magnetic principle: The O_2 content of expired air can also be determined on the basis of the paramegnetism of O_2 and its dependence on temperature. The other atmospheric gases are, in contrast to O_2, weakly diamagnetic and are repelled by a magnetic field. If the atmospheric O_2 is brought into the field of a powerful magnet, it collects in a manner corresponding to the direction and density of the lines of force. If an electrically heated wire is brought into the magnetic field (preferably at the point of greatest change in density of the lines of force) the paramagnetism of the O_2 decreases as a result of the heating. The heated O_2 is displaced by the older, still more strongly paramagnetic O_2. There arises thus a constant flow, a "magnetic wind," whose speed is proportional to the O_2 content of the air mixture. The cooling of the heating-wire caused by the O_2 flow leads to a measurable change in its electrical resistance. The measurement of the change in resistance permits direct determination of the O_2 content in volume %. The precision depends greatly on the maintenance of a constant temperature in the measuring chamber and amounts to about ± 0.1 to 0.2 volume %. The analysis devices developed by Rein also depend on the paramagnetism of O_2. These devices have a setting time that is relatively small (≈ 15 seconds). A special model is said to give a reading in only eight seconds and an extra-special one in only two seconds. In practice, however, this time is extended through the time taken for the amount being analyzed to flow through the expiration tube, the mixed-gas bottle, perforated tube and gas-analysis tube. Bearing in mind the reading delay, this method is well suited for continuous measurement and recording of O_2 content during and after ergometric performance. The Oxytest apparatus, from Hartmann & Braun, of Frankfurt am Main, is likewise based on the temperature-dependence of the paramagnetism of O_2. But it has certain advantages over the previously mentioned devices, namely, its extremely short reading delay (< 150 milliseconds) and the linearity of its indications throughout the reading range.

Interferometric gas analysis: This depends on the differential light-refraction indices of gases, which, depending on the known thickness of the layer and the concentration of the gas being analyzed, lead to displacements in the pattern of the interference bands as compared with that caused by a known gas used for comparison. By means of an optical compensator, whose

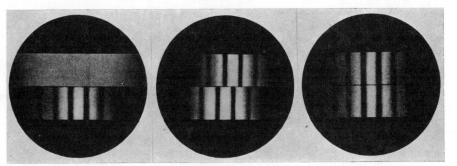

Fig. 100. Interference lines on interferometric gas analysis.

setting is calibrated in percentages of the gas being analyzed, the interference patterns of the gas being analyzed and the known comparison gas can be superimposed (Fig. 100). Interferometers for the analysis of O_2 and CO_2 are supplied by Zeiss of Jena. Their degree of precision may run to ± 0.1 volume % of O_2. (For further data on interferometric measurements, see F. Löwe: *Optische Messungen des Chemikers und des Mediziners*, Dresden and Leipzig: Steinkopff, 1954.) Unfortunately the method is not applicable for continuous recording during ergometric performance.

Mass-spectrometric gas analysis: The molecules of the gas to be analyzed are ionized in a high-vacuum tube through electron-emission of a heated tungsten wire, accelerated in an electrical field and deflected from their path in a magnetic field, the deflection corresponding to their mass and charge. The ions thus separated can be caught up in Faraday cages and their number determined electrically. Mass spectrometers for gas analysis have been developed in the United States by Hipple and Neuert. Mass spectrometers need less than 1 cubic centimeter of gas for analysis, have a very low reading-delay time of only 0.2 second and are extremely accurate. To be sure they are at present extremely expensive, but at the same time they are superior to the other methods for continuous gas analysis in ergometric performance since they can analyze several gases at the same time.

1.2 O_2 Measurement in Closed Systems

The subject inspires a closed system of air at constant volume and pressure. The temperature is held constant by means of a thermostat and cooling system. A spirometer bell coupled into the system shows all volume changes brought about by the subject and also by other factors on a kymograph with calibrated recording paper. From the rise in the breath curve or O_2 curve in

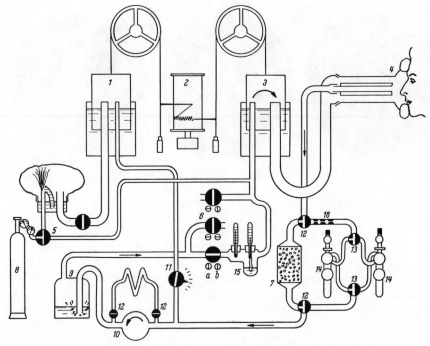

Fig. 101. Schematic drawing of the Knipping spirograph (assembly-stage C).

a unit of time, the magnitude of the O_2 consumption can be determined. The O_2 content of the air in the system can be kept constant during the ergometric performance by various means.

In the Knipping spirograph (Figs. 101 and 102), there is employed a two-bell system with communicating pipes. This makes possible a continuous, regulable introduction of O_2 while equal amounts of system air are being removed. CO_2 is absorbed continuously in a container of soda lime. To avoid resistance to breathing, the system air is kept flowing by means of a pump having a regulable minute volume. Since the system air is driven through the breathing mask at great speed there is no significant rebreathing up to moderate performances. A gas-changing device makes it possible to fill the system with high-concentration O_2 mixtures in a brief time. A kymograph permits recording at various paper speeds.

Fleisch's Metabograph makes use of a coupled double spirometer (see schematic representation in Fig. 103). In this two-chambered spirometer, the pumping minute volume need be only half as great for the same minute volume as in a simple spirometer in order to avoid rebreathing. The pumping performance of 270 liters per minute thus corresponds to 540 liters in an

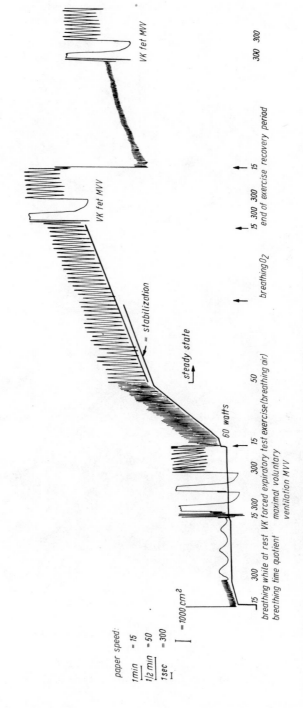

Fig. 102. Spirogram from a Knipping spirograph at a work load of 60 watts (after *Bolt*).

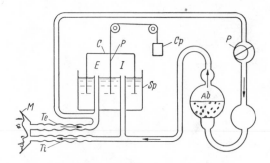

Fig. 103. Schematic drawing of a coupled double spirometer (after *Fleisch*).

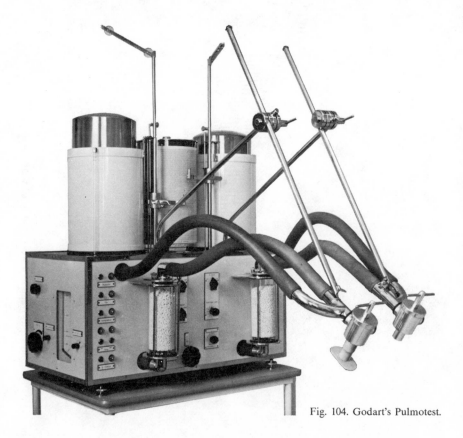

Fig. 104. Godart's Pulmotest.

ordinary spirograph. By this means, maximal minute volumes of more than 100 liters are possible without rebreathing. In addition, the resistance to breathing is reduced considerably and the time for absorption of CO_2 is doubled. The O_2 consumption in the system is measured and replaced in partial volumes of 20 cubic centimeters by a pump controlled by a system of electrical contacts. The device makes it possible to record continuously and electrically the tidal volume and rate, O_2 equivalent, CO_2 production and respiratory quotient. A gasometer attached to the system makes it possible to fill it with O_2 mixtures of various concentrations and even with other gas mixtures.

The Pulmotest, produced by the firm of Godart-Statham Medizinische Geräte GmbH, Bremen, Germany (Fig. 104), likewise consists of two complete spirometer systems with two pumps, with a maximal ventilation of 300 liters. The volume changes in both spirometers are recorded on a kymograph working at a speed of 30, 60 or 120 mm per minute. The O_2 consumption of the subject in one system is automatically replaced from the other O_2-filled system by means of an electrically-controlled valve. From the one air-filled system, it is possible to switch to the other for O_2 breathing by simply turning a three-way cock. Special larger CO_2 absorbers are available for ergometric experiments. To stabilize the temperature, an additional device has been developed with a water-cooling system, which reportedly can maintain the temperature constant at 21 °C even at maximal performances. Because of the small basic volumes in both systems, the instrument is especially suited for determinations of residual air by the gas-dilution method.

1.2.1 Sources of Error in Closed Systems

The great influence of temperature changes on the volume in closed systems can become a considerable source of error. With a rise in temperature of only 1 °C, which is unavoidable in some apparatus, especially at intensive performances, the volume of each 10 liters of air in the system is elevated by 34.1 cubic centimeters. With greater system volumes and elevated temperatures, errors of more than 100 cubic centimeters based on O_2 consumption may occur.

Distortions of the respiratory position during ergometric performance more in the inspiratory and expiratory reserve volume can also lead to considerable errors in calculations of the O_2 values. They must be measured by multiple recording of the lowest expiration point at the start of and during the performance and be taken into consideration, but this interrupts and disturbs the natural respiratory rhythm.

A considerable source of error in closed systems is rebreathing of CO_2 caused by insufficient air-moving capacity on the part of the pump. It leads to an abnormal increase in the tidal volume and the respiratory equivalent, and a drop in performance. Only with pump capacity that at every moment of the respiratory cycle is greater than the respiratory time volume can rebreathing be prevented. In great to maximal ergometric performances, we must reckon with maximal forced expiratory volume per second of 5 to 8 liters, i.e., in order to permit maximal ergometric performances, the pump must have a capacity of 300 to 480 liters per minute.

At such great pump capacities, however, considerable respiratory resistances develop and the absorption time for CO_2 becomes very short. Also, the use of closed systems with great pump capacity makes it necessary to use inspiration and expiration tubes of large diameters, which get in the way in hand-cranking exercises and cut down on the performance achievement. Despite these problems, apparatus with pumping capacity above 300 liters per minute must be used high intensity performances of more than 150 watts.

The air-tightness of the system must be checked before each experiment. Once the connection to the patient has been closed, loading the spirometer bell must not lead to any reduction in the system volume detectable on the spirometer dial. The glass cocks must be cleaned now and then with benzene and lightly brushed with special stopcock lubricant.

For the absorption of CO_2, the best substance to use is "indicator lime," which takes on a blue coloration when heavily saturated with CO_2. It must then be renewed before the next experiment. Insufficient absorption of CO_2 leads to an increase in the minute volume of respiration and a drop in the O_2 consumption and maximal performance.

1.3   Various O_2 Fractions and Their Calculation

The amount of O_2 absorbed in the lungs per unit of time is designated as "oxygen consumption." It is determined by the nature of the performance, its magnitude and many endogenous and exogenous factors. Some of the most important contributing factors are partial alveolar O_2 pressure, total alveolar surface area, pulmonary and cardiac output, O_2 transport capacity of the blood, arteriovenous O_2 difference, etc. In closed systems, the O_2 consumption can be read directly on the calibrated recording paper, bearing in mind the changes in system temperature. The readings are to be reduced according to Table 75 (pp. 408–411) to 0°C and dryness at 760 mm HG barometric pressure (STPD = standard temperature pressure dry). In open systems, the O_2 consumption can be calculated from the difference in O_2 content of the inspired and expired air as found by chemical or physical analysis and from the respiratory time volume.

In the analysis of totally dried air (dried by hygroscopic substances such as, for example, calcium chloride), the O_2 content measured in the expired air can be subtracted from the constant O_2 content of dry air of 20.95% (21% is sufficiently precise for all practical purposes). In the analysis of nondried air, it must be taken into account that its O_2 content is less than 21%, decreasing as the volume percent of water vapor the air contains increases.

There is no need to analyze for the water-vapor content of the inspired air, however, since even in damp air the quotient

$$\frac{\text{volume } \% \text{ of } O_2}{\text{volume } \% \text{ of nitrogen}}$$

remains unchanged. It amounts to 0.265. But the determination of the CO_2 content of the expired air is also necessary. The O_2 content of the inspired air can accordingly be calculated in the following way:

$$\left[100\% - \left(\begin{matrix}\text{volume-percent } O_2 \\ \text{(expired air)}\end{matrix} + \begin{matrix}\text{volume percent } CO_2 \\ \text{(expired air)}\end{matrix}\right)\right] 0.265$$
$$= \begin{matrix}\text{volume-percent } O_2 \\ \text{(inspired air)}\end{matrix}$$

Example: $100\% - (17\% \, O_2 + 5\% \, CO_2) = 78\% \, (N_2)$

$$78 \times 0.265 = 20.67\% \, O_2 \text{ (inspired air)}$$
$$\begin{matrix}20.67\% \, O_2 \\ -17.00\% \\ \hline O_2 \text{ consumption } (\%) = 3.67\% \, O_2\end{matrix}$$

With an inspired minute volume of respiration of, for example, 50 liters, a temperature of 20°C and 750 mm Hg. barometric pressure, the O_2 consumption is calculated (reduced according to Table 75) as follows:

$$50 \text{ liters} \times 0.8981 \times 3.67\% = 1648 \text{ cm}^3 \, O_2 \text{ consumption (STPD)}$$

The O_2 consumption rising at the start of an equivalent endurance performance up to a given level is designated as the onset O_2 consumption. The onset phase of the O_2 consumption is briefer in a vascular and respiratory system with high performance capacity and lasts longer in one of lower capacity. It is calculated by adding the O_2 consumption of the individual minutes of the onset period or by planimetric measurement of the onset O_2 area of a graphic representation.

If the O_2 requirement (O_2 consumption) needed for a performance and the complete oxidation of lactic acid and pyruvic acid is greater than the O_2 consumption at the moment, there arises in the organism an O_2 debt. The intermediate metabolic acid products which have arisen in the anaerobic phase of the muscular metabolism can then not be entirely oxidized. Consequently the levels of lactic and pyruvic acid in the blood rise in proportion to the O_2 debt. In the onset phase of any performance there arises an O_2 debt, because the O_2 consumption does not keep pace with the muscular performance. The O_2 debt may reach extremely high levels if during performance the O_2 requirement is continuously greater than the possible O_2 consumption. The O_2 debt accumulated during an exercise is made up by breathing during the rest period. The O_2 debt is calculated by subtracting the resting O_2 consumption from the recovery O_2 consumption.

The recovery phase lasts until the return of O$_2$ consumption to the resting figure. By adding up the O$_2$ consumption for the individual minutes of the recovery time, we obtain the total recovery O$_2$ consumption. In graphic registrations, the recovery O$_2$ amount can also be determined planimetrically from the paper. If, for example, the recovery time is twelve minutes, then we must subtract the resting O$_2$ consumption of twelve minutes from the total recovery O$_2$ in order to calculate the O$_2$ debt.

Recovery O$_2$ consumption (12 min)	9000 cm^3 O$_2$
Resting O$_2$ consumption (12 min)	3000 cm^3 O$_2$
O$_2$ debt	6000 cm^3 O$_2$

The O$_2$ utilization, to use Herbst's term for it, namely,

$$\frac{O_2 \text{ consumption in cm}^3/\text{min (STPD)}}{\text{minute volume of respiration in liters/min (BTPS)}}$$

tells how much O$_2$, in cubic centimeters, has been removed from the breathed air.

The so-called respiratory equivalent tells how much air is required to absorb one cubic centimeter of O$_2$ (Rossier and Méan).

$$\text{Respiratory equivalent} = \frac{\text{minute volume of respiration in cm}^3 \text{ (BTPS)}}{O_2 \text{ consumption in cm}^3 \text{ per minute (STPD)}}$$

Both quotients enable an evaluation of the respiratory economy. It certainly is more in keeping with the physiological conditions for the calculation of the respiratory equivalent or the O$_2$ utilization to start out from BTPS conditions or even from the uncorrected values (measured at equal apparatus temperatures), as several authors do. However, for reasons of standardization according to the international agreements of Atlantic City (1950), Paris (1954) and Luxembourg (1955), the minute volume of respiration is to be calculated under BTPS conditions but O$_2$ consumption under STPD. This has met with general acceptance.

2.   Physiological Basis

At the start of an exercise, O$_2$ consumption, respiration rate and minute volume of respiration rise in the form of an almost parabolic curve. The duration of this onset phase is directly proportional to the magnitude of the exercise and inversely proportional to the performance capability of the circulatory and respiratory systems. In the onset phase, the O$_2$ consumption lags considerably behind the O$_2$ consumption adequate for the exercise. Consequently, there arises an O$_2$ debt (O$_2$ deficit—Hill's term) in the orga-

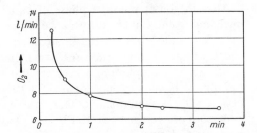

Fig. 105. The O_2 consumption for various durations of performance and equal running speed (20 km per hour) (after *Christensen* and *Högberg*).

nism, with a proportional increase in the lactic acid level in the muscles. For the same exercise level, more O_2 is consumed in the onset phase than later on. Since with predominantly anaerobic energy release, the efficiency of the muscle is low, the O_2 deficit arising in the onset phase is greater than the difference between the O_2 consumption adequate to the exercise and the actual consumption in the onset phase. Therefore the O_2 consumption for the first minute of a uniform exercise is always greater than for the second and succeeding minutes (see Fig. 105, after Christensen and Högberg). If an equal steady-state exercise performance is repeated after a pause lasting for less than 30 minutes, the O_2 consumption for this second exercise is somewhat less (Simonson and Hebestreit). This may be caused by the brief onset phase with predominantly anaerobic metabolism and greater efficiency in the overheated organism.

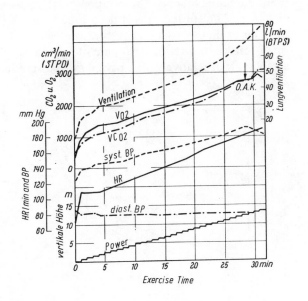

Fig. 106. O_2 consumption and other cardiorespiratory functions during increased exercise on the treadmill; mean values of 28 tests on 14 volunteers (*Balke*).

After the onset phase, a phase of equal O_2 consumption is reached at unchanging endurance performance which, since Hill, has been referred to as "steady state." In the steady state at equal performance, O_2 consumption and O_2 requirement remain the same. In increasing steady state exercise stages, O_2 consumption and minute volume of respiration of the exercise run almost linearly proportional (Fig. 106). Linear relationships also exist between O_2 consumption and heart rate in a range of $\approx$100–170 per minute in persons of average age (see Fig. 39). On this regularity are based indirect methods of determining the O_2 consumption from the HR during performance (see Fig. 55). In the recovery phase, the O_2 debt built up during the exercise is made up for in hard breathing. The still elevated O_2 consumption serves for the oxidation of the lactic and pyruvic acids that were produced during the exercise. The duration of the recovery time is, like that of the onset time, directly proportional to the magnitude of the performance and inversely proportional to the performance capacity. After very strenuous maximal performances, O_2 consumption may remain slightly above the basal value for from 24 to 48 hours (Herxheimer, Wissing and Wolff).

For consumption of equal amounts of O_2, different minute volumes are required, depending on morphological and physiological factors in the circulatory system and respiratory organs as well as exogenous factors, especially the partial O_2 pressure and the magnitude of the performance. With rapid breathing and low volume of respiration, the O_2 utilization from the inhaled air is low or the minute volume of respiration for the consumption of a particular volume of O_2 is large. With large tidal volume at low frequency on the other hand the O_2 utilization reaches higher values, a considerably smaller minute volume of respiration being necessary for the consumption of 1 liter of O_2. In the case of deep breathing a relatively large amount of fresh air of high partial O_2 pressure is mixed in the lungs with a relatively small reserve and residual volume of low partial O_2 pressure. The mixed alveolar air of relatively high partial O_2 pressure makes possible a great O_2

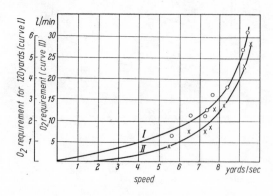

Fig. 107. The relation of O_2 consumption to running performance (after *Hill*).

utilization or a small respiratory equivalent. The O_2 utilization usually increases with increasing performance, falling again after individual border values are exceeded. Considerably higher figures for O_2 consumption or lower respiratory equivalents can be achieved by trained individuals. In cases of hyperventilation very low figures for O_2 utilization are reached, while with hypoventilation they are high.

In short, intense performances above maximal steady state performance (for example, short and medium distance runs) the O_2 debt grows steadily during performance, sometimes to a borderline value which forces the athlete to stop or reduce the degree of exertion. The lactic acid level of the blood can reach very high values. Such performances with mounting O_2 debt are called "unsteady state performances."

The O_2 consumption climbs in the case of unsteady-state performances in the form of an exponential curve (Fig. 107, after Hill), because with the rising anaerobic portion of the muscular metabolism and increasing performance the efficiency drops exponentially. Even protracted maximum performances (for example, in a 10,000-meter race) are achieved with slowly increasing O_2 deficit. If, at maximal ergometric performance, the O_2 consumption remains constant, the O_2 debt may increase. Such a case is distinguishable from an actual steady-state performance only by means of comparative measurement of the O_2 debt in the recovery phase, through continuous reading of the lactic acid level and (sometimes) by a respiratory quotient >1 during the performance.

3. Physiological Averages and Ranges of Variation in O_2 Consumption

Numerous investigators using different methods have found different figures for O_2 consumption during performance (Fig. 108 after Knipping, Valentin, Bolt and Venrath). These differences depend on:

a) Differing subject populations
b) Differing mechanical properties of the ergometers used
c) Physiological range of variation in the O_2 consumption at equal performances
d) Errors in calibration and mistakes in measurement.

Averages and $\pm 1\sigma$ range for the O_2 consumption in 100 men aged 20 to 40 at a power of 1 watt per kg of body weight (55 to 80 watts of hand cranking) are shown in Figure 109. The corresponding figures for pedaling while seating and reclining can be calculated from Figure 114. The corre-

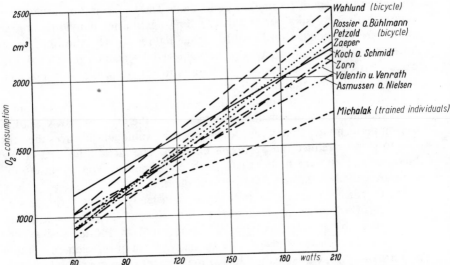

Fig. 108. O$_2$ consumption in the steady state of ergometric power in relation to the performance in watts as given by various authors (after *Knipping, Bolt, Valentin* and *Venrath*).

sponding figures for 1 watt per kg in children and teenagers are given in the graphic presentation in Figure 110 (after Dressler and Mellerowicz). The O$_2$ consumption figures for pedaling while reclining (30 revolutions per minute) at submaximal powers of 50, 100 and 150 watts in male subjects aged 20 to 40 are presented in Figure 111 (after Reindell and Kirchhoff). Figure 112 shows the O$_2$ consumption and its standard deviations at powers from 3 to 23 kpm per second for pedaling while seating in 66 untrained male subjects (after Hollmann and Heck). In Figure 113 are shown schematically the relationships of ergometric powers, various physical powers and O$_2$ consumption (after Hüllemann).

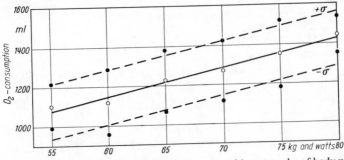

Fig. 109. O$_2$ consumption (STPD) during exercise of 1 watt per kg of body weight in 100 men aged 20 to 40. Handcrank ergometer, 35 rpm, closed system (after *Dransfeld* and *Mellerowicz*).

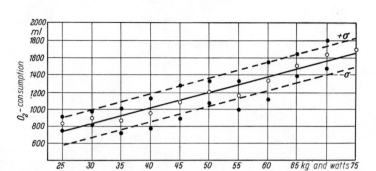

Fig. 110. O_2 consumption (STPD) at a power of 1 watt per kg of body weight in 188 males aged 7 to 18 (crank height 1 meter, crank length 30 cm, 30 rpm, closed system) (after *Dressler* and *Mellerowicz*).

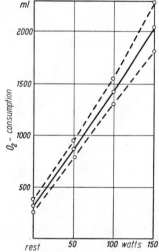

Fig. 111. O_2 consumption (STPD) at powers of 50, 100 and 150 watts. Pedaling while reclining 30 rpm, in 80 subjects aged 20 to 40 (after *Reindell* and *Kirchhoff*).

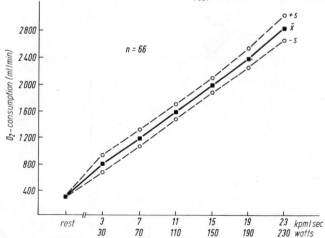

Fig. 112. O_2 consumption at powers of 3 to 23 kpm per second, pedaling while seating, at 60 rpm in 60 untrained male subjects (after *Hollmann* and *Heck*).

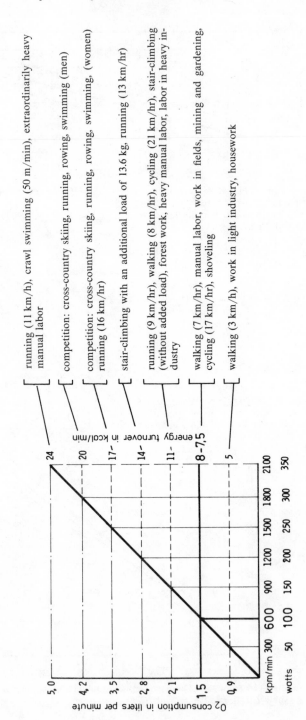

running (11 km/h), crawl swimming (50 m/min), extraordinarily heavy manual labor

competition: cross-country skiing, running, rowing, swimming (men)

competition: cross-country skiing, running, rowing, swimming, (women) running (16 km/hr)

stair-climbing with an additional load of 13.6 kg, running (13 km/hr)

running (9 km/hr), walking (8 km/hr), cycling (21 km/hr), stair-climbing (without added load), forest work, heavy manual labor, labor in heavy industry

walking (7 km/hr), manual labor, work in fields, mining and gardening, cycling (17 km/hr), shoveling

walking (3 km/h), work in light industry, housework

energy turnover in kcal/min

O$_2$ consumption in liters per minute

Fig. 113. Schematic representation of the relationships of ergometric powers, various physical performances and O$_2$ consumption (after *Hillemann*).

Fig. 114. O₂ consumption (STPD) in the steady state at 100 watts of hand cranking while standing, pedaling while seating and reclining in 36 untrained male subjects aged 20 to 40, hand-crank length 33.3 cm, pedal length 16.6 cm, and 35 rpm (after *Mellerowicz* and *Nowacki*).

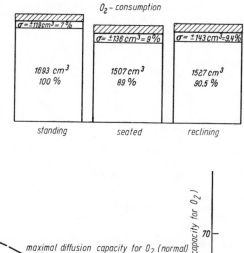

Fig. 115. The *vita maxima* figures for O₂ consumption and cardiac output equivalent figures in the course of aging. The curve in the upper part of the chart shows the development of the maximal diffusion capacity for O₂ with advancing years. The distribution area for the maximal O₂ consumption was obtained after the study of more than 500 normal individuals (after *Bolt, Knipping, Valentin* and *Venrath*).

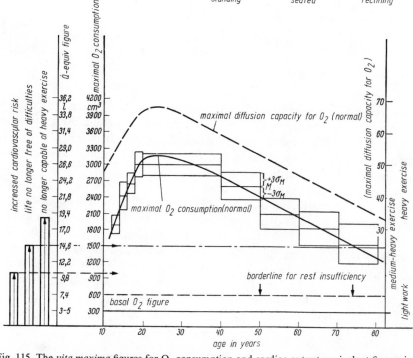

The averages for O₂ consumption as well as the ±1σ range in 36 untrained male subjects at 100 watts of ergometric exercise while standing, seated and reclining are shown in Figure 114 in graphic representation. At equal physical powers, the biological performances differ depending on the nature of the muscular exercise and the O₂ consumption.

The determination of the onset time of the O₂ consumption is also of interest for the evaluation of the cardiopulmonary performance capacity.

Table 21. The average values for the maximal O$_2$ consumption according to age group among normal individuals and the statistically verified distribution range (hand-crank ergometer, breathing O$_2$, step-by-step increments of 30 watts per minute).

Number of subjects	Age classes	Maximal average O$_2$ consumption in cm^3	3σ in cm^3	Exercise minute-volume of respiration average in liters:	3σ in liters
30	12 and 13	1860	±200	53	± 8.3
30	14 and 15	2450	±260	73	±12.0
30	16 and 17	2680	±200	89	±14.5
30	18 and 19	3020	±230	111	±12.0
50	20–40	3020	±180	108	±11.3
30	40–50	2630	±280	99	±14.9
30	50–60	2140	±310	91	±15.2
30	60–70	1850	±340	84	±17.2
30	70–80	1600	±410	79	±17.4

(after *Valentin, Venrath, Mallinckrodt* and *Gürakar*)

Brief onset times or warming times indicate a high performance cardiopulmonary system, longer ones indicate weakness of the system. An increase in the onset time is probable with increasing age. The normal figures for the onset time for various performance capacities and various age and sex groups have not as yet been defined.

Averages for the maximal O$_2$ consumption are shown in Table 21 and Figure 115. Of course, it must be noted that these figures were obtained with hand-cranking exercise at stepped increases in the O$_2$ consumption at one minute intervals and with O$_2$ breathing in Knipping's spirograph. They are valid, actually, only for this order of experimentation. However, they give figures of practical value as long as the conditions under which they were obtained are kept in mind. The maximal steady-state O$_2$ consumption figures (on Fleisch's Metabograph) are shown in Table 22 (after *Reindell* et al.). The considerably lower figures for the maximal O$_2$ consumption can be

Table 22. Maximal steady-state O$_2$ consumption at pedaling exercise while reclining, 60 rpm (closed system, Fleisch's Metabograph, after *Reindell* et al.).

Age group	Number	Weight in kg.	O$_2$ in cm^3	O$_2$ in cm^3/kg
10–11	42	35.5	1125.5	31.7
12–13	41	45.0	1430.8	31.8
14–15	42	52.3	1689.9	32.4
16–17	49	63.0	2181.7	34.6
18–19	51	67.5	2668.7	39.6
20–29	50	68.2	2373.0	34.8
30–39	50	70.5	2008.0	28.5
40–49	31	75.0	1847.8	24.6
50–59	30	75.5	1642.6	21.7
athletes	108	61.0	3202.6	52.5
athletes aged over 30	10	66.0	3288.5	49.8

explained by the pedaling work, in which fewer muscle groups are brought into play, as well as by the methodology of the study. Besides, these maximal O_2 consumption figures were obtained with air breathing, a more natural circumstance.

4. Endogenous and Exogenous Conditions Affecting O_2 Consumption During Performance

4.1 Dependence of the O_2 Consumption on Constitutional Factors

At equal power levels, O_2 consumption varies within a certain physiological range depending on constitutional factors. The constitutional differences in O_2 consumption are caused by the varying economy of the muscular, circulatory and respiratory work involved in the ergometric performance.

The maximal O_2 consumption is determined to a large extent by constitutional factors. The most important endogenous determinants are maximal circulatory performance, maximal respiratory performance, O_2 transport capacity of the blood, capillarity and oxidative capacity of the musculature as well as the amount of muscle mass used.

4.2 The Dependency of O_2 Consumption on Sex

For physically equal power productions, women use approximately the same amounts of O_2 as men (net performance O_2). No significant differences have been proved. The total O_2 consumption is assumed to be somewhat less in consequence of the lesser body weight. At approximately equal O_2 consumption, however, the O_2 consumption reserves in women are considerably smaller. The maximal average steady-state O_2 consumption figures in men would represent unsteady-state performances in women, with steadily increasing O_2 deficit.

The average maximal O_2 consumption is considerably lower in women than in men. In the case of 44 female physical education students aged 20 to 25, Åstrand found an average O_2 consumption of 2.9 liters at maximal bicycle power, compared with 4.1 liters for men; this is roughly 70% of the male value. The relative O_2 consumption in women, in milliliters per kg, however, amounted to 83% of the value for men (48.4 ml/kg/min:58 ml/kg/min).

These results can not be regarded as entirely representative, since they were obtained from a selection of well-trained subjects. But they do show good agreement with the results of Venrath and Hollmann (Fig. 116). The latter found in women on the average a maximal O$_2$ consumption that was lower by a third than that in men. Thalemann found in studies on 100 untrained healthy women the following figures for maximal O$_2$ consumption, using standardized methodology:

Group 1, aged 20–29, 1969 ml O$_2$/min (STPD) $\pm 1\sigma$ = 272 ml

Group 2, aged 30–39, 1770 ml O$_2$/min (STPD) $\pm 1\sigma$ = 456 ml

Group 3, aged 40–49, 1734 ml O$_2$/min (STPD) $\pm 1\sigma$ = 318 ml

Group 4, aged 50–60, 1559 ml O$_2$/min (STPD) $\pm 1\sigma$ = 333 ml

It can be assumed from available data that the maximal O$_2$ consumption in women averages relatively (per kg of body weight) approximately 20% and absolutely about 30% below that of men.

4.3   The Dependence of O$_2$ Consumption on Age

Maximal O$_2$ consumption increases in children and teenagers approximately in proportion to their weight as they grow older; i.e., calculated per kg of body weight, the maximal O$_2$ consumption in teenagers and men aged 20 to 30 is approximately the same. According to the studies by Åstrand on moderately trained subjects, it amounts to about 57 to 59 ml/kg of body weight in pedaling while seated (Fig. 117). By the 30th year, O$_2$ consumption decreases again (Fig. 115 and Tables 17 and 21).

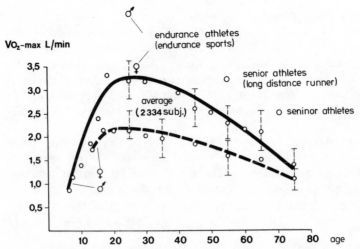

Fig. 116. Maximum O$_2$ consumption between 10 and 70 years of age. 85% of tested persons practiced sports (——— males; — — — females) (by *Venrath* and *Hollmann*).

Fig. 117. Maximal O$_2$ consumption per kg of body weight (pedaling) in 63 individuals aged 7 to 18 and 44 men aged 20 to 30 (after *Astrand*).

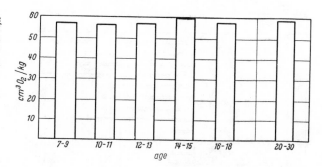

It is not surprising that teenagers of various ages and weights need about equal amounts of O$_2$ for equal ergometric power. The O$_2$ consumption during performance at equal submaximal ergometric exercise is clearly dependent on the magnitude of the exercise and the economy of motion, but conditions of development, weight, and stature are of importance only insofar as they affect the economy of motion in the course of the ergometric exercise. On the other hand, for example, the heart rate among teenagers of various ages is very variable even at equal power levels. It is overwhelmingly influenced by constitutional factors such as degree of development, the relation between body weight and power, cardiac volume, regulatory behavior, etc., as well as conditional factors. For example, a younger, underweight teenager requires about the same amount of O$_2$ as older, heavier teenagers for an equal ergometric power that he accomplishes with about equal economy of motion. But he needs a much higher HR with lower O$_2$ pulse. However, at relatively equal power—for example, 1 or 2 watts per kg of body weight—his O$_2$ consumption is less and the steady state HR is about equal (Mellerowicz and Lerche).

4.4   The O$_2$ Consumption in Trained Individuals During Performance

In all kinds of sports where the performance is essentially dependent on the coordination and motion technique, the trained individual needs less O$_2$ for the same power production (Fig. 118). Results from numerous authors are in agreement on this (Liljestrand and Lindhardt; Knoll; During; etc.). The lower O$_2$ consumption of the trained is also due to a greater economy of cardiorespiratory performance. The lower O$_2$ consumption is to be traced to greater economy of motion in the trained individual (for example, the avoidance of superfluous accompanying motions). In the majority of those trained in endurance performance there is established a predominant vol-

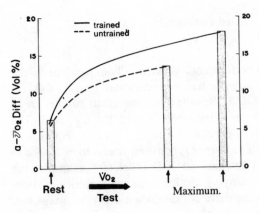

sport		speed m	10 20 30 40 50 60 70 80 90 100 110 cm³
SWIMMING	little trained	20	
		30	
		40	
		40	
	well trained	20	
		30	
		40	
		40	
SKIING	not trained	80	
		90	
	little trained	100	
		120	
	well trained	190	
		190	

Fig. 118. O₂ consumption for 1 kg of weight moved 100 m distance in different sports (*Chiari*).

ume-work on the part of the heart and lungs, in which the relationship between the heart's O₂ consumption and its own performance, and very probably the relationship of the O₂ consumption of the respiratory muscles to the amount of O₂ absorbed, is small. Besides, with a large A-VO₂Δ in trained individuals, the volume performance of the heart and its O₂ consumption during performance may be reduced (see Fig. 119, after Mathews and Fox).

The question has not been entirely satisfactorily cleared as to whether the lower O₂ consumption of the trained individual depends also on a greater degree of efficiency in muscular contraction itself, that is, a more economic muscular metabolism. Beznak assumes an improving of the biochemical mechanism of the muscular fibers through training as the main cause of the lower O₂ consumption.

Fig. 119. Comparable presentation of A-VO₂Δ in relation to O₂ consumption and performance in trained and untrained subjects (after *Mathews and Fox*).

If this assumption on Beznak's part is justified, the trained individual would need likewise less O_2 for muscular exercise which he performs with the same economy of motion as an untrained individual. This might be investigated, for example, with some very simple form of activity which does not permit any great variations in economy of motion, such as hand cranking or pedaling. The trained subject would of course have to be one not specially trained for this form of motion.

Studies of O_2 consumption at equal ergometric power in trained and untrained persons have resulted in no statistically significant differences. This is understandable for the following reasons:

a) In bicycle ergometric exercise while reclining the economy of motion of the trained individual, even a trained bicycle racer, probably is no greater than that of the untrained. Ergometric pedaling exercise while reclining is for reasons inherent in the mechanics of motion hardly comparable with pedaling while sitting on a bicycle.

b) In the ergometer exercise while reclining and wearing a face mask with breathing valve, all of which is new to the trained individual, there is a significant psychic alteration for the subject, and his natural respiratory economy is being more or less disturbed.

c) Thus, the lower O_2 consumption of the trained individual as a result of a (perhaps) more economic muscular metabolism might be lower compared with the O_2 saving through greater motion economy. Possibly not more than 1 to 5% is saved; that would amount to 10 to 150 cm^3 saved out of 1000 to 3000 cm^3 of O_2 absorbed. These figures lie, however, within the range of possible error of the usual spiroergometric methods. As a matter of fact, Kirchhoff, Reindell and Gebauer found a somewhat lower O_2 consumption in high-power athletes compared with individuals of average performance capacity, namely:

at 100 watts, 1410 cm^3 of O_2 : 1438 cm^3
at 150 watts, 1944 cm^3 of O_2 : 2043 cm^3

(in a total of 120 subjects, 40 high-performance athletes and 80 untrained individuals).

d) The statistically insignificant difference in O_2 consumption between trained and untrained individuals proves nothing. Possibly it merely shows that such a difference was not precisely provable with the always more or less faulty methodology being used and in the group of subjects at the moment under consideration. A relatively small difference can be hidden by a relatively great margin of error in the methodology, or a broad distribution of the variable over too small a number of subjects could produce a null result. It is impossible to measure finer distinctions by relatively coarse methods.

In summary, it may be said that:

1. The trained person (especially the trained endurance performer) definitely has a lower O$_2$ consumption in his own particular sport at equal performance than the untrained person (of approximately the same constitution, weight, etc.).
2. The lower O$_2$ consumption can be traced to greater economy of:
   a) motor performance
   b) circulatory performance
   c) respiratory performance
   d) perhaps muscular metabolism.
3. In ergometric exercise that is simpler from the motor point of view (for which the trained person is not specially trained), a less-meager O$_2$ consumption is to be expected through factors 2b, 2c and 2d, which, however, may lie within the margin of error of the customary spirographic methods. The chance of spotting this slight O$_2$ difference is greatest with the Scholander and Haldane gas-analysis methods. The difference can also be negated by psychic alterations in the subject through the more or less oppressive methods of examination. Nevertheless, the greater economy of the circulatory performance and respiratory work in the trained individual under equal ergometric exercise levels is definitely provable.

There is no doubt about the fact that trained endurance performers (long-distance runners, oarsmen, bicycle racers, etc.) can absorb much greater quantities of O$_2$ during physical exertion of great magnitude than can the untrained. While untrained men aged 20 to 40 can absorb approximately 3000 cm^3 of O$_2$ per minute at maximal exercise levels, highly trained endurance performers of high capacity have been known to attain levels of more than 6000 (Mellerowicz and Nowacki, etc.).

4.5   The Dependence of the O$_2$ Consumption on the Type of Physical Performance

At equal physical power, the O$_2$ consumption depends on the biological performance, which can vary in relation to the degree of efficiency of movements. Thus, at a power of 100 watts, O$_2$ consumption is greatest (100%) with hand cranking while standing, and considerably less during pedaling while seating (89%) and reclining (90.5%) (see Fig. 114, after Mellerowicz and Nowacki). Higher maximal O$_2$ consumption figures can also be achieved during hand cranking while standing than in pedaling while reclining (Galle). The maximal O$_2$ consumption is very probably also quite dependent on the muscular mass involved and its capillarity as well as numerous conditioning factors.

**4.6   The Dependence of the O_2 Consumption on Ambient
Temperature and Barometric Pressure**

Slight temperature differences of 18° to 24°C in the examination room (in
open systems) have no significant effect on O_2 consumption at submaximal
or maximal power. On the other hand, endurance performance and maximal O_2 consumption are reduced at temperatures of >25–30°C.

Maximal O_2 consumption decreases in regular proportion to the partial
O_2 pressure as barometric pressure decreases. The physical and psychic performance reserves fall to critical levels in direct proportion to a decrease in
O_2 consumption, and values below these critical levels are not compatible
with life. Altitude training can increase the O_2 transport capacity of the
blood and the circulatory and respiratory capacity, and thus the physical
and psychic performance capacity at low partial O_2 pressures can be considerably increased.

5.   Pathophysiology of O_2 Consumption During and After Exertion

At equal submaximal power, O_2 consumption in the steady state is approximately the same or a trifle higher in individuals with respiratory, cardiac
and hematogenic insufficiency than in healthy untrained individuals (Fig.
120, after Schmutzler and Mellerowicz). However, the respiratory equivalent is usually elevated (see Chapter XI).

The onset time for O_2 consumption is usually prolonged, depending on
the kind and magnitude of the insufficiency (Fig. 120). With prolonged
onset time, the O_2 debt and total O_2 consumption increase. The recovery
time for O_2 consumption is prolonged.

Maximal O_2 consumption is reduced in pathological cases, depending
again on the type and magnitude of the cardiac, respiratory or hematogenic
problems. The determination of $\dot{V}_{O_2}$ is therefore a suitable method for ascertaining the pathology quantitatively.

The most important causes of respiratory insufficiency are:

1. Mechanical (restrictive or obstructive) hindrances to breathing; for example, pleurisy, stenotic processes of the bronchial system (such as goiter,
   bronchial carcinoma, thoracic deformities, bronchial spasm, etc.)
2. Disturbances of the pulmonary diffusion in pneumoconioses, pulmonary
   fibrosis, Boeck's disease, pneumonias, tubercular conditions, pulmonary
   edema, pulmonary sclerosis

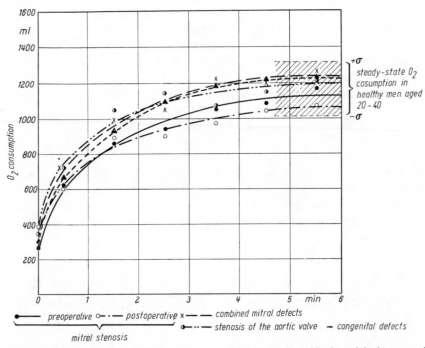

Fig. 120. O₂ consumption (STPD) at a power of 1 watt per kg of body weight in cases of acquired or congenital (noncyanotic) heart defects (after *Schmutzler and Mellerowicz*) as compared with norms (after *Dransfeld and Mellerowicz*). The O₂ consumption is not reduced in submaximal performances at the steady state. However, the onset time and recovery time are prolonged, depending on the nature and magnitude of the exertion. The O₂ deficit is increased and the maximal O₂ consumption reduced.

3. Reduction of O₂ utilization of the blood in reduced peripheral capillarity, atelectasis, pneumothorax, exudates and transudates of the pleura, postoperative conditions after segmental resection, lobectomy, thoracoplasty, etc.

4. Increase in the functional dead air space of the residual air and respiratory reserve volume in emphysema, bronchiectasis, stenotic breathing, etc.

5. Central or peripheral disturbances of the respiratory regulation in consequence of neoplasma, vascular processes, and inflammatory processes in the region of the respiratory centers as well as phrenic paresis, etc.

6. Cardiovascular causes: hyperventilation in right heart insufficiency, congenital shunt, vascular shunt in the pulmonary circulatory system, etc.

7. Reduction in partial O₂ pressure in the inhaled air through breathing low-O₂ air.

In cases of cardiac and hematogenic insufficiency, pathological changes, especially reductions in the O_2 consumption during exertion, may be caused by:

1. Myocardial insufficiency of various etiologies
2. Increased pressure in cases of stenosis
3. Increased volume in cases of valvular insufficiency and congenital shunt
4.˙Hindrance of the heart in pericarditis and its consequences, tumors of the thoracic cavity, scar processes, elevation of the diaphragm of various etiologies, etc.
5. Reduction in the O_2 transport capacity of the blood
6. Reduction of O_2 utilization of the blood in reduced peripheral capillarity
7. Hypertonic regulatory situations of the minor or major circulatory systems
8. Tachycardia of various etiologies, disturbances in the formation and transmission of stimuli, etc.

When the performance limits are exceeded, an excessive O_2 consumption, or "spirographic O_2 debt," may under certain conditions occur. This was found in the course of spiroergometric studies by Uhlenbruck and by Knipping in many patients with pulmonary and cardiac disease upon switching over from air to O_2 breathing. This must not be confused with Hill's "oxygen deficit," also known as oxygen debt, which sets in at the start of every prolonged performance and increases further in unsteady-state performances.

The spirographic O_2 debt can sometimes be caused by undersaturation of the blood with O_2 (to about 20 to 30%). An O_2 debt, on the other hand, develops with anaerobic muscular work with an increasing level of lactic acid in the blood and reduction of the standard bicarbonate, even without undersaturation of the blood with O_2. Because of methodological difficulties, it was at first not possible to prove regular relationships between the spirographic O_2 debt and the arterial undersaturation. After studies by Valentin, Worth, Gasthaus, Lühning and Werner, and on the basis of theoretical considerations, however, quantitative relationships between spirographically measured O_2 debt and arterial hypoxemia must be assumed. With an O_2 capacity in the blood of about 1000 cubic centimeters and a maximal steady-state O_2 consumption of about 3,000 to 4,000 cubic centimeters and an arterial undersaturation of 20 to 30%, saturation deficits of more than 600 cubic centimeters per minute (theoretically as much as about 900 cubic centimeters) are possible.

All forms of pulmonary insufficiency more or less favor the occurrence of arterial undersaturation and a spirographic O_2 debt (Fig. 121). This is especially true of:

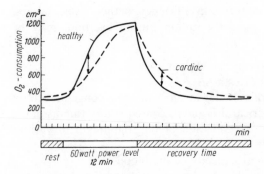

Fig. 121. Buildup of O_2 debt during work in a cardiac patient and its satisfaction in the recovery period (after *Landen*). Usually the recovery time is also prolonged.

1. Disturbances to pulmonary diffusion in cases of pneumocyanosis, tubercular processes, pulmonary fibrosis, Boeck's disease, pneumonia, pulmonary edema, pulmonary sclerosis, etc.
2. Reduction of the pulmonary diffusion surface area in cases of pneumonia, atelectasis, pneumothorax, exudates or transudates of the pleura, postoperative conditions after segmental resection, lobectomy, thoracoplasty, etc.
3. Partial by-passing of the pulmonary circulation in cases of right-left shunt, arteriovenous aneurysm, arteriovenous anastomosis of the minor circulation, etc.
4. Reduction of the partial O_2 pressure when breathing O_2-poor air.

Arterial undersaturation and spirographic O_2 debt may also be the result of a primarily cardiac-caused respiratory insufficiency (in cases of pulmonary edema due to left-heart insufficiency).

Cases of arterial hypoxemia and spirographic O_2 debt in O_2 saturation, however, also occur even in healthy individuals during great exertion. The less the magnitude of the performance and the greater the spirographic O_2 debt, the more probable is a pathological etiology. The greater the magnitude of the exercise and the smaller the spirographic O_2 debt, the more probable it is that we are faced with a physiological spirographic O_2 debt.

For an exact demarcation of the physiological from the pathological O_2 debt, we need extensive studies of healthy sex and age groups at minor, medium and major exercise levels. Only a knowledge of the average behavior of the spirographic O_2 debt and its physiological range of variation at different exercise levels will afford a more precise definition of the pathological spirographic O_2 debt.

After studies by Hollmann, Venrath and Tietz, we must reckon with an individual range of distribution on the order of $\pm 10\%$ for the figures on O_2 consumption in the steady state. For this reason, spirographic O_2 debt can not be assumed to exist unless figures at least exceed 10% of the O_2 consumption in air breathing.

6. The Evaluation of the O_2 Consumption in Ergometric Performance

At submaximal exercise levels, no reliable conclusions can be drawn as to the physical performance capacity of the subject merely from the magnitude of the steady-state O_2 consumption. On the other hand, with simultaneous determination of heart rate, the calculation of the O_2 pulse and its comparison with the physiological averages and standard deviations is valuable for the evaluation of the cardiac performance capacity (see Chapter VII).

A considerable delay in the onset time of the O_2 consumption as compared with the physiological averages and standard deviations points in the direction of cardiac and pulmonary insufficiency of varying etiologies. The onset time (for equal exercise levels) probably increases as we grow older. If the onset time is brief, the cardiovascular system is probably robust.

The O_2 debt increases considerably as the onset time lengthens. If the O_2 debt and recovery time for O_2 consumption are both high compared with physiological data for equal exercise levels, therefore, it is a rather sure sign of cardiac, pulmonary or hematogenic performance deficiency.

Magnitude of the maximal O_2 consumption is a reliable measure of the cardiac, pulmonary, hematogenic and general physical performance capability. Any insufficiency in one of the conditioning factors leads to reduction in O_2 capacity.[1]

In judging each individual case, it is important to bear in mind the margin of error in method (about 10%), type of ergometric exercise, rpm, time of day, maintainence of basal conditions under exercise levels, age, sex and state of training.

---

[1] For medical reasons in pathological cases and for subjective reasons in compensation cases, it is not always possible or advisable to determine the maximal O_2 consumption.

References

Apor, P., S. Szabo-Wahlstab, M. Miklos: Zusammenhänge zwischen einigen aeroben und anaeroben Parametern. In: 3. Internationales Seminar für Ergometrie. Berlin: Ergon-Verlag, 1973.

Åstrand, P. O.: Experimental studies of physical working capacity in relation to sex and age. Kopenhagen: Munksgaard, 1952.

Åstrand, P. O.: Progress in Ergometry. In: Ergebnisse der Ergometrie. Köln: Wissenschafts-Verlag, 1974.

Åstrand, P. O. and K. Rodahl: Textbook of Work Physiology. McGraw-Hill Co. New York 1977.

Balke, B.: Arbeitsphysiologie 15, (1954) 311.

Beznak, Durig and Knoll: zit. nach Prokop: Habil.-Schrift. Wien 1952.

Brauer, H.: Zschr. Kreisl.forschg. 44, (1955) 770.

Chiari, O.: Sportverletzungen, Sportschäden. Wien: Hölder-Pichter-Tempsky, 1950.

Christensen, E. H. and P. Högberg: Arbeitsphysiologie 14, (1950) 249.

Dirken and Heemstra: after E. Opitz and H. Bartels. In: Handbuch der physiologisch-pathologisch-chemischen Analyse. Heidelberg. Springer, 1955.

Dirken and Orie: in Firma Lode, Groningen (Holland), Oosterstraat 38.

Dransfeld, B. and H. Mellerowicz: Zschr. Kreisl.forschg. 48, (1959) 901.

Dressler, F. and H. Mellerowicz: Zschr. Kinderhk. 85, (1961) 31.

Fleisch, A.: Neue Methoden zum Studium des Gasaustausches und der Lungenfunktion. Leipzig: Thieme, 1956.

Galle, L.: Diss. (Berlin, Freie Universität). Der Sportarzt 10, (1962) 332.

Herbst, R.: Dtsch. Arch. Klin. Med. 162, (1928) 33.

Hertle, F. H.: Der Aussagewert der alveolo-arteriellen Sauerstoff-Druckdifferenz (AaD O₂) im Arbeitsversuch. In: 2. Intern. Seminar für Ergometrie. Berlin: Ergon-Verlag, 1967.

Hertz, C. W.: Die ergometrische Begutachtung von Gasaustauschstörungen. In: 1. Internationales Seminar für Ergometrie. Berlin: Ergon-Verlag, 1965.

Herxheimer, H., E. Wissing and E. Wolff: Zschr. exper. Med. 52, (1926) 447.

Hill, A. V.: Muscular Movement in Man. New York: McGraw-Hill, 1927.

Hollmann, W., H. Valentin and H. Venrath: Münch. med. Wschr. 39, (1959) 1680.

Hollmann, W. and H. Heck: Ärztliche Fortbildung 1, (1972) 62.

Hüllemann, K. D.: Leistungsmedizin—Sportmedizin. Stuttgart: Thieme, 1976.

Knipping, H. W., W. Bolt, H. Valentin and H. Venrath: Untersuchung und Beurteilung des Herzkranken. Stuttgart: Enke, 1955.

Kofranyi, E. and H. F. Michaelis: Arbeitsphysiologie 11, (1941) 141.

Landen, H. C.: Die funktionelle Beurteilung des Lungen- und Herzkranken. Darmstadt: Steinkopff, 1955.

Liljestrand, G. and A. Lindhardt: Skand. Arch. Physiol. 39, (1920) 167.

Löllgen, H., F. H. Hertle and R. Stufler: Lungenfunktionsgrößen und maximale Sauerstoffaufnahme. In: 3. Internationales

Seminar für Ergometric. Berlin: Ergon-Verlag, 1973.

Mathews, D. K. and E. L. Fox: The Physiological Basis of Physical Education and Athletics. Philadelphia: W. B. Saunders Company, 1976.

Mellerowicz, H. and D. Lerche: Zschr. Kinderhk. 81, (1958) 36; Internat. Zschr. angew. Physiol. einschl. Arbeitsphysiol. 17, (1959) 459.

Mellerowicz, H. and P. Nowacki: Zschr. Kreisl.forsch. 50, (1961) 1002.

Rein, H. and M. Schneider: Physiologie des Menschen. Berlin-Göttingen-Heidelberg: Springer, 1957.

Reindell, H. and H. W. Kirchhoff: Dtsch. med. Wschr. 81, (1956) 592 u. 1048.

Robinson, S.: Arbeitsphysiologie 10, (1938) 251.

Rossier and Méan: after P. H. Rossier, A. Bühlmann and K. Wiesinger: Physiologie und Pathophysiologie der Atmung. Berlin-Göttingen-Heidelberg: Springer, 1956.

Schmutzler, H., H. Mellerowicz and E. Carl: Zschr. Kreisl.forschg. 49, (1960) 445.

Schönholzer, G., G. Bieler, H. Howald: Ergometrische Methoden zur Messung der aeroben und anaeroben Kapazität. In: 3. Internationales Seminar für Ergometrie. Berlin: Ergon-Verlag, 1973.

Scholander and Evans: after E. Opitz and H. Bartels. In: Handbuch der physiologisch-pathologisch-chemischen Analyse. Berlin-Göttingen-Heidelberg: Springer, 1955.

Shepard and Sperling: after E. Opitz and. H. Bartels. In: Handbuch der physiologisch-pathologisch-chemischen Analyse. Berlin-Göttingen-Heidelberg: Springer, 1955.

Simonson, E. and H. Hebestreit: Klin. Wschr. 8, (1929) 2146, after H. Herxheimer: Grundriß der Sportmedizin. Leipzig: Thieme, 1933.

Thalemann, Ch.: Diss. Freie Universität Berlin 1969.

Tlusty, L.: Beitrag zur Frage der Leistungsbreite älterer Menschen. In: 2. Internationales Seminar für Ergometrie. Berlin: Ergon-Verlag, 1967.

Valentin, H., H. Venrath, H. v. Mallinckrodt and M. Gürakar: Zschr. Altersforschg. 9, (1955) 291.

Valentin, H., G. Worth, L. Gasthaus, W. Lühning and K. Werner: Arch. Gewerbepath., Berlin 16, (1957) 86.

Venrath, H. and W. Hollmann: Sport in prophylaxe u. Rehabilitation von Lungenerkrankungen. Therapiewoche 14, 683 (1965).

X. Respiratory Time-Volumes in Ergometric Performance

1. Measurement of Respiratory Time-Volumes

1.1 Measurement of Respiratory Time-Volumes in Open Systems

1.1.1 Measurement with Spirometers

The simplest way to measure the respiratory time-volume in ergometric performances is to collect the expired air in a Douglas bag (see page 165) and then measure it in spirometers. The simplest spirometers consist in principle of two sliding, concentric cylinders, one fitting airtight into the other. The airtight closure can be achieved by filling the inner cylinder with water. The air to be measured can be blown into the spirometer through a filling tube. The one cylinder is then raised a certain amount by the air blown in. From the radius of the cylinder, r, and the height by which it has been raised, the volume of air introduced can be calculated ($V = \pi r^2 h$).

Corresponding to the calculated volume of the cylinder at various lifts, the one measuring cylinder can be calibrated to indicated volume. In order to avoid errors in measurement caused by the inherent weight of the measuring cylinder, the latter should be kept small and be made of light plastic or aluminum or else be counterbalanced by a counterweight via a pulley (Fig. 122). Such simple spirometers are well suited for measuring vital capacity. To measure great respiratory time-volumes several measurements or larger spirometers are required. The temperature of the breathed air must be taken for conversion to BTPS or STPD figures (page 406–411).

1.1.2 Measurement of Respiratory Time-Volumes with Gasometers

a) Measurement with wet gasometers
Wet gasometers (Fig. 123) use a measuring drum with several chambers of determined volume, into which the volume of gas to be measured flows

199

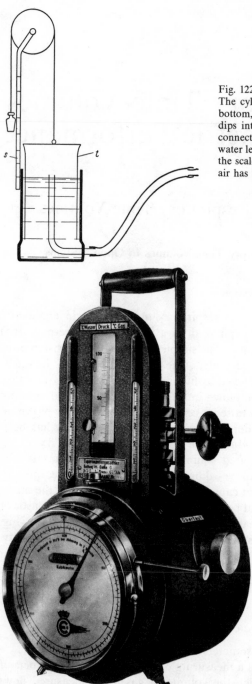

Fig. 122. Schematic drawing of a spirometer. The cylindrical spirometer bell, open at the bottom, is balanced by a counterweight and dips into a water bath. The breathing tube connects with a pipe leading up above the water level inside. After proper calibration of the scale, s, it is possible to judge how much air has been breathed in or out (after *Rein*).

Fig. 123. Experimental wet gasometer produced by Elster & Co., AG, of Mainz, Germany. It is equipped with a manometer (which can be switched off) to read resistances from 0 to 100 mm of water as well as two thermometers to measure the temperature of the fluid and air. The large pointer and the rolling counter can be set to zero by hand. Screw feet and a spirit-level enable the counter to be placed absolutely horizontal.

alternately in on one side and out at the other. The intake and outlet lie above a blocking liquid (water or low-viscosity oil).

A turning motion is imparted to the measuring drum by the pressure difference in the filling and emptying of the chambers. In this way an always equal chamber volume is displaced by the entering flow and is measured. The revolutions of the drum (and therefore the number of times the chambers fill to a known volume) are continuously recorded by a counting device calibrated in liters. The temperature of the gas in the measuring drum has to be measurable in order to obtain the BTPS or STPD figures.

In measuring the inspiratory volumes, it is sufficient to keep account of the ambient room temperature. Wet gasometers are manufactured for minute-volumes up to 200 liters or more. Even in the case of noncontinuous flow, a precision of measurement of ±0.5% is said to be obtained. The resistance to flow is reported to be only 5 to 8 mm of water at a flow of 100 to 200 liters per minute.

b) Measurement with dry gasometers

A dry respiratory gasometer well suited for ergometric studies (Fig. 124) was developed by the Max Planck Institute for Work Physiology in Dortmund from earlier models by Zuntz, Kofranyi and Michaelis. Two equal chambers in the device are separated into halves by means of an intermediary membrane of leather. As one chamber is filled, the other is emptied. The leather

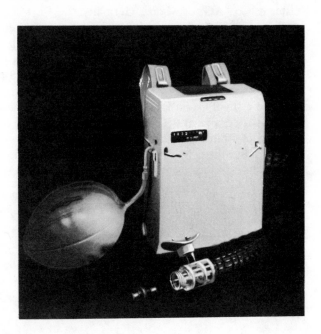

Fig. 124. The portable respiratory gasometer of the Max Planck Institute for Work Physiology in Dortmund, Germany.

membranes transmit their movements via a system of levers to a crank shaft. The latter turns continuously in one direction, thus operating two sliding valves which alternately fill and empty the halves of the chamber and at the same time operate a counting device. A double-membrane pump that works with each phase of the gasometer cycle exhausts 3 to 5‰ of the breathed air, as desired. For measuring the gas temperature at any given moment, there is a thermometer built in. A carrier consisting of two shoulder straps makes it possible to wear the gasometer like a knapsack. It weighs 3.5 kg.

The rubber bags used to collect the samples of air permit CO_2 and O_2 to diffuse to a considerable degree depending on the differences in their partial pressures. Filling the rubber bag with exhaled air two or three hours before the start of the experiment reduces the error due to this factor. As soon as possible after the conclusion of the experiment, samples of the air should be drawn off for analysis by means of glass pipettes with mercury closure. The diffusion-caused error must be determined for various differences in partial pressure and various storage periods and the results allowed for. The accuracy of measurement of this respiratory gasometer is reportedly ±1% for up to 60 liters of respiratory minute-volume. The resistance to breathing at 50 liters minute-volume amounts to 10 to 20 mm of water, while at performances of greater magnitude and respiratory minute-volumes above 50 liters and second-volumes above 5 liters considerable breathing resistance is encountered.

Dry gasometers well suited for ergometric studies are also supplied by Elster & Co., AG, of Mainz, Germany.

The calibration of the gasometer is accomplished either with a very accurately calibrated experimental gasometer or with a so-called "cubicator" (precision spirometer), which in principle resembles the spirometer in Figure 122. The calibration of gasometers can be performed very accurately with weighed amounts of a known gas. For this purpose, for example, are required a small O_2 flask and a precision weighing scale. Since 1 liter of O_2 weighs 1429 grams at 0°C and 760 mm Hg., the size of a calibrated volume (say, about 10 liters) at a given temperature at known pressure (using conversion tables) can be calculated from the weight loss of the O_2 flask.

1.1.3   Measurement of Respiratory Time-Volumes and the Speed of Flow of Expired Air with Pneumotachographs

Pneumotachographs record the changes in speed of flow of breathed air in a small-diameter tube, dependent on the differing time-volumes. From the pneumotachogram and the calibration curve of the device, the second-volumes can be calculated. The time-volumes can be calculated by planimetry from the area between the curve and the zero line or by electronic integrating procedures.

In principle, pneumotachographs are based on Poiseuille's Law. The speed of flow in laminar movement in a fine, stiff tube is directly proportional to the pressure loss per unit of length. If the pressure difference between two points in the tube is recorded, there results a differential curve, the pneumotachogram (Fig. 126). The ordinates of the curve are directly proportional to the speed of the flow of breath and the respiratory time-volume.

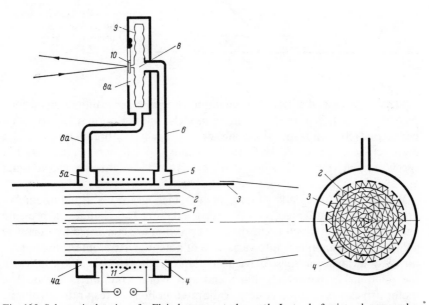

Fig. 125. Schematic drawing of a Fleisch pneumotachograph. Instead of using a large number of fine tubes, a corrugated nickel sheet is rolled up together with a smooth nickel sheet, both 0.05 mm thick, in the form of a spiral. This produces air canals (1) with a cross-section of about 0.8 mm and 32 mm long. The resulting cylinder is fitted into a brass tube (2). In order to transmit the pressure difference, there is a further layer of corrugated sheet applied to the brass tube (2) and enclosed by another brass tube (3). This outer tube (3) has small holes (4) around its circumference to release the pressure. All these holes open into a ring-shaped channel (5) which is soldered on airtight and from which a rubber tube (6) leads to a differential manometer (8). 20 cm from the channel (5) is another similar soldered-on channel (5a) which leads the pressure at a second ring of holes (4a) via a tube (6a) to the left side (8a) of the differential manometer. The two chambers (8) and (8a) are separated by a membrane made of corrugated sheet metal. When in Figure 125 the air is flowing from right to left, the pressure in ring-canal (5) will be greater than that in (5a), membrane 9 will bulge out toward the left, and the light ray reflected from mirror (10) will be deflected upward. If on the other hand the air flows from left to right, the pressure in ring-channel (5a) will be greater than in (5), the membrane will bulge toward the right and the light ray will be deflected lower. Note that the membrane responds to pressure difference, not to absolute pressure. As long as the air flow speed does not exceed a certain limit, laminar flow predominates and thus strict proportionality prevails between air speed and deflection. Once this limit is exceeded, a slight turbulence occurs which becomes evident in the zig-zag nature of the recorded curve.

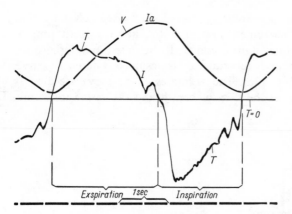

Fig. 126. Pneumotachogram T and spirogram V in a human subject. The horizontal line T = 0 is the zero line of the pneumotachogram. During inspiration, curve T lies above this line. The ordinate values of curve T show at any instant the speed at which the air is flowing through the pneumotachograph. Curve V represents the volume of breathed air: it increases during the total expiration phase and decreases during inspiration (after *Fleisch*).

Fleisch developed a practical pneumotachograph according to this principle (Fig. 125). It is available in three models: one for normal (up to 1 liter per second) human respiration, one for medium-heavy breathing (up to 2.5 liters per second) and one for forced breathing (up to 6 liters per second). For special ergometric studies, only the models for the higher second-volumes are of value.

Wolff's IMP (integrating motor pneumotachograph) is a pneumotachograph especially adapted for ergometric studies. The changes in pressure and speed of flow which occur during expiration are converted by means of a differential manometer into variations of potential. After intensification by means of a transistor, these drive a small integrating electric motor in which the relationship between voltage and speed of revolution is linear. The motor drives a revolution counter calibrated in liters of respiratory volume. The respiratory time-volume is thus immediately readable. The apparatus is also equipped with a small pump for automatically collecting minute samples of the breath (capable of settings from 0.3 to 2 ml) out of 1 to 3 liters of expired air. Special containers are supplied for holding the collected samples. The small, plastic sample-bag is suspended in an aluminum canister, and the intervening space can be filled through a closable opening in the canister and can be filled with expired air. When the sample bag is filled, the interstitial air in the metal canister is pressed out through a valve. In this way differences in the composition of the sample can be reduced to a minimum.

1.2   Measurement in Closed Systems

Closed systems are usually equipped with devices for continuous graphic recording of the respiratory volumes. They make it possible to observe changes in the breathing level, i.e., shifts in respiratory volume in the range of the inspired or expired reserve volume. The precise measurement of temperature in the system is necessary on a continuous basis during an ergometric performance in order to make it possible to reduce the recorded figures to 37°C, 760 mm Hg, full humidity saturation of the air (BTPS) or to 0°C, 760 mm Hg and dryness (STPD).

1.3   Thoracography

The respiratory movements of the thorax can be timed and recorded by means of a thoracograph. The latter can be slipped into a strap applied around the thorax. The respiratory changes in the circumference of the thorax can thus be recorded and measured mechanically or electrically. A thoracogram affords the possibility of determining the respiration rate, the change in thoracic circumference during respiration and an approximation of the respiratory quotient. Determinations of the respiratory time-volume are not possible from a thoracogram, since it does not include the action of the diaphragm.

2.   Physiology of the Regulation of the Respiratory Time-Volume During Physical Activity

In the onset phase at the start of an exercise, the respiratory time-volume and O_2 consumption are regulated in an almost parabolic curve. The respiration rate and the respiratory volume increase into the range of the inspiratory and expiratory reserve volume, either entirely or as far as possible, to meet the O_2 requirement of the moment. The duration of the onset phase is determined by numerous endogenous and exogenous factors. It is briefer in more robust respiratory and circulatory systems. In near-maximal work, the onset time of respiratory time-volume and O_2 consumption is lengthened.

After the steady state is reached, respiratory time-volume and O_2 consumption are balanced with the immediate O_2 requirement of the organism. At this point, as a rule, an economical relationship between respiration rate and depth of breathing sets in, with relatively low O_2 consumption in the respiratory muscles (in relation to total O_2 consumption). Uneconomical forms of breathing are:

1. Rapid breathing during exercise with low respiratory volume ("frequency-type"). In this type, the mixed relationship between low respiratory volume (with high partial O_2 pressure) and the expiratory reserve volume and residual volume (with low partial O_2 pressure) is most unfavorable. The O_2 utilization of the breathed air is small here. The O_2 consumption of the respiratory musculature itself is probably high.

2. The unsatisfactory participation of the diaphragm, which can also have an unfavorable effect on the respiratory economy. In this connection, we must reckon with unsatisfactory aeration of the caudal lobes of the lungs and minimal utilization of the atmospheric O_2.

3. Forced breathing at unphysiological pressure, in which the natural respiratory rhythm and the free course of ventilation are disturbed, with temporarily closed vocal cords. O_2 consumption in the respiratory muscles is elevated. O_2 consumption of the inspired air is elevated, O_2 utilization of the inspired air is reduced. Venous delivery of blood to the right heart is strangulated. In the arteries of the minor and major circulatory systems, the blood must be ejected against an increased level of resistance.

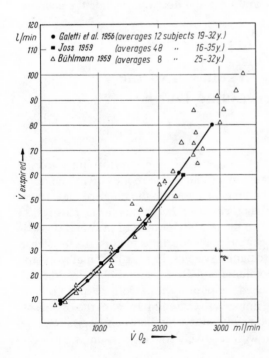

Fig. 127. Relationship between respiratory time-volume and O_2 consumption. Spirometrically measured averages by Galetti et al. (1956) and Joss (1955) as well as the individual figures from an independent series of studies with an open experimental arrangement (after *Bühlmann*).

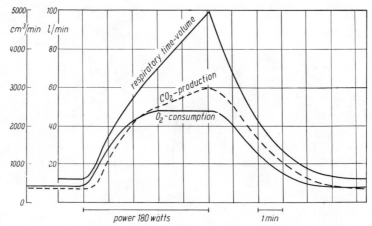

Fig. 128. Respiratory time-volume, O_2 consumption and CO_2 production in an unsteady-state performance to the point of exhaustion (after *Joss*).

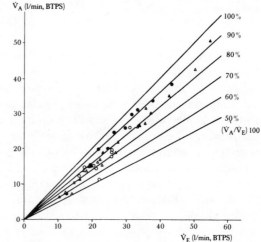

Fig. 129. Alveolar efficiency as a function of performance in exercise on the bicycle ergometer (after *Stegemann* and *Heinrich*).
$\dot{V}_A$ = (alveolar ventilation).
$\dot{V}_E$ = (expired volume/min).

In increasing steady-state stages, respiratory time-volume and O_2 consumption increase in almost linear proportion to the magnitude of the performance up to maximal steady-state performance (Fig. 127). The maximal-performance respiratory minute-volume lies approximately 1/3 below the maximal voluntary ventilation (Fig. 128).

The ventilatory pressure and volume work of the respiratory musculature is performed against flow resistances, tissue viscosity and elasticity of the respiratory apparatus, and increases as ergometric performance intensifies. The economy of respiratory work and alveolar ventilation and its degree of efficiency thus increases (Fig. 129).

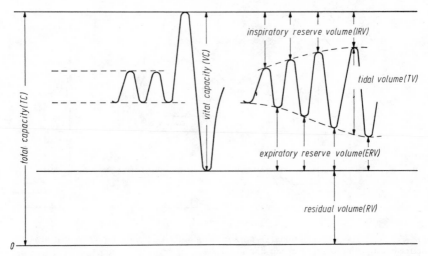

Fig. 130. Schematic representation: tidal volume (AV), inspiratory reserve volume (IRV), expiratory reserve volume (ERV), residual volume (RV), vital capacity (VK) and total capacity (TC) (after *Comroe*).

Upon exceeding the maximal steady-state limit, the performance can be further intensified with additional anaerobic muscular exercise, elevated lactate level in the blood and growing O_2 deficit. At the same time, O_2 consumption increases a bit more. The respiratory time-volume increases further together with a drop in O_2 utilization when the steady-state limit of performance is exceeded. In this range, lying beyond the maximal steady-state power, arterial undersaturation of the blood may occur even with increasing hyperventilation and falling O_2 utilization of the atmospheric air (see Chapter XVI). However, the maximal ventilation is not reached by healthy individuals even at utmost physical exertion.

The O_2 deficit built up during the exercise in the onset phase or in steady-state performance shows itself in protractedly elevated respiratory time-volume in the recovery phase. It sinks in characteristic curve form (see Fig. 141a) until it reaches its resting value. Between the magnitude of the performance, the performance capacity and the recovery time of the respiratory time-volume there are regular relationships.

Respiratory time-volume, O_2 utilization of the inspired air and O_2 consumption increase for a short time after the conclusion of brief, intense, unsteady-state performances of 30 to 60 seconds (after Reindell and Roskamm).

The extraordinarily complex regulation of respiration during performance takes place in the respiratory center. According to available studies, a distinction can be made between an inspiratory center, an expiratory center (in the medulla oblongata) and a pneumotactic center (in the pons). These centers are connected with the diencephalon, the frontal lobe and other parts of the brain. The adaptation of respiratory rate, tidal volume, respiratory time-volume and O_2 consumption to current performance requirements is effected through chemical and physical stimuli, namely:

1. The P_{CO_2} of the blood
2. The pH of the blood
3. The P_{O_2} of the blood
4. Temperature stimuli
5. Reflex control via the sensory receptors of the pulmonary vagus
6. Reflex control via the sensory receptors in respiratory muscles, joints and ligaments of the rib cage
7. Possibly sensory receptors in the skeletal muscles.

The CO_2 pressure of the blood affects specific CO_2 receptors in the region of the respiratory center. Changes in the pH of the blood also affect the cells of the respiratory center itself. As O_2 pressure falls, specific chemoreceptors in the carotid body and in the thoracic aorta (Heymans), which are connected to the respiratory centers, are stimulated and respiratory time-volume is increased (Fig. 131). Through peripheral or central temperature stimuli, respiration may also be influenced via the heat-regulatory center in the diencephalon. Through breathing solely through the nose at the maximal range of physical exertion, respiratory time-volume and O_2 consumption are reduced as compared with mouth-breathing (Fig. 132). Quantity and quality of respiration at any given time result from the summation of a large number of stimuli, to which must be added emotional and psychic effects.

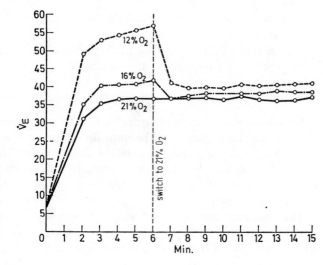

Fig. 131. The magnitude of ventilation in constant exercise after switching to atmospheric air after low-O_2 air (after *Hollmann* and *Grünewald*, unpublished).

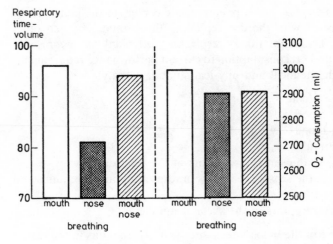

Fig. 132. The effect of separate nose and mouth breathing on the respiratory time-volume and O_2 consumption in the course of an exercise of 23 kpm per second performed by two subjects on a bicycle ergometer (after *Liesen* and *Hollmann,* unpublished).

3. Physiological Averages and Range of Variation of the Respiratory Time-Volume

The figures found for respiratory time-volume by various investigators diverge considerably (Fig. 133, after Knipping, Bolt, Valentin, and Venrath). These considerable discrepancies are caused by:

1. Differences in the groups of subjects (constitution, age, sex and state of training)
2. Various mechanical properties of the ergometers used (varying crank length, crank height, rpm, etc.)
3. The nature of the ergometric performance (hand cranking while standing, pedaling while seated and reclining)
4. Differences in conditions under which the studies were done
5. Errors in calibration and reading the apparatus used, etc.

In order to obtain more comparable results in ergometry, the mechanical properties of the ergometers, the rpms for various ranges of power, and the experimental conditions ought to be standardized (see Chapter III). In comparing data obtained with averages found by various investigators, the conditions under which the various results were obtained should always be taken into account.

The averages and the $\pm 1\sigma$ range of respiratory time-volume in 100 healthy men aged 20 to 40 at a power of 1 watt per kg of body weight are shown in Figure 134. The corresponding figures for pedaling while seated

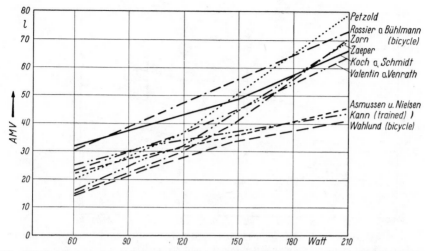

Fig. 133. Respiratory time-volume in the steady state in comparison to power in watts reported by various authors (after *Knipping, Bolt, Valentin* and *Venrath*).

and reclining can be calculated from Figure 12 in Chapter 1. The figures for 1 watt per kg of body weight for children and teenagers are given in Figure 135.

Respiratory time-volumes for pedaling while reclining in 80 healthy subjects aged 20 to 40 are shown in Figures 136a and b. From these figures can be calculated the approximate corresponding figures for hand cranking while standing and pedaling while reclining using the data in Figure 13, Chapter I.

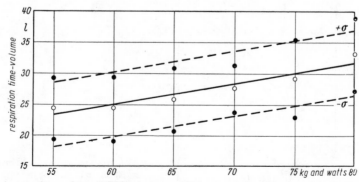

Fig. 134. Respiratory time-volume (BTPS) at a power of 1 watt per kg of body weight in 100 men aged 20 to 40 at hand cranking under standard conditions (after *Dransfeld* and *Mellerowicz*).

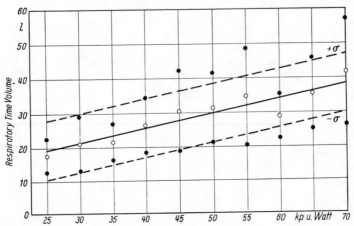

Fig. 135. Respiratory time-volumes of 185 boys aged 7 to 17 at a power of 1 watt per kg of body weight at hand cranking exercise (after *Dressler* and *Mellerowicz*).

In 10 untrained male subjects aged 20 to 40 at maximal power (in increasing exercise levels), comparative figures were obtained for respiratory time-volume in Table 23, after Galle and Mellerowicz. Table 23 shows that considerably lower respiratory time-volumes are attained at maximal power in pedaling while reclining than in hand cranking while standing or pedaling while seated.

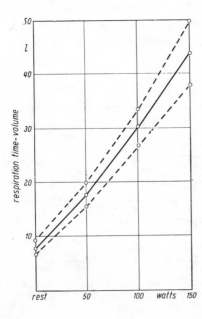

Fig. 136a. Respiratory time-volume and its standard deviations in 80 healthy men aged 30 to 40 for pedaling at 50, 100 and 150 watts while reclining (after *Reindell et al.*).

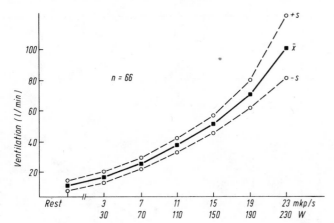

Fig. 136b. Respiratory time-volume during cycling in sitting position of 3–23 kpm with 60 rpm of 66 untrained male volunteers, third decennium (after *Hollmann* and *Heck*).

Table 23. Maximal respiratory time-volume

At hand cranking, standing	82.4	liters	(100 ± 13%)
At pedaling, sitting	80.1	liters	(97 ± 12%)
At pedaling, reclining	73.0	liters	(88.5 ± 15%)

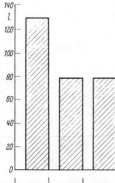

1	AGW/max. AMW in liters (average)	131	76	77
2	respiratory volume in cm³ (average)	2268	2400	2415
3	respiration rate per min (average)	57.7	31.6	31.5
4	depth of breathing in relation to vital capacity (average in %)	53.9	57.1	57.4
		hyper-ventilation	3 min exercise	10 min exercise

Fig. 137. Comparison of the maximal voluntary ventilation figures and maximal working respiratory time-volume at three- and ten-minute exercises to the point of exhaustion (averages for 38 healthy individuals of various ages and sexes, after *Heine, Benesch* and *Hertz*).

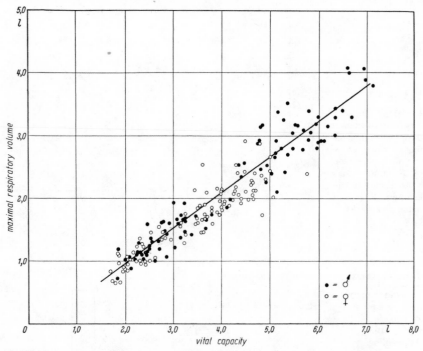

Fig. 138. The maximal respiratory volume in relation to vital capacity (pedaling while seated) (after Åstrand).

Maximal values for the respiratory time-volume, tidal volume and respiration rate in various age groups are shown in Figures 137 and 138, Table 23, and also Figures 201 and 202. Expect readings 20–30% lower for women.

4. Endogenous and Exogenous Factors Controlling the Respiratory Time-Volume

The respiratory time-volume in equal physical exertion varies, depending on constitutional factors, within a certain range of physiological variation. The respiratory time-volume (for equal physical exertion) is controlled by the following factors:

1. Differences in motion economy and degree of efficiency and also differences in rpm in ergometric exercise
2. Differences in respiratory economy, which find expression in greater or lesser O_2 utilization from atmospheric air. A high respiratory equivalent and a corresponding increased respiratory time-volume are present in uneconomical high-frequency respiration.
3. Such morphological factors as character and surface area of the alveolar membranes and pulmonary capillaries also determine respiratory equivalent and the respiratory time-volume.

The maximal respiratory time-volume in ergometric performance is determined mainly by the magnitude of vital capacity and performance capacity of the respiratory musculature, which can be considerably improved by training.

In physically equal performances of 6 to 21 kpm per second, respiratory time-volumes in women and men are approximately the same, according to Hollmann. This is especially true of the net performance respiratory time-volume. Having on the average somewhat lower resting respiratory time-volume, women must be expected to have somewhat lower total respiratory time-volume (in submaximal performance.) Comparative studies to this end on a sufficiently broad sample of untrained men and women are yet to be done. At exercise levels high enough to be unsteady-state performance for women, respiratory minute-volume (with already decreasing O_2 utilization) can be somewhat greater than in men.

Maximal respiratory time-volume is on the average considerably lower in women than in men. According to comparative studies by Åstrand and Hollmann, which were carried out on trained men and women, the figures for women were about 30% below those for men.

Maximal respiratory time-volume in children and teenagers increases with age in almost direct proportion to weight (according to Åstrand). Accordingly, their respiratory time-volume per kg of body weight is approximately equal at maximal performance. A progressive decline in maximal respiratory time-volume, corresponding to maximal O_2 consumption (page 188), is also to be expected after about age 30. The behavior of respiratory time-volume at various age levels at equal submaximal performances is shown in Table 24 and Figure 139.

Table 24. Respiratory time-volume in subjects aged 20 to 40 vs. those aged 50 to 70 at equal power in hand cranking (after *Hollmann, Venrath* and *Valentin*).

	aged 20–40 (30 subjects)	aged 50–70 (30 subjects)	Sigma difference and t-value *Koller*
40 watts	26.21	27.31	Sigma-diff. 1.90 l, t = 5.71
70 watts	33.81	38.11	Sigma-diff. 2.70 l, t = 8.11

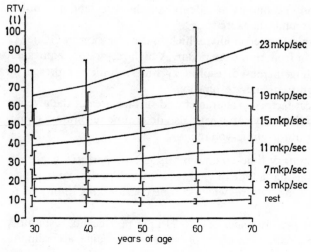

Fig. 139. The effect of age on respiratory values of male persons from the third to the seventh decennium during increased exercise on a bicycle ergometer (after *Hollmann, et al.,* 1970).

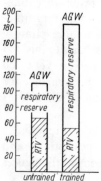

Fig. 140. Maximal voluntary ventilation, respiratory reserve and respiratory time-volume at a power of 120 watts in a subject in untrained condition and again after 1-1/2 years of endurance training (after *Hollmann*).

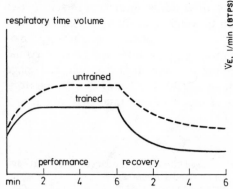

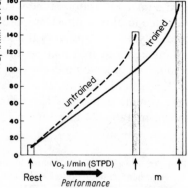

Fig. 141a. Comparative schematic presentation of respiratory time-volume of an untrained and an endurance-trained person during and after equal power.

Fig. 141b. Comparative representation of respiratory time-volume in trained and untrained individuals (after *Mathews* and *Fox*).

Through training (middle-distance running and endurance training), maximal respiratory time-volume can be considerably increased. At equal athletic performances (e.g., 3000-meter run in 12 minutes) the respiratory time-volume of the trained runner is lower (Figs. 140 and 141a and b). At equal ergometric power, the respiratory time-volume in trained individuals is only slightly lower. The differences become greater, however, at higher power (according to Kirchhoff, Reindell and Gebauer). This reveals economy of breathing during exertion on the part of the trained individual.

At equal powers, the respiratory time-volume depends on the kind of biological performance and the respective degree of efficiency. Thus, the average respiratory time-volume in 36 males aged 20 to 40 at a power of 100 watts amounted to 37.6 liters (100%) in hand cranking while standing, 31.2 liters (83%) in pedaling while seated and 33.5 liters (89%) while reclining. At maximal ergometric exercise while reclining, 10 subjects were able to attain only 88.5% of the maximal respiratory time-volume attained at hand cranking while standing (100%), and only 97% at pedaling while seated, according to Galle and Mellerowicz.

Slight temperature differences in the examination room apparently have no effect worth mentioning on the respiratory time-volume during ergometric performance. On the other hand, very high and very low temperatures may have a greater effect, though this is not yet known.

As the barometric pressure falls, respiratory time-volume at equal physical and biological performances decreases in regular relationship to the magnitude of the partial O_2 pressure.

5. Respiratory Time-Volumes During Performance in Pathologic Conditions

While at rest and during submaximal power production, respiratory time-volume can, in the presence of various forms of cardiac, respiratory and hematogenic insufficiency, be greater with less utilization of O_2 than in healthy individuals (Fig. 142). An increase in respiratory time-volume during and after submaximal performance is found in cases of:

1. Disturbances of pulmonary diffusion in pneumocyanosis, pulmonary fibrosis, Boeck's disease, pneumonia, tubercular processes, pulmonary sclerosis, etc.
2. Increase in residual air and expiratory reserve volume in, for example, emphysema, increase in functional dead air space, extensive pulmonary cysts and after embolisms

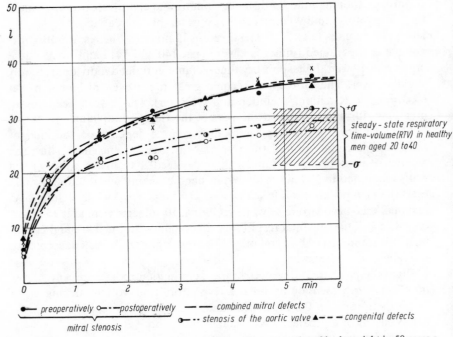

Fig. 142. Respiratory time-volume during exercise of 1 watt per kg of body weight in 50 cases with congenital and acquired heart defects (after *Schmutzler* and *Mellerowicz*).

3. Central disturbances in respiratory regulation as a result of neoplasms, vascular conditions, inflammation in the neighborhood of the respiratory centers
4. Insufficiency of cardiac performance in left-heart insufficiency and pulmonary edema and in hyperventilation resulting from right-heart insufficiency
5. Partial bypassing of the pulmonary circulation in congenital right-left shunt, arteriovenous aneurysms and anastomosis of the minor circulation and in vascular short circuit of nonparticipating parts of the lungs
6. Reduction of partial O_2 pressure in inspired air when breathing O_2-poor air.

When O_2-undersaturation of the blood and spirographic O_2 deficits occur (in disturbances of pulmonary diffusion, left-side cardiac insufficiency, lack of O_2, and extremely heavy exertion in healthy individuals), the respiratory time-volume is regulatively increased. The O_2-saturation deficit of the blood can be made up by breathing O_2 and a reduction of excessive respiratory time-volume can thus be effected (Chapter IX). A lesser reduction in respi-

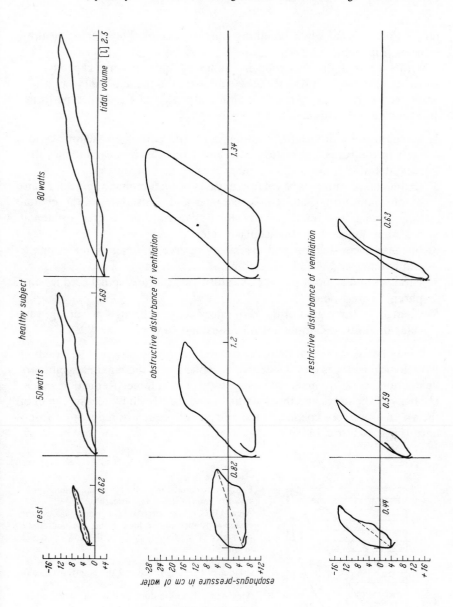

Fig. 143. Pressure-volume diagrams from a healthy subject, a patient with obstructive disturbance of ventilation and a patient with restrictive disturbance of ventilation at rest and during exercise (after *Zeilhofer* and *Rupprecht*).

ratory time-volume when breathing pure O_2 occurs, however, in healthy subjects (Fig. 145).

With even a slight restriction in pulmonary performance capacity, the maximal voluntary ventilation value is lowered and the maximal respiratory time-volume (respiratory minute-volume at maximal endurance performance) is reduced. This can be caused by:

1. Mechanical hindrance to breathing in pleural pathology, stenotic conditions in the bronchial system (e.g., goiter or bronchial carcinoma), thoracic deformity, abdominal tumor, obesity, meteorisms, etc.
2. Reduction of pulmonary volume in cases of pneumonia, tubercular conditions, lung tumor, atelectasis, exudates and transudates of the pleura, lung edema, pneumothorax, postoperative conditions after segmental resection, lobectomy, thoracoplasty, etc.
3. Increase in residual air and expiratory reserve volume, in, for example, emphysema and stenotic breathing.
4. Paralysis and atrophy of the respiratory musculature, spinal cord lesions, phrenic paresis, etc.
5. Changes in the region of the respiratory centers through poisoning, vascular diseases, inflammation processes and tumors.

It may be assumed that there are interrelationships between the extent of pathological changes and the degree of reduction in the maximal voluntary ventilation value or maximal respiratory time-volume. Reduction in the elasticity of the lungs and thorax, which can be detected by measurement of the volume-pressure coefficient (compliance), frequently reduces performance (Figs. 143 and 144).

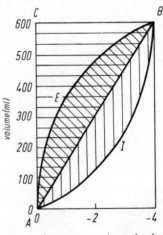

esophagus-pressure in cm of water

Fig. 144. Schematic presentation of the volume-pressure diagram of drawing a breath:
Area AIBC Total exercise performed against the elastic resistance of the lung tissue, the non-elastic resistance of the lung tissue, and the flow-resistance of the air passages.
Area AIB Exercise done against the non-elastic resistance of the lung tissue and the flow-resistance in the air passages during inspiration.
Area ABC Exercise done against the elastic resistance of the lung tissue during inspiration.
Area BEA Exercise done against the non-elastic resistance of the lung tissue and the flow resistance in the air passages during expiration (expiration requires no active exercise, but occurs passively through elastic retraction of the expanded lungs).
From: Documenta Geigy, Wissenschaftliche Tabellen, 7th ed., by permission from Ciba-Geigy AG, Basel, Switzerland.

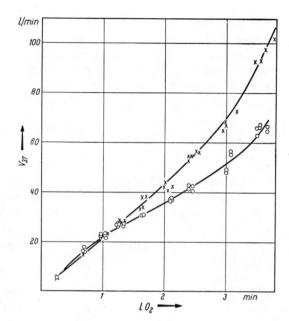

Fig. 145. Respiratory time-volume in breathing normal air and pure O$_2$ (BTPS) (after *Asmussen* and *Nielsen*).
X—X breathing air.
O—O breathing 100% O$_2$

6. The Evaluation of Respiratory Time-Volume in Ergometric Performance

Respiratory time-volume is usually altered by psychic factors at the start of an examination with an open or closed system while at rest. Often there is hyperventilation, less frequently hypoventilation. Respiratory quotients above 0.9 indicate hyperventilation; low RQs of about 0.7 point to hypoventilation. As a rule, not until after several minutes of breathing while at rest does normal respiratory time-volume set in, with a respiratory quotient and a respiratory equivalent within the normal range of variation. This period of adjustment can be shortened by calming the patient, suggesting that he not breathe self-consciously and, insofar as possible, that he not think at all.

During the exercise, the comparison between the measured respiratory time-volumes and the respiratory equivalent on the one hand and their averages and physiological range of variation on the other provides information as to whether there is a pathological change in ventilation and how extensive it is.

A reduction far exceeding the ordinary in respiratory time-volume while breathing pure O$_2$ indicates an arterial undersaturation of the blood.

At increasing power levels, the respiratory time-volume at first increases in almost linear proportion to the exertion. Upon exceeding the maximal steady-state power, respiratory time-volume climbs more steeply with falling O_2 utilization, accompanied by an increase in respiration rate and decrease in respiratory volume.

6.1 Respiratory Volume at Maximal Physical Endurance

At maximal physical exercise, the subject does not breathe with his total vital capacity but with only about 50 to 60% of vital capacity (Fig. 138). A somewhat greater range of variation of maximal volume ventilation in relation to vital capacity was revealed in male subjects aged 6 to 91 in studies by Robinson (Table 25). The relative figures for maximal voluntary ventilation compared to vital capacity are reduced by obstructive disturbances in ventilation but not by restrictive disturbances.

Vital capacity is the quantity of air (BTPS) that can be expired with the greatest effort after maximal inspiration (see Fig. 130, after Comroe). Even after maximal expiration, a residual volume remains in the lungs. To measure vital capacity, spirometers, gasometers and spirographs with faultless calibration should be employed.

Among the numerous data for calculation of the ideal vital capacity, those of Anthony seem to be the soundest and the most useful for practical purposes:

$$\text{vital capacity} = \text{basal metabolism in cal}/24 \text{ hrs} \times 2.3 \; \male$$
$$\text{vital capacity} = \text{basal metabolism in cal}/24 \text{ hrs} \times 2.1 \; \female$$

Table 25. Respiratory volume at maximal exercise (on treadmill) and its relation to vital capacity on the part of male subjects aged 6 to 91 (after *Robinson*).

Group	No.	Age Avg.	Age Extremes	Wt. in kg Avg.	Wt. in kg Extremes	max. volunt. ventilation (lit) Avg.	max. volunt. ventilation (lit) Extremes	max. volunt. vent. 100 / vital capacity Avg.	max. volunt. vent. 100 / vital capacity Extremes
I	8	6.0	5.7– 6.6	20.2	17.6–27.0	0.54	0.41–0.68	45.5	34–69
II	10	10.5	8.2–12.6	29.5	35.3–39.1	0.92	0.73–1.12	43.5	31–52
III	11	14.1	13 –15	55.8	41.7–67.4	1.88	1.48–2.34	52.0	40–63
IV	12	17.4	16 –19	68.4	55.1–88.0	2.66	2.27–2.91	55.8	52–69
V	11	24.5	20 –29	72.5	61.2–84.4	2.93	1.86–4.13	56.0	44–77
VI	10	35.1	32 –38	79.4	60.7–93.5	2.88	2.33–3.59	59.4	55–69
VII	10	44.6	41 –48	74.7	63.5–81.2	2.53	1.71–3.	56.3	45–68
VIII	9	51.8	48 –57	70.6	62.2–81.6	2.34	2.02–2.45	53.0	42–69
IX	8	63.0	59 –71	67.5	54.3–79.	2.33	1.89–2.82	59.6	55–72
X	3	75.0	73 –76	67.5	61.2–75.6	1.64	1.40–1.93	50.8	43–58
XI	1	91.0		66.4					

Table 26. Basal metabolism (Harris-Benedict standard) for determination of the normal (total) number of calories per hour (after Roth, P., Metabolic Compendium, 1924). The table is based on the following equation: Men: $W = 66.474 + 13.751 \, G + 5.0033 \, H - 6.7550 \, A$; Women: $W = 65.50955 + 9.5634 \, G + 1.8496 \, H - 4.6756 \, A$, ($W$ = total calories in 24 hours, G = weight in kg, H = height in cm, A = age in years). The normal number of calories per hour is obtained by adding the figures from Chart 1 to the corresponding figures from Chart 2. Uneven weights in Chart 1 must be interpolated.

Chart 1. Calories by weight according to Genscht.

Weight in kg	Total calories per hr Men	Women	Weight in kg	Total calories per hr Men	Women
10	8.5	—	72	44.0	56.0
12	9.7	—	74	45.2	56.8
14	10.8	—	76	46.3	57.6
16	12.0	—	78	47.5	58.4
18	13.1	—	80	48.6	59.2
20	14.3	—	82	49.7	60.0
22	15.4	—	84	50.9	60.8
24	16.6	—	86	52.0	61.6
26	17.7	37.6	88	53.2	62.4
28	18.8	38.4	90	54.3	63.2
30	19.9	39.2	92	55.5	64.0
32	21.1	40.0	94	56.6	64.8
34	22.2	40.8	96	57.8	65.6
36	23.4	41.6	98	58.9	66.4
38	24.5	42.4	100	60.1	67.2
40	25.7	43.2	102	61.2	68.0
42	26.8	44.0	104	62.4	68.8
44	28.0	44.8	106	63.5	69.6
46	29.1	45.6	108	64.7	70.4
48	30.3	46.4	110	65.8	71.2
50	31.4	47.2	112	67.0	72.0
52	32.6	48.0	114	68.1	72.8
54	33.7	48.8	116	69.3	73.6
56	34.9	49.6	118	70.4	74.4
58	36.0	50.4	120	71.6	75.2
60	37.2	51.2	122	72.7	76.0
62	38.3	52.0	124	73.9	76.8
64	39.5	52.8	126	75.0	77.6
66	40.6	53.6	128	76.1	78.4
68	41.8	54.4	130	77.2	79.2
70	42.9	55.2			

These statements are based on the relationships of vital capacity to weight, stature, age and sex. Basal metabolism according to the tables of Norris and Benedict (Table 26) is thus only a mathematical figure, without direct causal relationship to vital capacity. In cases of severe obesity it seems advisable to use the standard weight and/or the approximate ideal weight (see the Geigy tables of 1955) in the calculation. According to Anthony, it is necessary to reckon with a range of distribution of ±25% of the norm.

Chart 2. Calories by age and height.

Men

Centi-meters	20	25	30	35	40	Age 45	50	55	60	65	70
150	25.6	24.2	22.8	21.4	20.0	18.6	17.2	15.8	14.4	13.0	11.6
155	26.6	25.5	23.8	22.4	21.0	19.6	18.2	16.8	15.4	14.0	12.6
160	27.7	26.3	24.9	23.6	22.1	20.7	18.3	17.9	16.5	15.1	13.7
165	28.7	27.3	25.9	24.5	23.1	21.7	20.3	18.9	17.5	16.1	14.7
170	29.8	28.4	27.0	25.6	24.2	22.8	21.4	20.0	18.6	17.2	15.8
175	30.8	29.4	28.0	26.6	25.2	23.8	22.4	21.0	19.6	18.2	16.8
180	31.9	30.4	29.1	27.6	26.2	24.8	23.4	22.0	20.6	19.2	17.8
185	32.9	31.5	30.1	28.7	27.3	25.9	24.6	23.1	21.7	20.3	18.9
190	34.0	32.5	31.2	29.7	28.3	26.9	25.5	24.1	22.7	21.3	19.9
195	35.0	33.6	32.2	30.8	29.4	28.0	26.6	25.2	23.8	22.4	21.0
200	36.1	34.6	33.2	31.8	30.4	29.0	27.6	26.2	24.8	23.4	22.0

Women

Centi-meters	20	25	30	35	40	45	50	55	60	65	70
150	7.7	6.7	5.7	4.7	3.8	2.8	1.8	0.9	0.0	−1.0	−2.0
155	8.1	7.1	6.1	5.1	4.2	3.2	2.2	1.2	0.2	−0.7	−1.7
160	8.5	7.5	6.5	5.5	4.5	3.6	2.6	1.6	0.6	−0.4	−1.3
165	8.8	7.8	6.9	5.9	4.9	4.0	3.0	2.0	1.0	1.0	−0.9
170	9.2	8.2	7.3	6.3	5.3	4.3	3.4	2.4	1.4	0.5	−0.5
175	9.6	8.6	7.6	6.7	5.7	4.7	3.7	2.8	1.8	0.8	−0.2
180	10.0	9.0	8.0	7.0	6.1	5.1	4.1	3.3	2.2	1.2	0.2
185	10.3	9.4	8.4	7.5	6.5	5.5	4.5	3.5	2.6	1.6	0.6
190	10.8	9.8	8.8	7.8	6.8	5.9	4.9	3.9	3.0	2.0	1.0
195	11.2	10.2	9.2	8.2	7.2	6.2	5.3	4.3	3.3	2.4	1.4
200	11.5	10.5	9.6	8.6	7.6	6.7	5.7	4.7	3.7	2.7	1.8

Table 27 gives a survey of vital capacity of healthy children. A good practical rule of thumb that agrees well with statistical data is a predicted vital capacity of:

about 50 to 70 ml/kg of body weight (for healthy men of average age)
about 40 to 60 ml/kg of body weight (for healthy women of average age).

Vital capacity is reduced by pathological conditions leading to reduction in pulmonary volume, an increase in residual air and paralysis of the respiratory musculature (Chapter X, 5). The vital capacity may thus be hampered restrictively in cases of mechanical impedance to expansion of the lungs and thorax; for example, through adhesions of the pleura, thoracic deformity, cirrhotic conditions in the lungs, etc. In cases of obstructive disturbances of ventilation resulting from increased resistance to air flow in the bronchial system (for example, stenotic conditions, bronchial asthma, bronchitis, etc.), the vital capacity is usually not reduced.

On the other hand, in these cases of obstructive disturbance, the one second forced expiratory volume (the maximal volume of air expired in one second from the maximal inhalation position) is reduced in relation to vital

Table 27. Vital capacity in healthy children (after *Stewart*).

Age in years	Boys Number	Avg. ht. in cm	Vital capacity in cm³ Average	Σ	Range	Age in years	Girls Number	Avg. ht. in cm	Vital capacity in cm³ Average	Σ	Range
4	6	103.4	792	—	500– 900	4	9	95.4	664	—	350– 850
5	20	106.8	927	—	600–1150	5	26	106.4	888	—	600–1200
6	62	112.2	1154	182	800–1600	6	62	111.5	1085	163	700–1600
7	112	116.9	1290	194	900–2200	7	81	114.4	1228	181	900–1800
8	98	121.8	1468	220	1050–2100	8	76	121.0	1401	199	800–1950
9	110	129.9	1715	246	1200–2300	9	73	127.0	1513	229	1000–2250
10	87	133.4	1872	262	1400–2650	10	117	132.1	1672	273	900–2400
11	113	137.8	1991	270	1300–2800	11	119	135.9	1799	241	1250–2550
12	114	142.4	2182	340	1300–3300	12	135	144.0	2053	343	1400–2900
13	132	148.7	2458	430	1700–4000	13	162	151.4	2349	409	1550–3600
14	177	154.8	2712	484	1400–4300	14	192	156.6	2607	361	1900–3800
15	155	159.9	3145	551	1850–4400	15	131	157.8	2702	413	1900–3700
16	67	167.2	3425	573	2100–4300	16	29	160.1	2778	—	2050–3500
17	23	171.4	3776	—	2400–4500	17	7	162.6	2943	—	2250–3400

capacity. About 70% of vital capacity may, according to Tiffeneau, Hirdes and van Veen, be taken as the lower borderline of normality. In restrictive disturbance to ventilation, not the relative but only the absolute second-capacity is found to be reduced.

6.2 Respiratory Time-Volume During Maximal Physical Endurance Performance and the Maximal Voluntary Ventilation

At maximal physical endurance performance, the subject breathes not with maximal voluntary ventilation (MVV), that is, the maximal possible respiratory time-volume in voluntary hyperventilation, but at only about 60 to 70% of the MVV (Fig. 137). More precise statistically based figures on the relationship for various age and sex groups and for pathological conditions of the cardiopulmonary system are not yet available. Even at maximal endurance performance, there is still theoretically a considerable respiratory reserve of about 30 to 40%. It is, however, in practice just as impossible to utilize it fully as it is to equal in a 10,000-meter race the top speed of a 100-meter dash.

In measuring the MVV, the patient is required to breathe as rapidly and as deeply as possible during a period of six to ten seconds while standing. The really top MVV can not be achieved with too-deep and too-rapid breathing. In these cases, the respiratory volume must be corrected to about 50% of vital capacity and respiration rate to about 60 per minute. According to studies by Heine, Benesch and Hertz, the highest values for respiratory time-volume are achieved at a respiratory volume of about 40 to 60% of vital capacity and a respiration rate of about 60 to 70 per minute.

To measure the MVV, spirograph systems, pneumotachographs and open systems with gasometers, all being as free of sluggishness of operation as possible, can be used. The precision of calibration must be checked even under the ventilation conditions of the determination of the respiratory borderline value with rapidly changing respiratory time-volumes. The cross section of mouthpieces must be at least as great as that of the trachea (1.5 to 2.7 cm in diameter, according to Kopsch). The resistance to breathing resulting from spring pressure must be kept as small as possible in order to limit methodological deviations to a minimum. In repeated determinations of the MVV, standard deviations of about ±5 to 10 liters were found (Larmi; Needham et al.). The accurate reproducibility of the MVV therefore assumes a ready will on the part of the patient.

Ideal values for the MVV are given by various authors:

Bartels, Bücherl, Hertz, Rodewald, Schwab: predicted VC × 33
Matheson, Spies, Gray, Barnum: predicted VC × 32.8
Rossier, Bühlmann, Wiesinger: predicted VC × 40;

"VC" standing of course for "vital capacity."

Starting with predicted vital capacity and second-capacity, Bartels et al. give the following empirically obtained tables (Tables 28 and 29) for calculating the predicted MVV. In the case of the figures calculated for the MVV from the predicted vital capacity, age and sex are also taken into consideration when starting out from Anthony's and Harris-Benedict's data (page 223). According to Bartels et al., deviations of less than 30% can not be regarded as pathological. The maximal voluntary ventilation is reduced both by restrictive and obstructive disturbances to ventilation. On the other

Table 28. For calculation of the predicted maximal voluntary ventilation at various respiratory rates.

Respiratory rate	K
30	24
35	26
40	28
50	30
60	32
70 to 100	33

K = factor by which the predicted vital capacity is to be multiplied.

Table 29. For calculation of the maximal voluntary ventilation from the second-capacity.

Respiratory rate:	K^1
60 to 120	40
50	37
40	35
35	32
30	33

K^1 = factor by which the absolute second-capacity is to be multiplied to obtain the maximal voluntary ventilation at the selected respiratory rate.

hand, vital capacity need not be reduced in obstructive cases, although the relative volume of air expired in one second is substantially decreased. In restrictive ventilation pathology, the absolute volume of expired air is decreased. However, the relative second-capacity is considerably reduced, while with restrictive interference with ventilation the absolute second-capacity is limited.

References

Anthony, A. J.: Dtsch. arch. klin. Med. 167, (1930) 120.

Asmussen, E. and M. Nielsen: Acta physiol. Scand. 27, (1952) 217; 35, (1955) 73.

Åstrand, P. O.: Experimental studies of physical working capacity in relation to sex and age. Kopenhagen: Munksgaard 1952.

Åstrand, P. O. and K. Rodahl: Textbook of Work Physiology. McGraw-Hill Comp. New York 1977.

Bartels, H., E. Bücherl, C. E. Hertz, G. Rodewald and M. Schwab: Lungenfunktionsprüfungen (Methoden und Beispiele klinischer Anwendung). S. 72 and 79, Berlin-Göttingen-Heidelberg: Springer, 1959.

Böhlau, V. and J. Nöcker: Sport als Mittel der Gesunderhaltung. Theorie and Praxis der Körperkultur 1956, Proceedings of Conferences of the Arbeitsgemeinschaft für Sportmedizin d. DDR, held 10.–12. Nov. 1955 in Weimar.

Bühlmann, A.: Schweiz. Zschr. Sportmed. 7, (1959) 128.

Cara, M.: Poumon 8, (1953) 371.

Christensen, E. H.: Arbeitsphysiologie 5, (1932) 463.

Comroe, J. H.: Fed. Proc. 9, (1950) 602.

Dransfeld, B. and H. Mellerowicz: Zschr. Kreisl.forschg. 48, (1959) 901.

Dressler, F. and H. Mellerowicz: Zschr. Kinderhk. 85, (1961) 31.

Fleisch, A.: Neue Methoden zum Studium des Gasaustausches und der Lungenfunktion. Leipzig: Thieme, 1956.

Galle, L. and H. Mellerowicz: Der Sportarzt 10, (1962) 332.

Harris-Benedict, after P. Roth: Metabolimetric Compendium 1924 (taken from the Geigy-Tabellen 1955).

Heine, F., W. Benesch and C. W. Hertz: Zschr. Tbk., Leipzig 102, (1953) 273.

Heymans, C., after Rein-Schneider: Einführung i. d. Psycholog. d. Menschen. Springer: Berlin-Göttingen-Heidelberg: 1956.

Hirdes, J. J. and G. van Veen: Acta tbc. Scand. 26, (1952) 264.

Hollmann, W., W. Barg, G. Weyer and H. Heck: Med. Welt 21, (1970) 1288.

Hollmann, W. and H. Heck: Ärztl. Fortbildg. 1, (1971) 62.

Hollmann, W. and Th. Hettinger: Zentrale Themen der Sportmedizin. Springer: Heidelberg, New York 1977.

Hollmann, W.: Der Arbeits- und Trainingseinfluß auf Kreislauf und Atmung. Darmstadt: Steinkopff, 1959.

Hollmann, W., H. Venrath and H. Valentin: Zschr. Altersforsch. 13, (1959) 60.

Joss, E.: Helvet. med. acta 24, (1959) 26.

Kirchhoff, H. W., H. Reindell and A. Gebauer: Dtsch. Arch. klin. Med. 203, (1956) 432.

Knipping, H. W., W. Bolt, H. Venrath and H. Valentin: Untersuchung und Beurteilung des Herzkranken. Stuttgart: Enke, 1955.

Larmi, T.: Scand. J. Clin. Laborat. Invest. 6, (1954) 12.

Liesen, H. and W. Hollmann: in Zentrale Themen der Sportmedizin. Springer: Heidelberg, New York 1977.

Matheson, H. W., S. N. Spies, J. S. Gray and D. R. Barnum: J. Clin. Invest. 29, (1950) 682.

Mathews, D. K. and E. L. Fox: The Physiological Basis of Physical Education and Athletics. W. B. Saunders Company, Philadelphia 1976.

Mellerowicz, H. and P. Nowacki: Zschr. Kreisl.forschg. 50, (1961) 1002.

Needham, C., M. Rogan and J. McDonald: Thorax 9, (1954) 313.

Rauber-Kopsch, F.: Lehrbuch und Atlas der

Anatomie des Menschen. Leipzig: Thieme, 1922.

Rein, H. and M. Schneider: Einführung in die Physiologie des Menschen. Berlin-Göttingen-Heidelberg: Springer, 1956.

Reindell, H. and H. W. Kirchhoff: Deutsche medizinische Wochenschrift 81, (1956) 592.

Reindell, H. and H. Roskamm: Schweiz. Zschr. Sportmed. 7, (1959) 1.

Robinson, S.: Arbeitsphysiologie 10, (1939) 251.

Rossier, P. H., A. Bühlmann and K. Wiesinger: Physiologie und Pathophysiologie der Atmung. Berlin-Göttingen-Heidelberg: Springer, 1956.

Schmutzler, H., H. Mellerowicz and E. Carl: Zschr. Kreisl.forschg. 49, (1960) 445.

Stegemann, J. and K. W. Heinrich: Studien über den respiratorischen Totraum bei körperlicher Arbeit und bei künstlicher Beatmung. Westdeutscher Verlag, Köln 1967.

Stewart, C. A.: Amer. J. Dis. Child. 24, (1922) 451.

Tiffeneau, R. and A. Pinelli: Paris méd. 37, (1947) 624.

Wolff, H. S.: "IMP" published in England, in agreement with the National Research Development Corporation by J. Langham Thompson Ltd. Bushey Heath-Herts-England.

Zeilhofer, R. and E. Rupprecht: Klin. Wschr. 39, (1961) 184.

XI. The Ventilatory Equivalent in Ergometric Performance

by Paul Nowacki

1. Significance and Calculation of the Ventilatory Equivalent

The concept "ventilatory equivalent," introduced into clinical functional diagnostics by Brauer and Knipping, has gradually replaced other expressions such as "specific ventilation," "respiratory equivalent," etc.

The ventilatory equivalent (hereinafter abbreviated VEO_2) tells how many cubic centimeters of air have to be ventilated in order for 1 cubic centimeter of O_2 to be absorbed. It is calculated from the following formula:

$$\text{ventilatory equivalent} = \frac{\text{respiratory time-volume cm}^3 \text{ (BTPS)}}{O_2 \text{ consumption cm}^3/\text{min (STPD)}}$$

$$VEO_2 \text{ L/min} = \frac{\dot{V}E \text{ cm}^3 \text{ (BTPS)}}{\dot{V}_{O_2} \text{ cm}^3 \text{ (STPD)}}.$$

In its original formulation by Brauer and Knipping, the formula contained one additional factor, either the factor 100 in the numerator or the factor 10 in the denominator. The value thus obtained told how many liters of air must be ventilated in order for 100 cubic centimeters of O_2 to be absorbed. The suggestion that the additional arbitrary factors be eliminated was made in 1943 by Rossier and Méan and led to the present relation of the ventilation to 1 cubic centimeter of O_2. However, there is also something arbitrary about this newer formula, namely, the conversion of the two factors to two different sets of conditions in the one formula. The respiratory time-volume is converted to BTPS (body temperature pressure saturated), that is, to 37°C, 760 mm Hg and water vapor saturation at 37°C, while the O_2 consumption is converted to STPD (standard temperature pressure dry), that is, to 0°C, 760 mm Hg and dry. This decision was arrived at on October 15, 1955, by the commission of experts of the Montan Union. It would make better sense to calculate the O_2 consumption on the basis of the BTPS also. Hertz pointed this out as early as the 62nd session of the Gesellschaft für Innere Medizine in 1956.

Another relationship between ventilation and O_2 consumption was published in 1928 by Herbst. He calculated his "coefficient of O_2 utilization" according to the following relationship:

$$O_2 \text{ utilization} = \frac{O_2 \text{ consumption in cm}^3/\text{min}}{\text{respiratory time-volume in liters}}.$$

This quotient tells how many cubic centimeters of O_2 are absorbed from 1 liter of air. If we represent both quotients, VEO_2 and coefficient of O_2 utilization graphically, we see that they stand in a reciprocal relation to each other (Fig. 150). In the course of time, however, the concept of the VEO_2 has gained more and more ground.

The VEO_2 affords insight into the economy of respiration. The lower the figure, that is, the less air needed for the inspiration of 1 cubic centimeter of O_2, the more economic the respiration. The magnitude of the VEO_2 is dependent on constitutional factors, especially morphological condition of the respiratory system, age, sex, and especially the economy of ventilation. Data for this parameter with the subject at rest as found by various authors are collected in Table 30.

Of special interest is the respiratory economy during an ergometric performance, especially a work or sports event. As is shown in the following paragraphs, conclusions are possible concerning cardiopulmonary performance in the human body from the behavior of the ventilatory equivalent.

If we consider only O_2 consumption during a submaximal performance, significant differences between normal individuals and patients with heart

Table 30. Ventilatory equivalent while at rest, according to various authors.

Authors	VEO_2	Distribution
Anthony (1930)	29.0	23.0 – 37.0
Knipping and *Moncrieff* (1932)	24.4	16.8 – 37.0
Hurtado and *Boller* (1933)	26.6	s = 7.3
Kaltreider and *MacCann* (1937)	24.0	18.3 – 39.8
MacMichael (1939)	24.9	s = 4.0
Mattheson and *Gray* (1950)	25.1	s = 3.0
Comroe (1951)	23.0	22.0 – 25.0
Haab and *Fleisch* (1956)	24.4	s = 2.0
Mellerowicz and *Nowacki* (1961)		
standing	27.0	s = 2.3
sitting	27.0	s = 2.4
reclining	26.0	s = 2.0

and lung disease can hardly be detected. On the other hand, the VEO$_2$, in conjunction with the nature and magnitude of the damage, usually shows changes even in submaximal performance stages.

2. The Physiological Ventilatory Equivalent During and After Ergometric Exercise

The ventilatory equivalent at first falls to a minimum as submaximal performance increases (Figs. 146, 149, 150, 197, and 198).

The decline is dependent on the state of training of the cardiopulmonary system. Especially in individuals trained for endurance, a drop to a VEO$_2$ of 17 to 20 is noticeable in the first minutes of the work load.

A high ventilation economy at exhausting ergometer performance was shown by professional soccer players at the peak of their soccer training. Thus, the participants in the 1974 World Cup soccer championship in West Germany were able to maintain a VEO$_2$ of 20 to 23 even at performances of 4 watts per kg of body weight (Fig. 147).

Respiratory time-volume begins to increase relatively more than O$_2$ consumption at a performance intensity that varies with the individual. The rise

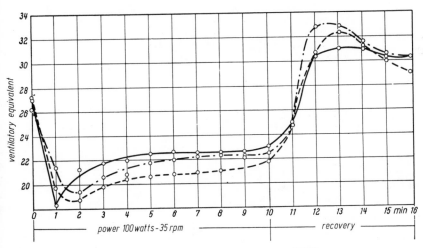

Fig. 146. The behavior of the average ventilatory equivalent $\frac{BTPS}{STPD}$ in comparative studies on hand cranking while standing and pedaling while seated at equal physical power (100 watts) during ten minutes of work and six minutes recovery in 36 untrained male subjects aged 20 to 40, ———— standing, — — — seated, —·—·— reclining (after *Mellerowicz* and *Nowacki*).

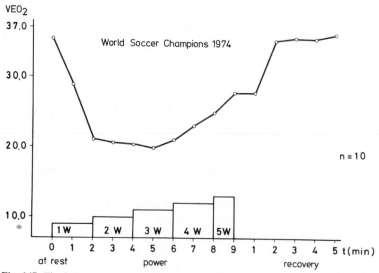

Fig. 147. The behavior of the average ventilatory equivalent of the participants in the world championship in soccer in 1974 (West German team, 10 individuals, all professional athletes) at exhausting physical exercise on the bicycle ergometer while seated (after *Nowacki*).

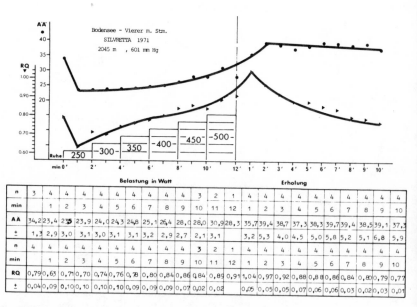

Fig. 148. The behavior of the average ventilatory equivalent and the ventilation respiratory quotient during exhausting pedaling while seated in increasing power levels in high-performance oarsmen at an altitude of 2045 meters (after *Nowacki*).

in VEO_2 is an indicator of a fall in respiratory economy. For absorption of equal amounts of O_2, greater volumes of air become necessary. This rise in the VEO_2 is a characteristic point in the maximal range of pulmonary and cardiac performance (performance point "A" in Figs. 197 and 198), and characterizes the maximal voluntary ventilation at which there is still optimal respiratory economy. It lies above the maximal pulse endurance performance level and below the maximal O_2 endurance performance level.

At comparable submaximal power stages, the VEO_2 of the trained individual is lower than that of the untrained individual and thus shows better ventilation economy (Fig. 149). The attainment of steady values in the neighborhood of 28 or exceeding the VEO_2 figure of 30 coincides with the point of exhaustion. Respiratory time-volume and maximal O_2 consumption have then attained their individual maximal magnitudes under conditions of performance metabolism. Parallel to this, the anaerobic capacity is completely exhausted, so that the exercise or athletic event must be interrupted (Table 38, Figs. 148 and 153).

Since the respiratory time-volume is, however, also dependent on subjective influences, VEO_2 is not always a reliable guide, especially in consultation of compensation cases at submaximal exercise levels.

Table 31. The functional dead space during exercise and its relation to respiratory volume (after *Rossier, Bühlmann* and *Wiesinger*).

Authors and methods	Cases	VO_2 in cm^3/min	VT in cm^3	VD in cm^3	$\dfrac{VD}{VT}$
Douglas and *Haldane* (1912)	1	2237	447	160	0.35
		1065	1535	320	0.21
		1595	2064	497	0.24
		2005	2524	549	0.22
		2543	3145	622	0.20
Aitken and *Clark-Kennedy* (1928)	1	1420	2371	295	0.12
Fractionated analysis of CO_2 in expired air		2050	3410	378	0.11
Houston and *Rilley* (1947)	2				
Arterial CO_2 tension,	a	272	667	160	0.24
microtonometry		862	1276	281	0.22
	b	297	596	235	0.39
		1538	1706	360	0.21
Rossier and *Bühlmann* (1957)	30	400	570	155	0.27
Arterial P_{CO_2}, pH		800	1050	260	0.25
and *Hasselbalch*-		1200	1400	229	0.23
Henderson formula		1600	1700	370	0.22
		2000	2020	470	0.23

Explanation of Symbols: VO_2 = O_2 consumption per minute during exercise
VT   = respiratory volume of a single breath
VD   = dead space

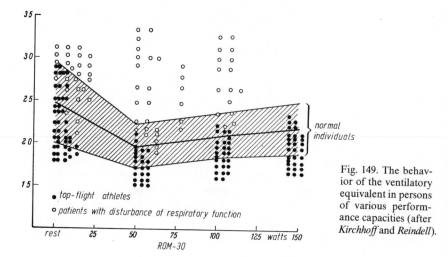

Fig. 149. The behavior of the ventilatory equivalent in persons of various performance capacities (after *Kirchhoff* and *Reindell*).

The magnitude of the respiratory dead space has an important influence on the ratio of respiratory time-volume to O_2 consumption. During exercise, the magnitude of the dead space actually increases absolutely, though its share in the respiratory volume decreases (Table 31).

The behavior of the VEO_2 and its standard deviations at ergometric powers of various kinds and intensities at various age levels is shown in Figs. 146 to 151 and Tables 32 to 35. In children and teenagers aged 6 to 18, according

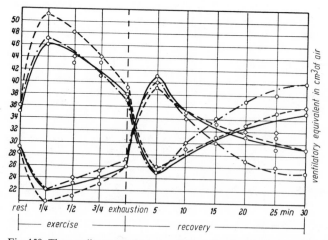

Fig. 150. The ventilatory equivalent and O_2 utilization during exercises increasing step-by-step (two minutes each at 50-watt increments) to the point of exhaustion, and the recovery phase: hand cranking while standing and pedaling while seated and reclining, 10 untrained male subjects aged 20 to 40 (after *Galle* and *Mellerowicz*).

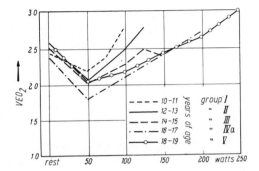

Fig. 151. Averages of the respiratory equivalent on the part of individual age groups (10 to 19) at rest and during exercise (steady-state) (after *König, Reindell, Keul,* and *Roskamm*).

Table 32. Ventilatory equivalent, O_2 consumption and respiratory time-volume ($\dot{V}_E$) in 92 males aged 16 to 70 at ergometric powers of 60 and 120 watts, pedaling while reclining, with Fleisch's metabograph (after *Joss*).

	Age group	Number	$\dot{V}_E$ in liters	O_2 in cm^3	VEO$_2$
At rest	16–25	27	8.8	311	28.4
	26–35	21	10.0	338	29.7
	36–45	17	10.5	335	31.3
	57–70	16	10.6	368	28.8
	56–70	11	11.8	362	32.6
60 watts	20	26	24.3	1050	23.1
	30	20	23.8	1068	22.2
	40	17	26.0	1059	24.4
	50	14	25.6	1043	24.5
	60	11	27.0	1106	24.5
120 watts	20	26	38.3	1764	21.7
	30	20	39.3	1757	22.4
	40	17	46.7	1778	26.2
	50	15	47.7	1803	26.5
	60	11	52.3	1822	28.7

to studies by Dressler and Mellerowicz, there are no significant differences in the behavior of the VEO$_2$ at relatively equal powers of 1 watt per kg of body weight in the several age and weight groups (Table 34). On the other hand, according to Åstrand and König et al., the VEO$_2$ declines at absolutely equal power in teenagers as development progresses (Fig. 151, Table 35). With increasing age, the VEO$_2$ continually increases (Tables 32 and 33). This is especially evident at high levels of performance.

The VEO$_2$ in women has to date not been studied with a sufficiently large number of subjects. However, it may be assumed that the VEO$_2$ in men and women does not differ significantly at submaximal power stages up to about 100 watts with approximately equal O$_2$ consumption and equal respiratory time-volume. This would be especially true of relatively (per kg body weight) equal power stages. However, a greater VEO$_2$ is to be anticipated in women at absolutely equal power stages of above about 100 to 120 watts.

Table 33. Ventilatory equivalent in men aged 40 to 64 at ergometric power of 40, 80, 120 watts pedaling while reclining at 60 rpm with Fleisch's metabograph (after *Aepli*).

Age group	Number	At rest	40 watts	80 watts	120 watts
41–50	28	28.9 ± 3.2	26.6 ± 2.9	27.2 ± 3.5	30.9 ± 5.4
51–55	14	28.9 ± 3.3	25.5 ± 3.7	24.7 ± 3.8	29.1 ± 6.5
56–65	26	28.7 ± 3.8	26.3 ± 2.2	27.1 ± 3.2	31.5 ± 4.5
Galetti					
19–32	—	25.3 ± 3.5	22.0 ± 1.9	22.5 ± 2.1	25.4 ± 2.9

When breathing air with an O_2 content higher than normal (up to pure O_2), the ventilatory equivalent becomes less because of high partial O_2 pressure in the alveoli, and the maximal O_2 consumption increases considerably (Tables 36a and b). With decreasing partial O_2 pressure (hypoxia, training at high altitude) the VEO_2 increases regularly (Tables 37 and 38) because a greater respiratory time-volume of air is required for the consumption of an equal amount of O_2.

Table 34. The ventilatory equivalent in the steady state at a power of 1 watt per kg of body weight in children and teenagers, arranged by age and weight groups (after *Dressler* and *Mellerowicz*).

Weight groups in kg	Boys				Girls			
	n	M	±σ	±ν	n	M	±σ	±ν
22.5–27.4	11	21.2	3.99	18.93	9	23.5	3.58	15.23
27.5–32.4	31	23.3	4.99	21.46	22	30.6	13.55	44.29
32.5–37.4	25	24.8	6.77	27.31	20	30.4	11.64	38.29
37.5–42.4	33	28.9	13.69	47.33	9	31.0	11.19	36.11
42.5–47.4	19	29.0	12.78	44.07	5	30.4	4.51	14.84
47.5–52.4	23	26.3	8.69	33.09	2	27.5		
52.5–57.4	19	30.3	13.99	46.62				
57.5–62.4	10	21.6	5.38	24.92				
62.5–67.4	9	24.5	8.09	33.02				
67.5–72.4	5	25.5	9.63	37.29				
Age groups in years								
7	4	24.7	3.52	14.24				
8	41	22.3	3.75	16.81				
9	20	21.2	3.83	18.07	20	31.3	12.6	38.54
10	18	28.3	11.33	40.00	26	30.6	11.67	38.15
11	20	32.9	3.89	42.23	16	25.3	17.30	28.86
12	12	28.4	10.76	37.84	4	34.1	11.24	32.97
13	31	27.8	12.19	43.81				
14	33	23.9	10.75	45.05				
15	15	23.4	5.22	22.32				
16	8	27.8	6.88	24.72				
17	9	26.3	6.62	24.82				
18	3	19.9	2.59	13.03				

Explanation of symbols: n　= number of subjects studied
M　= average
±σ = average quadratic deviation
±ν = coefficient of variation

Table 35. Averages, standard deviations and coefficients of variation of the ventilatory equivalent while at rest and during steady state work load (after *König, Reindell, Keul* and *Roskamm*).

		Rest	50 W	75 W	100 W	125 W	150 W	200 W	250 W
10–11 years	M	24.9	21.8	23.7	27.7				
I	s	6.1	3.4	3.8	4.8				
	v	24.3%	15.8%	16.4%	17.2%				
	n	49	49	36	12				
12–13 years	M	25.9	20.5	22.6	24.8	27.8			
II	s	2.0	2.4	2.4	2.3	3.2			
	v	8.0%	11.8%	10.9%	9.4%	11.5%			
	n	84	84	83	47	10			
14–15 years	M	25.2	20.1		22.7	24.9	23.7		
III	s	4.8	2.6		1.9	2.9	0.8		
	v	19.2%	13.1%		8.4%	11.6%	37.1%		
	n	47	47		41	18	5		
16–17 years	M	23.9	17.8		20.9		24.0	27.1	
IVa	s	4.9	2.9		1.8		2.9	4.9	
	v	20.6%	16.3%		9.0%		12.0%	18.2%	
	n	19	19		19		15	4	
IVb	M	25.1			20.6		23.2	24.1	
	s	3.7			2.6		3.1	2.2	
	v	15.0%			12.7%		13.7%	9.4%	
	n	19			19		19	7	
18–19 years	M	25.9	20.4		21.7		24.3	26.4	31.6
V	s	4.1	2.0		2.1		2.9	3.1	4.5
	v	15.8%	10.0%		9.6%		12.0%	11.6%	14.4%
	n	53	53		53		53	39	4

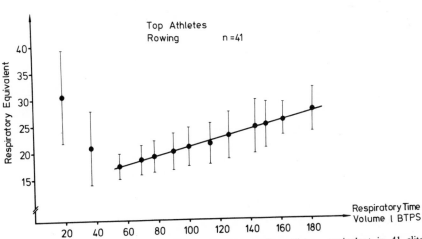

Fig. 152. Correlation between respiratory time-volume and ventilatory equivalent in 41 elite rowers during exhausting ergometric cycling in sitting position with increasing power (the routine power for rowers used by Nowacki starts with 250 watts, increases every two minutes by 50 watts, reaching the exhaustion stage between 450 to 500 watts).

Table 36a. Averages of 30 male subjects aged 20 to 30 under exercise increasing by the minute while breathing O_2 at exercise on a crank ergometer (after *Hollmann*).

Time	Load (watts)	$\dot{V}_{O_2}$ (ml)	3σ (ml)	$\dot{V}_E$ (L.ters)	3σ (Liters)	VEO_2
At rest workload	·/·	320		9.8		25
1 min	30	810	±141	20.0	± 5.7	20
2 min	60	1250	±144	24.1	± 5.3	20
3 min	90	1600	±152	28.2	± 4.9	18
4 min	120	1960	±156	36.3	± 4.9	19
5 min	150	2250	±165	43.5	± 5.7 ·	19
6 min	180	2750	±171	54.3	± 5.9	20
7 min	210	3230	±238	61.6	± 8.2	20
8 min	240	3490	±312	77.9	±11.2	22
9 min	270	3800	±334	86.7	±12.9	23
10 min	300	4140	±358	98.0	±13.7	24

Table 36b. Averages of the same subjects while breathing air.

Time	Load (watts)	$\dot{V}_{O_2}$ (ml)	3σ (ml)	$\dot{V}_E$ (Liters)	3σ (Liters)	VEO_2
At rest workload	·/·	330		9.1		23
1 min	30	880	±139	21.6	± 5.9	27
2 min	60	1340	±146	27.5	± 5.7	20
3 min	90	1640	±152	32.4	± 6.0	20
4 min	120	1920	±170	41.3	± 7.7	22
5 min	150	2370	±198	51.4	±10.5	22
6 min	180	2490	±203	65.2	±10.1	23
7 min	210	2720	±225	73.2	±10.3	24
8 min	240	3080	±310	81.0	±12.8	25
9 min	270	3470	±348	92.4	±13.5	26

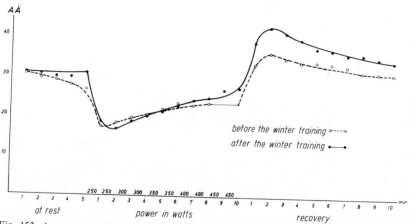

Fig. 153. Average ventilatory equivalent of 7 oarsmen at a maximal spiroergometry while seated, in mounting wattage stages, before and after an intensive winter training period (*Nowacki, Küchlin* and *Lütjohann*).

Between the respiratory time-volume (BTPS) and the ventilatory equivalent there is a highly significant correlation of 0.998 in top-flight athletes during exhausting ergometric exercise in increasing wattage stages. This correlation, represented in Fig. 152, is indicated by the decline in ventilatory equivalent figures until the second minute of the exercise. After that both parameters rise, constantly proportional to one another, approximately according to the expression

$$\bar{y} = 0.08224 \cdot \bar{x} + 12.77.$$

There is a further close correlation between CO_2 production and the VEO_2 of 0.985, and also between VEO_2 and respiration rate.

3. Performance Ventilatory Equivalent in Pathological Conditions

The most important causes of change in the ventilatory equivalent are:

1. Disturbances in pulmonary diffusion in cases of pneumoconiosis, pulmonary fibrosis, Boeck's disease, pneumonia, tubercular conditions, lung edema, pulmonary sclerosis, etc.
2. Reduction in the pulmonary diffusion area resulting from pneumonia, atelectasis, pneumothorax, exudates and transudates of the pleura, postoperative conditions after segmental resection, lobectomy, thoracoplasty, etc.
3. Increase in the functional dead space, residual air and expiratory reserve volume in emphysema, bronchiectasis, stenotic breathing, etc.
4. Mechanical restraints on breathing due to pleural adhesions, stenotic conditions of the bronchial tree, deformities of the thorax, etc.
5. Central or peripheral disturbances of respiratory regulation resulting from neoplasms, vascular conditions, inflammation in the region of the respiratory centers, paresis of the phrenic nerve, etc.
6. Cardiovascular causes: hyperventilation in right-heart insufficiency, congenital shunt, vascular shunts in pulmonary circulation, etc.
7. Reduction in the partial O_2 pressure in the inspired air (Tables 37a and b).

In all groups, the ventilatory equivalent is more or less increased depending on the etiology and its severity. An increase in the ventilatory equivalent contrary to the physiological values is often detectable first at lesser, then at greater performance levels. In restrictive disturbances to ventilation,

Table 37a. Ventilatory equivalent (calculated by us) and respiratory time-volume at various altitudes above sea level at equal O_2 consumption of 2 liters (after *Krestownikow*).

Altitude above sea level in meters	Respiratory time-volume in liters	O_2 in liters	VEO_2
0	48	2	24.0
2810	69	2	34.5
3660	83	2	41.5
4700	110	2	55.0

Table 37b. Ventilatory equivalent (calculated by us) and respiratory time-volume during physical exercise at various altitudes above sea level (after *Christensen*).

Altitude (meters)	Barometric pressure in mm Hg.	Work load kgm/min	O_2 (Liters)	Respiratory time-volume for $37°C$ in liters	Ventilatory equivalent VEO_2
0	760	1500	3.72	129.1	34.6
2810	543	1335	3.02	122.9	40.7
3660	489	1335	2.56	108.3	42.2
4700	429	910	2.19	136.0	62.0
5340	400	680	1.80	89.5	49.5

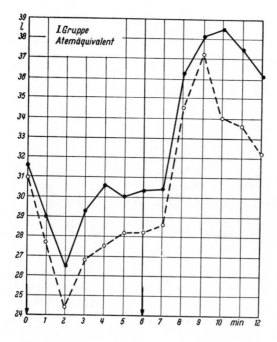

Fig. 154. The ventilatory equivalent of 14 heart surgery patients before and after an average of five weeks of rehabilitative training (interval training) standing at the crank ergometer at a power of 1 watt per kg of body weight (after *Smodlaka, Mellerowicz, Neuhaus, Paeprer* and *Schmutzler*).
—— before training, — — — after training

Table 38. Spiroergometric performance data on a world champion Olympic winning oarsman. during training at high altitude.

Maximale Spiro - Ergometrie im Sitzen (pneumotachographisch)

NAME _Berger_ Geb. _16. 10.49_ Untersuchungstag _4. 8. 71_ Luftdruck: _601 mm Hg_ Umrechnungsfaktoren
VORNAME _Peter_ Größe _196_ cm Ort _Silvretta 2040 m_ Temp.: _22°C_   STPD (0°): _0,6418_
VEREIN _RV Neptun Konstanz_ Gewicht _104_ kg Vitalkapazität: _7000 ml_ rel. Luftfeuchtigk.:   BTPS (37°):

Zeit min	Watt	RR	Hf	%O₂	%CO₂	RQ	AMV (ATPS)	AMV (BTPS)	AMV (STPD)	O₂ ccm	CO₂ ccm	O₂ Puls	AA	Af	AZV (BTPS)	O₂ Schuld	EKG	Bemerk.
0	Ruhe	130/90	60				O₂/kg										o.B.	
0	"	150/90	71	4,8	3,8	0,79	6,4	21,6	13,9	667	528	9,4	32,4	16	1350		o.B.	
1	250		120	7,4	5,0	0,68	20,9	45,6	29,3	2168	1465	18,1	21,0	14	3257		·	
2	250		124	7,4	5,4	0,73	31,3	68,5	44,0	3256	2376	26,3	21,0	19	3605		·	
3	300		134	7,4	5,6	0,76	34,0	74,4	47,8	3537	2677	26,4	21,0	19	3916		·	
4	300		135	7,4	5,9	0,80	36,1	79,2	50,8	3759	2997	27,8	21,1	19	4168		·	
5	350		145	7,4	5,9	0,80	41,6	91,2	58,5	4329	3452	29,9	21,1	20	4560		·	
6	350		148	7,2	5,9	0,82	45,8	103,2	66,2	4766	3906	32,2	21,7	23	4487		·	
7	400		156	7,4	6,0	0,81	48,2	105,6	67,8	5017	4068	32,2	21,1	24	4400		·	
8	400		165	7,0	5,8	0,81	50,8	117,6	75,5	5285	4379	32,0	22,3	26	4523		·	
9	450		168	6,5	5,6	0,86	53,9	134,4	86,3	5610	4833	33,3	24,0	29	4635		·	
10	450		172	6,1	5,3	0,87	57,8	153,6	98,6	6015	5226	35,0	25,5	34	4518		·	
11	500		176	5,6	5,1	0,91	77,6	177,6	114,0	6384	5814	36,3	27,8	40	4440		·	
12	500		180	5,5	5,0	0,91	64,4	189,6	121,7	6694	6085	37,2	28,3	45	4213		·	
13		240/80	160	4,8	5,0	1,04	44,1	148,8	95,5	4584	4775	28,7	32,5	36	3600		·	Erschöpfung
14		235/100	132	4,8	4,5	0,94	25,6	86,4	55,5	2664	2498	20,2	32,4	24	3600		·	
15		245/80	121	4,7	4,2	0,89	20,9	72,0	46,2	2171	1940	17,9	33,2	20	2933		·	
16		195/90	112	5,2	4,3	0,83	17,0	52,8	33,9	1763	1458	15,7	30,0	18	2550		·	
17		175/100	104	5,2	4,3	0,83	13,1	40,8	26,2	1362	1127	13,1	30,0	16	2320		·	
18		155/95	105	5,1	4,1	0,80	10,9	34,8	22,3	1137	914	10,8	30,6	15	2175		·	
19		150/90	103	5,0	4,0	0,80	10,7	34,8	22,3	1115	892	10,8	31,2	16	2280		·	
20		140/95	106	5,2	4,0	0,77	11,0	34,2	22,0	1144	880	10,8	29,9	15	2143		·	
21		145/90	108	5,6	4,2	0,75	10,4	30,0	19,3	1081	811	10,0	27,8	14	1846		·	
22		135/95	103	5,7	4,2	0,75	8,4	24,0	15,4	878	647	8,5	27,3	13				
23																		
24																		
25																		

17.022 l O₂ in 40' Erh.

Geb. = born
Untersuchungstag = date of examination
Luftdruck = barometric pressure
Umrechnungsfaktoren = conversion factors
Vorname = first name
Grösse = height
Ort = Location
Verein = club
Gewicht = weight
Vitalkapazität = vital capacity

rel. Luftfeuchtigkeit = relative humidity
Zeit = time (minutes)
Watt = watts
RR = BP
Hf = HR
RQ = RQ
amv = $\dot{V}_E$
AA = $\dot{V}EO_2$
Af = respiration rate
AZV = MVV

changes in the ventilatory equivalent may be entirely lacking.

Cardiovascular (Fig. 154) and hematogenic changes in the ventilatory equivalent occur in:

1. Right-heart insufficiency (primarily or secondarily cardiac in cor pulmonale) with stasis in circulation, increased pCO_2 and hyperventilation
2. Left-heart insufficiency of various etiologies with stasis in the pulmonary circulation and disturbances of the pulmonary diffusion
3. Congenital shunt with bypassing or overloading of the pulmonary circulation

4. Vascular shunts in the pulmonary circulation, arteriovenous fistulas of various etiology with deficient blood circulation in parts of the lungs
5. Reduced arteriovenous O_2 difference with deficient peripheral capillarity
6. Reduction in O_2 transport capacity of the blood
7. Polycythemia

The nature and extent of the changes determine the more or less considerable increase in ventilation equivalent above the normal borderline values. This excess may be latent with the subject at rest and not become clearly recognizable until there is an increase in ergometric performance.

References

Aepli, R.: Helvet. med. acta 26, (1959) 49.

Anthony, A. J.: Beitr. Klin. Tbk. 70, (1928) 452.

Åstrand, P. O.: Experimental studies of physical working capacity in relation to sex and age. Kopenhagen: Munksgaard, 1952.

Brauer, L. and H. W. Knipping: Beitr. Klin. Tbk. 101, (1949) 424.

Christensen, E. H.: after Krestownikow: Physiologie der Körperübungen. Berlin: Volk u. Gesundheit, 1953.

Dressler, F. and H. Mellerowicz: Zschr. Kinderhk. 85, (1961) 31.

Galle, L. and H. Mellerowicz: Der Sportarzt 10, (1962) 332.

Herbst, R.: Dtsch. Arch. klin. Med. 33, (1928) 129 and 257.

Hertz, C. W.: Verh. Dtsch. Ges. inn. Med. 62, (1956) 135.

Hollmann, W.: Ref. bei der Tagg. der Dtsch. Hochschulsportärzte, Münster 1960.

Joss, E.: Diss. Bern 1958.

Kirchhoff, H. W. and H. Reindell: Verh. 62. Kongr. Dtsch. Ges. inn. Med. 587 (1956).

König, K., H. Reindell, J. Keul and H. Roskamm: Internat. Zschr. angew. Physiol. einschl. Arbeitsphysiologie. 18, (1961) 393.

Krestownikow, A. N.: Physiologie der Körperübungen. Berlin: Volk and Gesundheit, 1953.

Mellerowicz, H. and P. Nowacki: Zschr. Kreisl.forsch. 50, (1961) 1003.

Nowacki, P.: Kassenarzt 13, (1973) 77–94.

Nowacki, P., J. Küchlin and U. Lütjohann: In Press.

Nowacki, P.: Sportmedizinische und leistungsphysiologische Aspekte des Ruderns. In: Adam, K., H. Lenk, P. Nowacki, M. Rulffs and W. Schröder, Rudertraining, Limpert Verlag, Bad Homburg, 251–646, 1977.

Rossier, P. H., A. Bühlmann and K. Wiesinger: Physiologie und Pathophysiologie der Atmung. Berlin-Göttingen-Heidelberg: Springer, 1958.

Rossier, P. H. and H. Méan: Schweiz. med. Wschr. 327 (1943).

Smodlaka, V., H. Mellerowicz, S. Neuhaus, H. Paeprer and H. Schmutzler: Zschr. Kreisl.forsch. 51, (1962) 152.

XII. CO_2 Production and Respiratory Quotient in Ergometric Performance

1. Methods of Measuring CO_2 Production

1.1 Measuring CO_2 in Open Systems

To measure CO_2 in expired air we may use in open systems total volume methods or sampling methods (see page 165).

1.1.1. Chemical Methods of Analysis for CO_2 (see page 167)

The Haldane-Scholander methods are well suited here.

1.1.2 Physical Methods of Analysis for CO_2

These are based on various physical properties of the atmospheric gases, such as differing heat conductivity, differing absorption of light rays and different mass. They take relatively little time and are preferable to the chemical methods for continuous recordings.

a) Analysis based on heat conductivity
The CO_2 content of expired air can be determined physically on the basis of the dependence of the heat conductivity of air on its composition (see page 169).

b) Measuring of CO_2 using the principle of infrared absorption
The procedure was developed in 1943 by Luft at the Badische Anilin- und Sodafabrik. CO_2 absorbs certain ranges of the infrared spectrum, certain absorption bands. This results in a diminution of the intensity of radiation

243

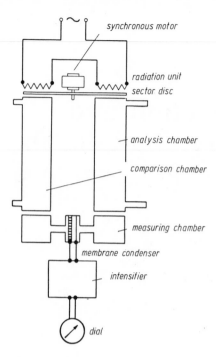

synchronous motor

radiation unit
sector disc

analysis chamber

comparison chamber

measuring chamber

membrane condenser

intensifier

dial

Fig. 155. Schematic diagram of the infrared absorption recorder. For explanation see text (after *Bartels, Bücherl, Hertz, Rodewald* and *Schwab*).

proportional to the concentration of CO$_2$. The heat radiation from two heating wires, wired in series, is sent through an analysis chamber and a comparison chamber. The heat radiation for each chamber is interrupted simultaneously at brief intervals by a sector disc. The expired air being analyzed in the analysis chamber absorbs the radiation more strongly than the gas in the comparison chamber. This results in a reduction in intensity of radiation proportional to the concentration of CO$_2$, which is indicated on a dial (Fig. 155).

The precision of the Uras instrument (Hartmann & Braun) is claimed by the manufacturer to be ± 0.2 volume percent (in a range of from 0 to 10% of CO$_2$). The recording lag inherent in the apparatus is $< .2$ second but this is considerably increased by the necessary drawing in of air for analysis.

c) Analysis of expired air for CO$_2$ using the interferometer (see page 170)

d) Analysis of expired air for CO$_2$ by mass spectrum (see page 171)

The framework of the present volume does not afford the framework for detailed reference to other methods. We refer the reader to Opitz and Bartels, *Handbuch der physiologisch-chemischen Analyse* and to *Lungenfunktionsprüfungen*, published by Springer-Verlag, 1959.

1.2   Measuring of CO_2 in Closed Systems (see page 171)

For binding CO_2 in a closed system, potassium, sodium or calcium hydroxide may be used in granular or liquid form. The amount of CO_2 bound can be determined titrimetrically by adding HCl or H_2SO_4 at certain intervals and measuring the amount of CO_2 driven off.

To measure the CO_2 it is possible to utilize the alteration in the electrical conductivity of potassium or sodium hydroxide resulting from binding of CO_2. The conductivity is measured by means of a Wheatstone bridge. The addition of fresh lime can be controlled in such a way that conductivity remains constant. Thus, CO_2 production of the subject can be measured by the amount and concentration of the inflowing lime. Fleisch's metabograph measures the formation of CO_2 according to this principle.

In closed systems, the requirements of CO_2 absorption are considerable, especially at more intensive performance levels (up to about 5000–6000 cm³ of CO_2 per minute). If the CO_2 content in the system increases by only 0.5 volume percent in the inspired air, there still results a significant increase in the volume of expired air. If chemical titrimetric measurement of the CO_2 is used, lime can be used for the absorption. It is more practical to use an indicator lime, which changes color if the CO_2 saturation exceeds a certain range. If insufficient CO_2 is bound, the lime must be replaced by a fresh supply. Whenever the volume of expired air is of inadequate magnitude, the possibility of insufficient CO_2 absorption must be borne in mind.

Because of this uncertainty in closed systems, open-system procedures (some of them pneumotachographic) have in late years been more popular in spiroergometric diagnostic exercise. (Nowacki)

2. CO_2 Production and Respiratory Quotient (RQ) During Ergometric Performance under Physiological Conditions

In the course of biological oxidation of carbohydrates, proteins and fats, large quantities of CO_2 are formed. According to studies by Zuntz (Table 39), in the combustion of 1 gram of carbohydrate, 830 cubic centimeters of CO_2 are formed. For fats the figure is 1430 and for proteins 770 cubic centimeters. Therefore, ascertaining CO_2 production affords insight into the quantitative processes in the intermediate metabolism.

During exercise, the production of CO_2 is greatest in those skeletal muscles being most actively used. The nonvolatile acids (especially lactic acid) collecting in the working muscle and blood cause CO_2 to be evolved faster

Table 39. The relationships involved in the combustion of carbohydrates, fats and proteins (after *Zuntz*).

	O_2 combustion in g/cm	CO_2 formed per g in cm³	RQ	Calories per gram	Calories per liter of O_2
Carbohydrates	830	830	1.0	4.2	5.05
Fats	2020	1430	0.7	9.4	4.68
Proteins	960	770	0.8	4.3	4.48

from the bicarbonates. The relationships of the lactic acid level and the pH of the arterial and venous blood to respiration time-volume, O_2 consumption and HR during increasing performance are shown in Fig. 156.

In arterial blood, the lactic acid level rises in regular relationship to magnitude and duration of the performance (Keul, Doll and Keppler). In the venous blood of the cubital vein (in cycling), however, the lactic acid level remains for a longer time at approximately the same level until a certain magnitude of exertion is reached, and only then climbs steeply. Muscles not

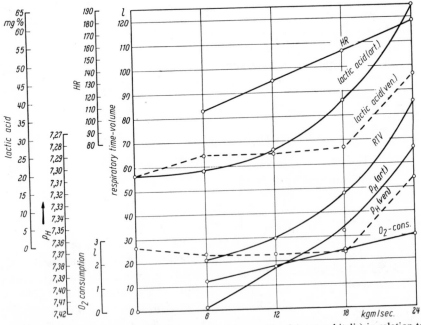

Fig. 156. Lactic acid and pH levels in arterial and venous blood (vena cubitalis) in relation to respiration time-volume, O_2 consumption and HR (ergometric pedaling in 40 male subjects aged 20 to 30) (after *Hollmann*).

participating in the exercise seem to cooperate in the elimination of lactic acid (Barr and Himwich). The liver is also involved. At maximal performance, very high levels of lactic acid in the blood can be reached, up to 150 to 170 mg% (Schenk; Krestownikow; etc.). According to Barr, Himwich and Green, 1 mg of lactic acid can displace 1.5 to 2.6 volume percent of CO_2.

We can not go into further detail at this point on the conditions of the CO_2 transport of the blood. Hemoglobin is the most important protein for CO_2 transport. However, most of the CO_2 is transported in the bicarbonates of the plasma. Because of the very good diffusion conditions for CO_2, there are no significant differences between alveolar and arterial CO_2 pressure.

In the air we inspire, there is usually 0.03 volume percent of CO_2. When expiring, while at rest, the volume percent amounts to about 3 to 4-1/2.

Before an ergometric examination, especially if the subject is already connected to the apparatus, most individuals incline to hyperventilation. Thus, there is more CO_2 production than normal. The quantity of CO_2 measured is considerably more than the amount resulting from the oxidation processes. Reassuring the patient can help shorten this period of psychic hyperventilation. The ergometric examination should not be started until CO_2 production has sunk again to a respiratory quotient (see below) between 0.80 and 0.90.

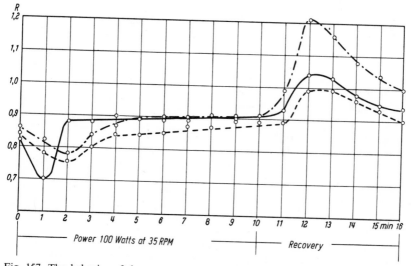

Fig. 157. The behavior of the average respiratory quotient in comparative studies of hand cranking while standing and pedaling while seated and reclining at equal power (100 watts) during ten minutes of exercise and six of recovery in 36 male untrained subjects aged 20 to 40 (after *Mellerowicz* and *Nowacki*). ——— standing, — — — sitting, —·—·— reclining.

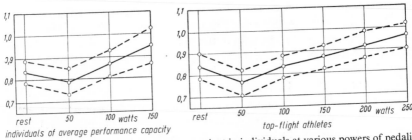

rest   50   100 watts 150   rest   50   100   150   200 watts 250

individuals of average performance capacity   top-flight athletes

Fig. 158. The behavior of the respiratory quotient in individuals at various powers of pedaling while reclining 30 to 60 rpm, in 80 subjects of average performance capacity and 40 top-flight athletes (after *Kirchhoff* and *Reindell*).

During the exercise in increasing steady-state stages, the formation of CO_2 increases in almost linear proportion to the magnitude of the exertion (Fig. 106). In comparison with O_2 consumption, the increase in CO_2 production is a bit steeper, until the two lines cross at a respiratory quotient of 1 (Fig. 160).

Generally, it can be taken for granted that, independently of age, sex and probably also of state of training, close correlations exist during an exhausting ergometric exercise between CO_2 production and various physiological performance parameters, such as heart rate, time-volume and absolute and relative O_2 consumption.

By measuring CO_2 production and calculating the respiratory quotient, physical performance capacity of the body can be judged with greater reliability even at low-wattage stages. Thus one is relieved of the need of always loading the subject to maximal performance. In compensation examinations, the desire of the examinee to undergo great exertion is usually not to be counted on.

The behavior of CO_2 production and respiratory quotient in an ergometric power of 100 watts at hand cranking while standing and pedaling while seated and reclining is shown in Figures 14, 15, and 157.

On the behavior of CO_2 production at various ergometric power levels and in various age groups, see Tables 38 and 40a and b to 45, and Figures 148, 157 and 160.

At equal powers, CO_2 production of trained individuals is somewhat less than that of the untrained (Tables 40a and 40b). Studies by Helbing, Mellerowicz and Nowacki on the behavior of CO_2 production by trained and untrained men showed a significantly quicker return of CO_2 production to the starting level among the more robust athletes. Thus, from the behavior of CO_2 production during recovery, conclusions can be drawn as to performance and recovery capacity of a subject. CO_2 production falls after a prolonged recovery period, usually to below the starting level. This is partly

Table 40a. The CO$_2$ production and respiratory quotient (RQ) on different ergometric powers (while reclining) of 80 males of 20 to 40 years of age (*Kirchhoff, Reindell* and *Gebauer*).

No. of persons	Power	CO$_2$ production	RQ
80	Rest	247 ± 47	0.84 ± 0.05
80	50 w/30 RPM	698 ± 73	0.79 ± 0.06
80	100 w/30 RPM	1249 ± 123	0.87 ± 0.06
66	150 w/30 RPM	1946 ± 218	0.95 ± 0.08
41	Rest	174 ± 31	0.83 ± 0.06
41	100 w/60 RPM	1290 ± 118	0.83 ± 0.06
32	150 w/60 RPM	1835 ± 72	0.88 ± 0.05
24	200 w/60 RPM	2575 ± 157	0.97 ± 0.07

Table 40b. The CO$_2$ production and RQ in gradually-increased ergometric power (while reclining) of 40 selected highly-trained athletes (*Kirchhoff, Reindell* and *Gebauer*).

No. of persons	Power	CO$_2$ production	RQ
40	Rest	274 ± 44	0.84 ± 0.06
40	50 w/30 RPM	667 ± 69	0.76 ± 0.06
40	100 w/30 RPM	1167 ± 155	0.83 ± 0.05
40	150 w/30 RPM	1683 ± 171	0.87 ± 0.06
40	Rest	289 ± 57	0.84 ± 0.07
40	100 w/60 RPM	1201 ± 102	0.80 ± 0.05
40	150 w/60 RPM	1786 ± 113	0.85 ± 0.06
31	200 w/60 RPM	2367 ± 217	0.91 ± 0.06
22	250 w/60 RPM	3187 ± 412	0.97 ± 0.06
9	300 w/60 RPM	4130	1.03

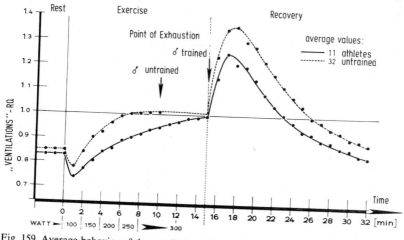

Fig. 159. Average behavior of the ventilation RQ during exhausting ergometric hand cranking exercise at increasing power levels (when 300 watts was reached the exercise proceeded until the point of exhaustion) and during the ensuing recovery phase. — — — — = 32 untrained men aged 20 to 40. ———— = 11 top-flight athletes aged 20 to 40 (after *Helbing; Mellerowicz* and *Nowacki*).

Table 41. CO_2 production and respiratory quotient at increasing ergometric performance (while reclining) in men aged 19 to 32 years (after *Galetti*) and men aged 40 to 65 (after *Aepli*).

Age Group	Number	Resting	40W	80W	120W
19 to 32	CO_2	271 ± 39	682 ± 38	1192 ± 89	1739 ± 125
	RQ	0.84 ± 0.09	0.87 ± 0.03	0.91 ± 0.04	0.95 ± 0.05
41 to 50	$28\ CO_2$	232 ± 33	715 ± 67	1245 ± 129	1878 ± 203
	RQ	0.93 ± 0.10	0.90 ± 0.06	0.96 ± 0.07	1.01 ± 0.07
51 to 55	$14\ CO_2$	229 ± 38	691 ± 69	1201 ± 119	836 ± 193
	RQ	0.93 ± 0.09	0.88 ± 0.06	0.94 ± 0.06	0.99 ± 0.07
56 to 65	$26\ CO_2$	218 ± 35	721 ± 74	1260 ± 154	975 ± 245
	RQ	0.93 ± 0.11	0.92 ± 0.0	0.97 ± 0.06	1.03 ± 0.07

to be explained on methodological grounds, since as a rule not enough time and patience are expended at the start of an examination to wait for the accelerated production of CO_2 resulting from hyperventilation to subside. Also, a relatively increased resynthesis of lactic acid to glycogen, liberating a good deal of alkali for increased binding of CO_2, may play a role.

Tables 38 and 40 to 42 provide an overview of the quantitative conditions of CO_2 production in various age and performance groups. Top-flight athletes may exhale up to, on the average, 38 ± 6 liters of CO_2 in ten to twelve minutes during an exhausting ergometric exercise period of increasing wattage stages of 250 to 500 watts. In an ensuing ten-minute recovery period, more than 16 liters of CO_2 may be produced. (From this it is also evident that closed systems, with their fixed absorption capacity, may quickly suffer from overdemand.)

The respiratory quotient is not merely a function of combustion processes, according to more recent studies by Rossier et al., as well as Bartels, Bücherl, Hertz, Rodewald and Schwab. It is also a function of the momentary ventilation conditions of the respiratory gases, CO_2 and O_2. This RQ, which plays a role in the respiratory physiology and in testing spiroergometric functions is called the "ventilation RQ."

Table 42. Quantitative representation of three cardiopulmonary performance parameters of the Bodensee four-oar scullers (world champions 1970, European champions 1969, 1971, Olympic champions 1972), at ergometric pedaling while seated; under hypoxic conditions (2045 meters above sea level, 601 mm Hg) on August 4, 1971, recorded pneumotachographically in the open system after Jäger or Würzburg (after *Nowacki, Krause, Ritter* and *Uthgenannt*).

	O_2 consumption	CO_2 production	Respiratory volume
V max 1/min	6.078 $\pm$ 0.666	5.442 $\pm$ 0.508	184.1 $\pm$ 26.8
Performance period 1/10–12 min	48.798 $\pm$ 8.782	38.227 $\pm$6.154	1257.5 $\pm$ 157.2
Recovery period 1/10 min	17.741 $\pm$ 1.817	16.402 $\pm$ 1.181	685.4 $\pm$ 129.4

Table 43. Average values for CO_2 production and its respiratory quotient in ten male subjects aged 20 to 40 in maximal ergometric performance while standing, sitting and reclining (after Galle and Mellerowicz).

		Exercise			Recovery/min			
	Rest	1/2	Exhaustion	5th	15th	20th	30th	
Standing CO_2 (cm³)	318	1990	3359	838	449	377	278	
RQ	0.87	0.93	1.07	1.30	0.97	0.88	0.83	
Sitting CO_2 (cm³)	311	1773	3248	717	422	340	262	
RQ	0.87	0.90	1.09	1.21	0.94	0.88	0.77	
Reclining CO_2 (cm³)	306	1571	2923	717	343	289	229	
RQ	0.89	0.93	1.04	1.24	0.86	0.79	0.69	

Compared to the "metabolic RQ," the ventilation RQ is calculated according to the following formula:

$$\text{ventilation RQ} = \frac{\text{exhaled } CO_2 \text{ in cm}^3 \text{ STPD}}{O_2 \text{ consumption in cm}^3 \text{ STPD}}$$

$$\text{metabolic RQ} = \frac{CO_2 \text{ production in cm}^3 \text{ STPD}}{O_2 \text{ consumption in cm}^3 \text{ STPD}}.$$

Only when breathing at rest and, occasionally, when exercising at the steady state is the amount of CO_2 formed equal to the amount expired and the O_2 intake equal to its consumption; and only under these conditions does the figure for the metabolic RQ correspond to the ventilation RQ. With changes in ventilation or metabolism, the time required for the establishment of a new equilibrium is dependent on the extent of the change and on the situation at the outset. If the changes in ventilation or metabolism are very great, however, then no balance is reached between the metabolic and ventilation RQs.

If conclusions are to be drawn from the RQ as obtained by gas analysis, it is essential that respiration be constant for an appreciable length of time. Failure to observe this principle has often led to misinterpretation of the RQ.

At the start of an exercise, the RQ falls in spite of increased production of CO_2. A number of authors have detected this, e.g., Rein; Fleisch; Knipping et al.; Kirchhoff and Reindell; Joss and Mellerowicz. Bartels, Bücherl, Hertz, Rodewald and Schwab believe that alveolar ventilation does not immediately reach the required level and the A-VO$_2\Delta$ increases faster than the A-VCO$_2\Delta$.

As intensity of performance increases, so does the respiratory quotient. The rapidity of this increase depends on intensity of the performance, age, sex and state of training of the subject.

A respiratory quotient of 1.0 is a useful criterion for a certain borderline physical performance. In normal individuals aged 20 to 40, the respiratory quotient reaches 1.0 at work loads of only 150 to 200 watts. Champion

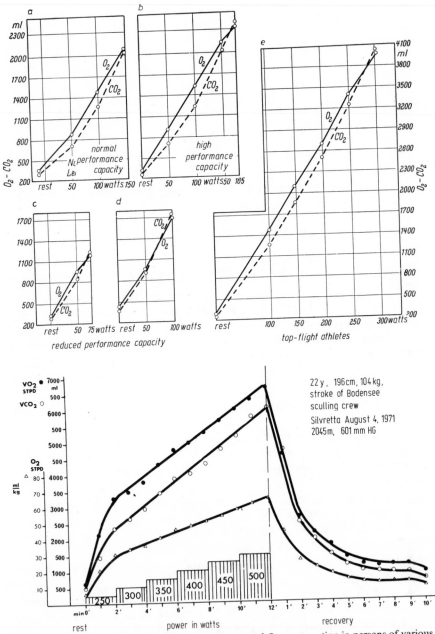

Fig. 160a–f. Individual examples of CO$_2$ production and O$_2$ consumption in persons of various performance capacity during ergometric performance (pedaling while reclining, Figs. 160a–e, after *Kirchhoff* and *Reindell*) and one top-flight oarsman under conditions of hypoxia (pedaling while seated, Fig. 160f, after *Nowacki et al.*).

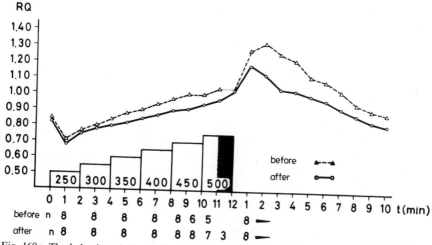

Fig. 160g. The behavior of the ventilation RQ at exhausting ergometric pedaling before and after a twelve-day altitude training course by the German National eight-oar crew in 1970 on the Silvretta Dam Lake at 2040 meters above sea level (after *Nowacki, Adam* and *Krause*).

athletes in sports of strength and endurance (Figs. 148 and 158) reach a ventilation respiratory quotient of 1.0 only at exercise levels between 400 and 500 watts, if the ergometric performance testing is done in conformity with the recommendations for examinations in record sports levels (Nowacki). An exercise above the respiratory quotient of 1.0 is, according to the studies, not possible for untrained children, men and women. Usually the performance is interrupted upon attaining respiratory quotient levels of 0.95 to 0.98, since the untrained are not accustomed to exercising to the point of exhaustion.

Athletes with a very high anaerobic capacity (pH drop below 7.1 to 6.9) are able to perform another two to four minutes beyond a respiratory quotient of 1.0 (Nowacki, Krause, Adam and Rulffs).

In international champion oarsmen there is a close correlation between the behavior of the heart rate and the respiratory quotient during exhausting pedaling performance.

Only at performance HR of more than 170 per minute does the respiratory quotient reach 1.0.

Joss found in his extensive studies that the increase in the respiratory quotient to 1.0 in increasing stages occurs sooner with increasing age. Christensen and Hansen saw an increase in the respiratory quotient to 1.0 when the O$_2$ consumption exceeded the 2-liter borderline in untrained individuals. In trained subjects, the same increase was not reached until a maximal O$_2$ consumption of 3 to 4 liters per minute was reached. According to studies by

Table 44. The respiratory quotient in 271 children and teenagers, all male, aged 10 to 19, at ergometric performances of various magnitudes (after *König, Reindell* and *Roskamm*).

Group			Rest	50 watts	100 watts	125 watts	150 watts	200 watts
I	9 subjects	x	0.87	0.84	0.93			
		s	0.13	0.08	0.10			
		v	15.0 %	9.7 %	11.9 %			
II a	9 subjects	x	0.91	0.78	0.92			
		s	0.20	0.12	0.09			
		v	22.2 %	15.9 %	9.9 %			
II b	9 subjects	x	0.85	0.78	0.90	0.90		
		s	0.11	0.09	0.09	0.06		
		v	12.9 %	12.5 %	10.3 %	7.2 %		
III a	12 subjects	x	0.91	0.78	0.96			
		s	0.25	0.11	0.10			
		v	27.9 %	14.6 %	11.8 %			
III b	15 subjects	x	0.94	0.78	0.88	0.94		
		s	0.22	0.12	0.06	0.10		
		v	24.2 %	15.7 %	7.5 %	11.1 %		
IV a	22 subjects	x	0.85	0.67	0.85		0.93	
		s	0.20	0.21	0.09		0.09	
		v	24.2 %	32.5 %	19.9 %		10.2 %	
IV b	10 subjects	x	0.08		0.84		0.87	0.95
		s	0.11		0.07		0.05	0.07
		v	14.6 %		8.3 %		6.4 %	7.7 %
V a	14 subjects	x	0.84	0.82	0.93		0.99	
		s	0.11	0.07	0.05		0.05	
		v	13.7 %	9.6 %	5.7 %		5.5 %	
V b	35 subjects	x	0.85	0.82	0.87		0.94	0.98
		s	0.28	0.09	0.07		0.06	0.06
		v	33.4 %	12.0 %	8.2 %		7.3 %	6.9 %

x = average   s = sigma   v = sigma in percent

Helbing, untrained women also reach a respiratory quotient of 1.0 much more quickly than trained women.

In physiological examination of aviators and astronauts, the respiratory quotient is used. Thus, at a certain gravitational load in a large centrifuge, respiratory quotients above 1.0 were found in young trained men. When they wore antigravity suits (clothing for protection against acceleration), the same load had less of an effect: the respiratory quotient failed to reach 1.0 (Babushkin, Isakow, Malkin and Usachev).

The rise in respiratory quotient to 1.0 during heavy labor and its performance-limiting character is no longer subject to any doubt after the studies by Rein; Furusawa et al.; Christensen and Hansen; Nöcker; Hollmann; Hill; Knipping et al.; Reindell et al.; Galetti; Joss; Aepli; and Mellerowicz and Nowacki. A number of authors were of the opinion that the rise to 1.0 was caused by the combustion of carbohydrates. An extreme rise in the lactic acid level in the blood must lead to extreme production and expulsion of CO$_2$, with an increase in the respiratory quotient to 1.0 and even higher.

Table 45. The respiratory time-volume and CO_2 production in liters and converted to grams at various conditions of rest and at various work power converted for one hour (from Johannes Müller, *Die Leibesübungen*, 4th ed., Teubner Verlag, Leipzig-Berlin, 1926).

Activity	Respiratory time-volume in liters	CO_2 production	
		liters	grams
Sleep	282	11.3	22
Reclining (awake)	400	16	31
Standing (comfort)	435	17.5	34
Standing (at attention)	475	19	37
Walking (leisurely)	1005	40.2	78
Descending a hill (25% grade)	1105	46	89
Walking (1 km/10 min)	1200	48	93
Cycling (15 km/hr)	1340	71	137
Hill-climbing (leisurely)	2000	80	155
Hill-climbing (strenuous)	3100	176	341
Fast swimming	2600	114	221
Record foot-race and record rowing	3600	318	618

Ice hockey league players, who are subject in the course of world championship events to brief spurts of high anaerobic exercise, also show the ability in exhausting spiroergometric work to perform for a long time at a respiratory quotient above 1.0 (Fig. 161, after Nowacki and Simai).

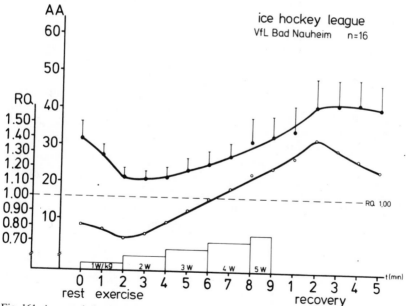

Fig. 161. Average behavior of ventilation RQ and respiratory equivalent in ice hockey league players during and after exhausting spiroergometric pedaling while seated (watts-per-kg method) (after *Nowacki* and *Simai*).

In labor performed over the course of several hours, the respiratory quotient reaches a point of decline, according to studies by Eckert; Krogh and Lindhard; Margaria; and Keller and Böhm. This is traced to increasing production of CO_2 from an increase in the combustion of fats. In the usual short-lasting ergometric examinations, no such change in the respiratory quotient is to be anticipated.

During recovery, the respiratory quotient goes on rising at first for a short time, depending on the type and magnitude of the performance, the subject's constitution, age, sex, state of training, etc. (Fig. 159). RQs of 1.5 and even 2.0 may be attained. Hansen found an RQ of 2.2 after a 100-meter dash. Continually increased CO_2 production after the performance, with more rapidly falling O_2 consumption, may be an explanation for this. Then, after a few minutes, there occurs a sharp drop in RQ, usually to below the starting level. At equal powers, the rise in RQ and the time lapse until return to resting level behave in inverse proportion to physical performance capacity.

After high-altitude training, the RQ was lower in submaximal exercise than before training; this depended on the psychological, aerobic and anaerobic physical capacities. Nowacki, Adam and Krause found in 1970, after twelve days of altitude training of the German eight-oar crew on Silvretta Dam Lake at 2,040 m, a highly significant increase in the exercise capacity, from $3,700 \pm 437$ to $4,125 \pm 354$ watts; a maximal O_2 consumption from $5,742 \pm 514$ to $6,552 \pm 432$ ml STPD; a maximal voluntary ventilation from 152.3 ± 13.4 to 175.5 ± 12.8 lit BTPS; and in ten minutes of recovery, an O_2 debt of 12.823 ± 2.300 to 15.755 ± 2.146 lit O_2 STPD. Training also postponed the attainment of an RQ of 1.0 (Fig. 160g).

In summing up, it may be said that the magnitude of the RQ during and after an ergometric exercise permits conclusions to be drawn as to performance capacity and state of training on the part of an individual. At submaximal performance stages one can predict whether a still higher exercise can be tackled. From the level of the RQ during recovery, the "degree of exertion" of a subject in an exercise can be approximately estimated. An increase in the RQ to 1.0 during the exercise shows the attainment of a certain borderline of performance in an individual. Continuation of the exercise is then possible only with the greatest will power for a short time, until exhaustion of the maximal anaerobic capacity.

3. CO_2 Production and Respiratory Quotient During Ergometric Performance under Pathologic Conditions

In the presence of pathological changes of various etiologies in the circulatory and respiratory apparatus, the CO_2 consumption and total CO_2 production are at equal submaximal steady-state stages, equal to or a trifle higher than in healthy untrained subjects. The maximal CO_2 consumption per unit of time is reduced in direct relationship to the nature and magnitude of the insufficiency. At increasing performance stages, higher RQs are reached sooner depending on the extent of the reduction in cardiopulmonary performance. The recovery times of CO_2 and the RQ are prolonged depending on the type and extent of the damage.

As the CO_2 level in the blood increases during ergometric performance, the expiration of CO_2 may be reduced by disturbances in pulmonary diffusion, reduction of pulmonary diffusion area, mechanical (obstructive or restrictive) interference with breathing, increase in residual air and expiratory reserve volume, central or peripheral disturbance of respiratory regulation, right-heart insufficiency with partial bypassing of the pulmonary circulation, hypochromic anemia, etc. The most important causal factors of respiratory and cardiac insufficiency are listed in Chapter IX, Section 5. Here, however, the diagnostic measures must concentrate more on blood gas analytical examination during and after the exercise (see the comprehensive bibliography in Hertz, C. W.: *Begutachtung von Lungenfunctionsstorungen*, Thieme, Stuttgart 1968).

CO_2 content and CO_2 pressure in the blood are also regularly dependent on the type and extent of the pathological changes in the circulatory system, lungs and blood. Detailed treatments of these points has been given by Rossier, Bühlmann and Wiesinger; and Bartels, Bücherl, Hertz, Rodewald and Schwab.

References

Aepli, R.: Helvet. med. acta 26, (1959) 49.
Babuschkin, W. J., P. K. Isakow, W. B. Malkin and W. W. Usatschew: Fiziol. z. SSSR. 44, (1958) 342.
Barr and Himwich: J. Biol. Chem. Baltimore 55, (1933), after H. Herxheimer: Grundriß der Sportmedizin. Leipzig: Thieme, 1933.

Bartels, H., E. Bücherl, C. W. Hertz, G. Rodewald and M. Schwab: Lungenfunktionsprüfungen.Berlin-Göttingen-Heidelberg: Springer, 1959.
Christensen, H. E. and O. Hansen: Scand. Arch. Physiol. 81, (1939) 137 and 152, 160, 172, 180.

258 CO₂ Production and Respiratory Quotient in Ergometric Performance

Eckert, A.: Zschr. Biol. 71, (1920) 137.

Fleisch, A.: Neue Methoden zum Studium des Gasaustausches und der Lungenfunktion. Leipzig: Thieme, 1956.

Furusawa, K.: Proc. Roy. Soc. London 5, (1925) 98.

Galetti, P. M.: Thèse des sciences. Lausanne 1956.

Galle, L. and H. Mellerowicz: Der Sportarzt 10, (1962) 332.

Hansen, E.: Arbeitsphysiologie 8, (1935) 151.

Helbing, G.: Inaug. Diss., Berlin, 1966.

Hertz, C. W.: Begutachtung von Lungenfunktionsstörungen, Thieme, Stgt. 1968.

Hill, Long and Lupton: Proc. Roy. Soc. London 96/97 (1924/25).

Hollmann, W.: Lecture given at a conference of the Dtsch. Hochschulsportärzte Nov. 1960 in Münster.

Joss, E. E.: Diss. Bern 1958.

Keller, W. and M. Böhm: Arbeitsphysiologie 17, (1958) 107.

Keul, J., J. Doll and Keppler: Muskelstoffwechsel. Barth, München 1969.

Kirchhoff, H. W., H. Reindell and A. Gebauer: Dtsch. Arch. klin. Med. 203, (1956) 423.

Kirchhoff, H. W. and H. Reindell: Verh. Dtsch. Ges. inn. Med. 62, (1956) 587.

Knipping, H. W. and Mitarb.: Beitr. Klin. Tbk. 79, (1932) 1; 92, (1939) 144.

König, K., H. Reindell, J. Keul and H. Roskamm: Arbeitsphys. 18, (1961) 393.

Krause, R.: Inaug. Diss., Lübeck 1971.

Krestownikow, A. N.: Physiologie der Körperübungen. Berlin: Volk und Gesundheit, 1953.

Krogh, H. and J. Lindhard: J. Physiol. 53, (1919/20) 431.

Margaria, R.: Reale Accad. Naz. dei Lincei 7, (1938) 6.

Mellerowicz, H. and P. Nowacki: Zeitschrift für Kreislaufforschung 50, (1961) 1002.

Nöcker, J.: Grundriß der Biologie der Körperübungen. Berlin: Sportverlag 1959.

Nowacki, P.: I. Internat. Seminar on Ergometry, Hrsg.: Mellerowicz, H. and G. Hansen, p. 92, Berlin, Ergon-Verlag 1965.

Nowacki, P.: Leistungssport 2, (1971) 37.

Nowacki, P., R. Krause, K. Adam and M. Rulffs: Sportarzt and Sportmed. 10, (1971) 227.

Nowacki, P.: Sportmedizinische und leistungsphysiologische Aspekte des Ruderns. In: Adam, K., H. Lenk, P. Nowacki, M. Rulffs and W. Schröder: Rudertraining, Limpert Verlag, Bad Homburg 251–646, 1977.

Rein, H.: Pflügers Arch. Physiol. 247, (1944) 576; Arch. exper. Path. Pharmak. 171, (1933).

Rein, H. and M. Schneider: Physiologie des Menschen, 11. ed. Berlin-Göttingen-Heidelberg: Springer, 1955.

Reindell, H. and H. W. Kirchhoff: Dtsch. med. Wschr. 15, 592; 17, 659; 26, (1956) 1048.

Rossier, P. H., A. Bühlmann and K. Wiesinger: Physiologie und Pathophysiologie der Atmung. Heidelberg: Springer, 1958.

Schenk: Münch. med. Wschr. 72 (1925), after H. Herxheimer: Grundriß der Sportmedizin. Leipzig: Thieme, 1933.

Zuntz, N.: Pflügers Arch. Physiol. 83, (1901) 557.

XIII. The Ergometric EKG

by Fritz Matzdorff

1. Indication

The Ergometric EKG (ergo-EKG) is one of the basic tests in functional diagnostics that can be carried out even in private practice. Its area of application is the proof or disproof of latent coronary insufficiency. The detection of this condition for forewarning of coronary disease has been steadily gaining in importance in the last two decades as the increase in cardiac infarction has assumed epidemic proportions. More and more young people of both sexes have been falling victim to this malady. Only improvement in early warning techniques in ambulant practice and intensification of preventive measures can hope to check this alarming trend.

Anamnesis and EKG with the subject at rest are not adequate for early warning of coronary disease. Coronary disease, which is almost always of arteriosclerotic origin and develops only after advanced stenotic coronary sclerosis, may lie latent for years. If there is sufficient blood flow in the coronary arteries while at rest, a disparity between blood supply and blood requirement will occur only on the off-chance of overexertion. A conventional EKG with the patient at rest is, therefore, as a rule unable to detect latent coronary insufficiency. Only in the event of characteristic angina pectoris symptoms triggered by physical activity, mental agitation or cold does anamnesis justify the diagnosis of coronary disease. There are, however, many patients with coronary disease who reveal a pattern of atypical or psychological complaints or no heart symptoms at all. Differential diagnosis of these atypical heart symptoms, in contradistinction to the common extra-cardiac symptoms very frequently ascribed to the heart, is extremely important in private practice.

In this connection, exclusion of the possibility of coronary insufficiency is perhaps of even greater value than its confirmation. The financial burdens that can result from falsely identifying symptoms and prescribing expensive coronary therapy are certainly greater than the cost of an ergo-EKG. More oppressive is the anxiety from false advice and unnecessary restriction on life style, movement and professional activity which may result from a diagnosis of supposed coronary disease.

Exercise therapy is often the only effective treatment for functional heart trouble, and therefore any limitation on physical activity can only have a deleterious effect. Even after a myocardial infarct it happens in a relatively high percentage of cases that heart conditions are revealed that are of psycho-vegetative and not organic etiology. These can make rehabilitation very difficult, frequently leading to unjustified interruption in wage-earning and even premature pensioning.

The ergo-EKG is therefore important in rehabilitation and sociological medical evaluation, since when properly carried out it can afford information about the seriousness of a coronary insufficiency and thus indicate how much physical exertion and rehabilitative training and participation in gainful employment is possible and safe. If, even under light exercise, typical angina pectoris symptoms and ST depression occur regularly, critical stenoses are very often present in several coronary vessels. Such patients are seriously threatened with infarct or reinfarct. Insofar as age and clinical findings permit, not too much time should be allowed to elapse before resorting to coronary angiography and, if found necessary, to an aortocoronary-bypass operation.

Compared with its importance in proving or disproving coronary insufficiency, the ergo-EKG's value in the diagnosis of arrhythmias is limited. The continuous EKG is the method of choice for detecting arrhythmias. Table 46 shows how frequently an ischemic reaction, arrhythmias or both were detected in myocardial infarct patients by means of an ergo-EKG and by means of a telemetry or a continuous EKG during the usual stresses of daily life. According to it, in comparison with a resting EKG, in only 9% more

Table 46. Comparison between telemetry, continuous, and ergo-EKGs in patients recovered from cardiac infarct.

Changes compared with resting EKG	Tele-EKG	Continuous EKG	Ergo-EKG
Unchanged	68%	24%	58%
Horizontal or downsloping ST depression > 0.1 millivolts	5%	12%	33%
Horizontal or downsloping ST depression + arrhythmia	3%	18%	2%
Arrhythmia	23%	46%	7%
Number of patients	224	336	1702

patients were arrhythmias found (mostly extrasystoles) in ergo-EKGs, but in telemetry EKGs in 26% and in continuous EKGs in 64% more. Ischemic reactions were about equally often detected in ergo-EKGs (35%) and continuous EKGs (30%), but considerably more rarely (8%) in telemetry EKGs.

The significance of the ergo-EKG in differential diagnosis between vegetatively and ischemically caused extrasystole is today the subject of dispute. The earlier view, that vegetatively caused extrasystoles disappear under exercise and ischemically caused ones occur under it or become more frequent is now in doubt, at least as regards younger people.

If an abnormal curve pattern is detectable even in a resting EKG, than the pros and cons of an exercise EKG must be weighed with care. In no case must an ergo-EKG be carried out without the knowledge gained from a previous rest-EKG. If even in the rest-EKG the ST segments or T waves are very much changed pathologically or blocks with discordant displacement of the ST-T section are detected, then only very rarely can an ergo-EKG afford any new insight. An ergo-EKG is contraindicated in the presence of manifest cardiac muscular insufficiency, cardiac dilation, more serious types of arrhythmia, aortic stenosis, cor pulmonale or aneurysms of the aorta or cardiac walls. An ergo-EKG should also be avoided in hypertension with blood pressure readings of 200/110 or above.

2. Value of Evidence

Statements as to the value of the ergo-EKG for diagnosis of coronary insufficiency are possible from a comparison with clinical and coronographic findings and with the course of the disease. However, it must be remembered that a comparison between morphology and function can never afford 100% agreement. Ischemic reactions and malaise in the cardiac region are not always caused by coronary insufficiency, angina pectoris is not always accompanied by coronary insufficiency, and not every case of coronary sclerosis has to result in coronary insufficiency. An ischemic heart muscle or an ischemic reaction in an ergo-EKG may also be caused by anemia, CO poisoning or deficient O_2 saturation resulting from heart defects or pulmonary disease. Insufficient blood supply can also arise from lowered perfusion pressure in aortic and mitral stenosis. These diseases must therefore be ruled out when a diagnosis of coronary insufficiency is made on the basis of an ischemic reaction in an ergo-EKG.

It has already been pointed out that the comparison between the complaint of heart symptoms and the results of an ergo-EKG is problematic and only to a limited extent permits conclusions about the value of the ergo-

EKG. Since more than half the cases of complaints of heart symptoms are of extracardial origin and often accompany milder degrees of coronary insufficiency with atypical heart symptoms, and since there are even cases of coronary insufficiency without angina pectoris, the absence of ST depressions in an ergo-EKG without angina pectoris is not necessarily due to false negative or false positive EKG findings.

In order to judge the diagnostic value of an ergo-EKG, a comparison with coronographic findings is advisable. If angina pectoris is also included in this comparison, the correlations between the results of the ergo-EKG and the coronographic findings are particularly good. Thus, Roskamm found in more than 90% of his cases a more than 50% stenosis of at least one cardiac artery in patients without cardiac infarct but with an ischemic ST depression during exercise and simultaneous presence of angina pectoris. In patients who had recovered from infarct of the posterior wall of the heart, and in whom there occurred under exercise an ischemic ST depression and angina pectoris, more or less severe stenosis in a second or even a third coronary vessel was detectable in more than 60%. On the other hand, in patients without ischemic ST depression and without angina pectoris, a significant stenosis could be verified in only 3%. The studies showed, moreover, that there was a close connection between the extent of the vascular affection and the extent of the ST depression during exercise or load stage in which an ischemic reaction and angina pectoris occurred. The more marked the ST depression and the lower the exercise at which the ST depression occurred, the more frequently was the involvement of more than one blood vessel or a left main branch stenosis observed (Table 47).

Table 47. (By *H. Roskamm*).

		ST-Depression (mv)	Watts	ST-Depression $\times$ 1000 / Watts
1 vessel involved	n = 18	0.117	80.3	1.46
2 vessels involved	n = 31	0.180	52.9	3.40
3 vessels involved	n = 30	0.280	44.7	6.26
Left main branch stenosis	n = 15	0.317	43.6	7.27

In addition to coronographic findings, the course of the disease after an ergo-EKG is an important criterion for judging the value of this method, especially as concerns prognosis. The catamnestic study published by Robb and Marks in 1964 on 1659 applicants for life insurance in the United States showed a four times higher total death rate in the case of individuals in whom an ergo-EKG revealed pathological conditions than in those with a normal one. The differences were still greater when only the coronary mor-

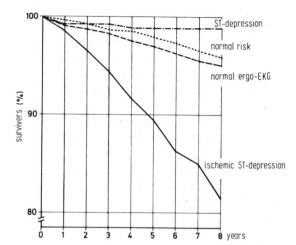

Fig. 162. Survival rate as a factor of the result of the exercise EKG. A pathological curve reduces the life expectancy considerably. It is noteworthy that the "ascending ST depression goes hand-in-hand with a better-than-average life expectancy" (after *Robb* and *Marks*)

tality rate was compared. The coronary death rate was actually seven times as great in the group in whom an ergo-EKG showed pathological findings as in the group with normal findings (see Fig. 162). An increased coronary death rate was observed only in individuals with descending or horizontal ST depression but not in those with isolated T changes or with ascending ST depression. In the latter were found even lower mortality than in individuals with normal ergo-EKGs. Moreover, the coronary death rate rose with increasing ischemic ST depression, and with a depression of more than 0.2 mV was almost thirteen times as high as with a depression of less than 0.1 mV.

For prognosis after healed cardiac infarct an ergo-EKG is also of great value, as shown by a catamnestic study we made on 447 men between the ages of 40 and 59, all at least six months after myocardiac infarct (Matzdorff).

Table 48. Frequency of reinfarction per 1000 infarct patients and per year in relation to the results of the ergo-EKG.

Ischemic reaction during and after exercise	Frequency of reinfarction per 1000 cardiac infarct patients and per year		
Ergo-EKG	Fatal reinfarction	Non-fatal reinfarction	Total reinfarction
None	7	23	30
At 100 watts or more	23	23	46
At 75 watts or less	37	35	72
Total number of ischemic reactions	30	29	59

According to this, the prognosis in infarct patients was overwhelmingly affected unfavorably by reinfarction, and infarct patients suffered reinfarction more frequently the less they tolerated exercise or the lower was the exercise at which an ischemic reaction occurred (Table 48).

The results can be explained very well on the basis of Roskamm's angiographic findings mentioned above and observations of the course of the disease after angiography made by Webster. According to the latter, the frequency of ischemic ST-depression at low exercise intensities and the coronary death rate increases with the number of coronary branches involved. As can also be seen from the frequency of reinfarction calculated in Table 48, the number of fatal reinfarctions was about 50% higher than the coronary death rate calculated by Robb and Marks of 21 per thousand per year in individuals without infarct but with an ischemic reaction in an exercise EKG.

3.   Methodology

Prerequisite to wide use of the ergo-EKG in practice is that the examination be on the one hand risk-free and performed as a routine procedure, but on the other that it permit with sufficient certainty not only the proof or disproof, but also the evaluation, of the degree of severity of a coronary insufficiency. Certain minimum requirements must, therefore, be fulfilled by the apparatus being employed and the methodology of its use, especially in regular practice. The nature and performance of the load are particularly important.

The exercise challenge of ten to thirty knee bends still widely used in Germany is not suited to the detection of a latent coronary insufficiency. Since, in knee bending, the magnitude of the exercise depends on the weight of the subject as well as the tempo and the manner of performance, and since older and more obese patients often perform the knee bends slowly and incompletely, no standardization is possible with this form of exercise, nor is any judgment as to the severity of a coronary insufficiency.

In contrast to knee bending, Master's two-step test and Kaltenbach and Klepzig's stair-climbing test is indeed standardized. Depending on age, sex and weight, the stair-climbing speed is varied in Master's test, and the speed and height of the steps are varied in the stair-climbing test. The stair-climbing test has an advantage over the Master test in that the subject need not turn around again and again during the workout and thus is avoided the dizziness often met with in the elderly. In addition, the patient uses both arms as well in the stair climbing test, thus employing additional muscles and improving the efficiency of motion. Both step tests have the advantage of being inexpensive and taking up little space. However, they have the disadvantage that the exercise can not be increased by stages during the course of testing to check the severity of a coronary insufficiency. Also, as with knee bending, it is not possible to measure the blood pressure while the patient is climbing the stairs, and an EKG can seldom be recorded with precision.

A standardized performance at increasing exercise levels is possible only with a treadmill or a bicycle ergometer. The treadmill commonly used in the English-speaking countries has various disadvantages, which we can not go into here. Since it is also more expensive and takes up more room than the bicycle ergometer, we can not recommend it in practice. The exercise on the bicycle ergometer while seated or reclining is certainly the best available form of exercise for an ergo-EKG. Mechanically braked bicycle ergometers with subdivisions into 10- to 25-watt increments are not beyond the means of the general practitioner. Bicycle ergometry permits not only the simultaneous and technologically sound recording of an EKG but also an increasing exercise level within a single exercise. This has several advantages. In the first place, ischemic ST-depressions quite frequently recover within a half to a full minute after an exercise (Table 49). This would not be detected with forms of exercise that do not permit a perfect recording until after the end of an exercise period. In the second place, the test need be increased only as far as the stage at which an ischemic reaction actually occurs. Thus, not too great a demand is made on the subject. Moreover, angina pectoris less often occurs since the ischemic reaction usually develops first. In the third place, serious EKG changes such as extrasystolic aberrations can be detected early and the test interrupted at once, thus avoiding further complications. In order to detect abnormal EKG changes quickly during the exercise and save recording paper, an oscilloscope for continuous checking of the EKG is particularly useful.

Table 49. Ischemic reactions in the ergometer EKG (≥ 0.1 mV).

Number	During load	Immediately thereafter	After 1 min	After 2 min	After 3 min
60	100%	93%	62%	45%	33%

We start generally with an exercise level of 50 watts at 50 rpm and increase by 25 watts every two minutes, or else by 10 watts every minute. The standardization suggestions for ergometric testing, published in 1964, recommend at least three stages of 25 watts, each lasting six minutes without recovery heart rate. Older untrained persons and cardiac patients, however, do not make it to the end of this exercise level because of fatigue in the thighs. The test would last 30 minutes with preparation and EKG checks before and after the exercise, and would be unsuitable for general practice just for this reason. Since with a total exercise period of a few minutes the appearance of an ischemic reaction depends mainly on the magnitude and less on the duration of a wattage stage, power stages of 25 watts for two minutes or 10 watts for one minute are also sufficient for the detection of a coronary insufficiency. If no EKG deviations are detected, the power production in individuals over 50 and in infarct patients is increased up to 125 watts, in younger patients without heart disease up to 150. The exercise is terminated early if pathognomonic EKG alterations occur or if, depending on age, the HR exceeds 180–200/min minus personal age, or the blood

Table 50. Ergo-EKG.

Indication:	Proof or disproof of latent coronary insufficiency and estimation of its severity.
Contraindications:	Manifest heart-muscle insufficiency, heart dilation (relative cardiac volume above 500 ml/m²), more serious arrhythmias, aortic stenosis, cor pulmonale, aneurysm of aorta or ventricle, hypertonia above 200/110 at rest, acute inflammatory heart and general diseases.
Form of exercise:	Step-by-step increasing exercise on the bicycle ergometer while reclining or seated, without recovery pauses. Exercise stages of 10 watts for one minute or 25 watts for two minutes. 50 rpm per minute. Start at 50 watts (±10–25 watts). Increase up to a heart rate of 180–200 minus age. Interrupt exercise in the event of: ischemic reaction of over 0.2 mV, serious arrhythmias, disturbances of conduction, blood pressure above 240/120, increase in stenocardia, dyspnea, pallor, cyanosis, or failure to maintain pace.
EKG leads:	Single-channel machines: V5, Nehb A or MC_5 Three-channel machines: V2, V4, V5 Four-channel machines: V2, V4, V5, V6 Six-channel machines: V2, V4, V5, I, II, III
When to record:	At rest; in the last 10 seconds of each exercise level; immediately, 1, 2, 3 and possibly 5 minutes after cessation of exercise.
EKG Criteria: Ischemic sign:	Descending or horizontal ST-depression of 0.1 mV or more, ST elevation of 0.2 mV or more, late neg U wave.
Abnormal, but not sure signs of ischemia:	Descending and/or horizontal ST-depression of less than 0.1 mV, PQ prolongation, clustered extrasystoles, QRS broadening to branch block, ST and T changes with branch block, T negativization.
Normal:	Ascending ST-depression, T leveling.
Nitrate test:	For differential diagnosis between ischemic and digitalis-caused ST-depression. Ischemic ST-depression disappears after nitrate (sublingual). Digitalis-caused ST-depression does not.

pressure 240/120 mm Hg. Even though precise measurement of blood pressure is difficult during the exercise, considerations of safety and the detection of hypertonic disturbances in regulation dictate that it not be dispensed with.

If these rules are observed, the step-by-step increase in exercise on the bicycle ergometer is without danger, even for cardiac patients. From 1961 until the end of 1975 we carried out about 15,000 ergo-EKGs, about 10,000 of them on patients with healed myocardial infarct, and had not a single serious incident.

Since an ischemic reaction as a rule develops earlier and more distinctly in the left precordial leads and the isoelectric line often varies very much in the extremity leads, the curves being overlaid by muscular currents, chestwall leads V4 to V6 are the most productive in the detection of latent coronary insufficiency. Simultaneous recording of several left precordial leads is recommended since in individual cases an ascending ST-depression can occur in V4 but a descending or horizontal ST-depression in V5 or V6, or an ST-depression in V4 only, not being definitely detectable in V5 or V6. If only a single-channel electrocardiograph is available, the Wilson lead V5 or the bipolar lead Nehb A (right parasternal second intercostal space-heart apex) or MC_5 (manubrium sternal position V5) should be recorded.

The electrodes are most simply attached with perforated rubber bands into which are inserted button electrodes covered with fabric and readily dampened with a spray bottle. In order to avoid accidental artifacts in the tracings as a result of body movements, the locating of the electrodes may vary from the rule. When the exercise is performed by a reclining subject, the chest wall electrodes are located as usual. The two arm electrodes, however, are attached to the upper arms, and the leg electrodes over the groins on the abdomen. When recording the Wilson leads during the exercise while seated, it is advantageous to attach the extremity electrodes on the back at shoulder-blade level, as described by Rosenkranz and Drews (see Fig. 163).

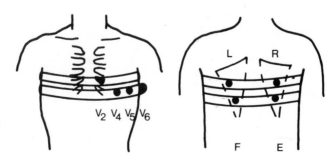

Fig. 163. Chest wall leads (after *Rosenkranz* and *Drews*).

V_2 V_4 V_5 V_6

L   R

F   E

At present, only horizontal or descending ST-depression of at least 0.1 mV and the occurrence of a late negative wave are valid as EKG criteria. In the case of old anterior wall infarcts, an ST elevation is in isolated instances observed in brief ischemic conditions. The ischemic ST-depression must be distinguished from the benign ascending ST-depression, which occurs mainly in tachycardias and therefore frequently shows up during exercise. The ascending ST-depression has no significance. PQ prolongation, QRS broadening and T changes occurring during exercise are, even though not normal, no certain indication of coronary insufficiency. In the evaluation of ergo-EKGs of patients on digitalis, one should be cautious in interpreting an ST-depression. The resting EKG may still be completely normal and the ST-depression due to digitalis not show up until an exercise load is applied. To distinguish a digitalis-caused ST-depression from an ischemic one in differential diagnosis by ergo-EKG, Ritter and Klepzig have recommended the nitrate test. After doses of nitrate in the case of ischemic ST-depression, there occurs a normalization of the ST segment and the U wave during exercise. In changes caused by digitalis alone, the normalization does not occur. In Table 50 are summarized once more the most important criteria in evaluating an ergo-EKG.

References

Kaltenbach, M. and H. Klepzig: Das EKG während Belastung u. s. Bedeutung für die Erkennung der Koronarinsuffizienz, Z. Kreisl. Forschung 52 (1963) 486.

Master, A. M.: The two-step-exercise electrocardiogram, a test for coronary insufficiency. Ann. Intern. Med. 32 (1950) 842.

Matzdorff, F.: Herzinfarkt–Prävention und Rehabilitation, München: Urban & Schwarzenberg, 1975.

Ritter, H. and H. Klepzig: Belastungs-EKG beim digitalisierten Patienten Med. Klin. 69 (1974) 794.

Robb, G. P. and H. H. Marks: Latent coronary artery disease, Determination of its presence and severity by the Exercise Electrocardiogram, Amer. J. Cardiol. 13 (1964) 603.

Rosenkranz, K. A. and A. Drews: Über undefinierte Ableitungsmethoden zur Registrierung von Brustwandelelektrokardiogrammen während dosierter körperlicher Belastung, Z. Kreisl. Forschung 53 (1964) 615.

Roskamm, H.: Die Interpretation der Untersuchungsergebnisse nichtinvasiver Methoden der Herzfunktionsdiagnostik aus dem Blickwinkel invasiver Untersuchungsergebnisse; Annual conference of the Deutsche Arbeitsgemeinschaft für Kardiologische Prävention und Rehabilitation i. V. held 18.–20. 3. 76 in Rotenburg/Fulda.

Webster, J. S., C. Moberg and G. Rincon: Natural history of severe proximal coronary artery disease as documented by coronary cineangiography, Amer. J. Cardiol. 33 (1974) 195.

XIV. Central Circulatory Dynamics in Ergometric Performance

by Horst Schmutzler

I. A knowledge of central hemodynamics—intracardial and intravascular pressures and volumes in the thoracic cavity—under conditions of physical exercise has been shown to be necessary to the solution of the following questions and problems:

1. Qualitative and quantitative relationships between pressures, volumes, contractility and performance under physiologic and pathophysiologic conditions
2. Assessment of myocardial insufficiency, pre-insufficiency, exercise insufficiency, compensation and decompensation, as well as performance capacity, performance limitation, performance reserves, adaptation and regulation
3. From the quantitative extent of the changes, as compared with the norm, can be gained a detailed understanding of the individual's circulatory dynamics, especially in the assessment of conservative, operative or rehabilitative therapeutic measures.

II. Ergometric examination methods should be standardized to be comparable and reproducible for both those with healthy circulation and those with compensated heart disease. The intensity of the exercise must therefore be neither too small nor too great. In pedaling on the ergometer while reclining, and with percutaneously applied catheters via the femoral vein or artery, the following two procedures for ergometric exercising have proved practical, depending on which and how many parameters are to be considered:

Table 51. Parameters of the central circulation in normal and pressured (mitral stenosis) instances. Averages and standard deviations ±1σ at rest and in the relative steady state of power of 1 watt per kg of body weight.

	Healthy subjects n = 6				Mitr. Sten. II n = 36				Mitr. Sten. III n = 34			
	R	±s	E	±s	R	±s	E	±s	R	±s	E	±s
mm Hg												
P LA s	17	2	23	4	21	4	42	8	31	8	59	10
LA d	6	2.6	7	2.6	11	3	24	7	18	5	36	7
LA m	9	2.9	16	3	16	3	31	6	23	5	46	7
PA s	26	2	36	3	31	4	57	11	50	13	105	24
PA d	13	1	16	3	57	3	33	7	26	6	53	13
PA m	18	2	24	4	22	2	41	6	34	10	72	15
RA s	8	2.3			8	2.7			8	2.8		
RA d	2	1.9			3	2.0			3	2.2		
RA m	3	2.1	4	2.6								
LV ad	2	1.8	5	1.7	5	2.6	7	4.4	4	2.9	7	3.0
LV ed	8	1.3	12	1.8	11	2.9	15	3.8	12	3.4	13	2.9
Ao s	137	16	159	25	124	12	146	24	123	11	140	17
Ao d	86	13	93	8	79	14	92	13	76	8	86	9
Ao m	103		115		94		110		91		104	
HQ l/min/m²	4.6	0.7	7.2	0.8	3.0	0.6	5.6	1.1	2.8	0.6	5.5	1.2
Vs ml/m²	58	14	59	12	39	9	47	15	41	10	44	13
HR	83	19	124	28	78	11	122	17	75	11	129	17

R	= Rest	RA d	= Right atrial diastolic
E	= Exercise	RA m	= Right atrial mean
P	= Pressure	LV ad	= Left ventricular beginning diastolic
P LA s	= Pressure left atrium systolic	LV ed	= Left ventricular end diastolic
LA d	= Left atrium diastolic	Ao s	= Aortic systolic
LA m	= Left atrium mean	Ao d	= Aortic diastolic
PA s	= Systolic atrial pressure	Ao m	= Aortic mean
PA d	= Diastolic atrial pressure	HZV	= Cardiac output
PA m	= Mean atrial pressure	Vs	= Stroke volume
RA s	= Right atrial systolic	HR	= Heart rate

1. A relatively equal, single-stage, submaximal performance of 0.5 or 1 watt per kg lasting at least 6 and at most 10 minutes, in which numerous continuous or repeated individual readings can be obtained at a sufficiently long-lasting relative steady state (Schmutzler, 1).
2. A stage-by-stage increasing submaximal exercise (e.g., 2-minute 25-watt or 1-minute 10-watt stages over a period of 6 to 10 minutes) during which fewer data can be gathered but those gathered can be pin-pointed in the several exercise levels.

The first procedure is attractive when a comprehensive picture of quantitative changes in circulatory dynamics is to be obtained with cardiac catheterization. Warm-up and recovery time behave proportionally to the magnitude of the exercise and inversely so to the individual's performance capacity. If no relative steady state sets in during uniform performance, then the performance limit has been exceeded. On the other hand, a relative steady state despite compensated circulation does not exclude the possibility of latent exercise insufficiency with elevated filling pressure and reduced contractility (Schmutzler, 2).

The second procedure for ergometric loading is suitable for qualitative and quantitative determination of coronary insufficiency by using an EKG (Kubicek, etc.) and measurement of left ventricular filling pressure by means of the application of a catheter (after Grandjean). The average filling pressure of the left ventricle can be measured as average pulmonary capillary pressure or diastolic pulmonary arterial pressure, the norms while at rest being regarded as perhaps 9 ± 3 mm Hg and, during a performance of 1 watt per kg of body weight, 16 ± 3 mm Hg (Schmutzler, 2) (see also Table 51).

III. Under normal conditions, with balanced vegetative tonus, the various parameters of the cardiovascular system are in dynamic equilibrium. At the center stands the regulation of pressure and volume, for the maintenance of circulatory sufficiency. Generally, the mode of reaction of a healthy heart and that of a compensated defective heart to an acute submaximal exercise can be regarded as similar. The agreement in regulation is shown by the fact that readings on the resting equilibrium during a short or long warm-up

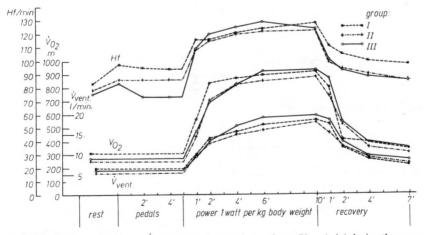

Fig. 164. HR, O_2 consumption ($\dot{V}_{O_2}$) and respiratory time-volume (V_{vent}/min) during the course of examination in individuals with healthy circulation (Group I) and those with pulmonary hypertension (mitral stenosis, Groups II and III).

(depending on the magnitude of the exercise level) achieve a relative steady state and carry out the same reaction in reverse after the exercise terminates (Fig. 164). The absolute readings may be subject to individual variation due to magnitude and duration of the exercise intensity, body posture, state of training and age.

The effects of various bodily postures on the resting and exercise readings of various circulatory factors are shown in Figure 165.

Table 51 affords an overview of pressure and volume data in individuals with normal pulmonary circulation and in those with pulmonary hypertension (see also Donald). The percentages of change in the criculation of normal individuals under relatively equal submaximal power of 1 watt per kg of body weight, compared with their resting values, are presented in Figure 166a. In all three groups the pressures in the pulmonary artery, left atrium and systemic arteries react simultaneously and similarly under graded exercise, even if with differing intensity (Schmutzler, 2). On the other hand, pure volume overloads of the pulmonary circulation (regurgitation defects) up to three times the norm cause no greater pressure overload than in those with

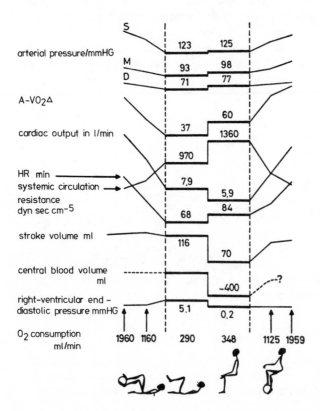

Fig. 165. Effects of various postures on the resting values and the reaction during exercise (pedaling ergometer) on three different circulatory factors. (Illustration is from Gauer and Thron's *Handbook of Physiology,* vol. 3, sec. 2, *Circulation*).

Table 52. Relationship between pressure and volume in the pulmonary circulation in patients with regurgitation defects, at rest (R) and in the relative steady state (E) of a power of 1 watt per kg of body weight (VSD = ventricular septal defect, ASD = atrial septal defect.

| | VSD n = 7 | | | | Ductus arteriosus n = 7 | | | | ASD n = 13 | | | |
| | R | | E | | R | | E | | R | | E | |
		±s		±s		±s		±s		±s		±s
Pulmonary arterial pressure avg. mm Hg	16.3	3.2	22.1	6.2	14.9	3.7	20.6	6.9	16.8	2.6	27.2	6.4
Pulmonary circulation MV 1/min	8.7	1.3	16.5	2.7	9.8	1.3	16.4	1.8	14.8	3.7	24.4	4.0

healthy circulatory systems. Only if the volume is still further increased is any increased pressure-loading recorded (Table 52) (Schmutzler et al.; Ekelund and Holmgren). Figures 166b and 166c present the relationships between cardiac output (Q) and O_2 consumption ($\dot{V}_{O_2}$) or pressures in the pulmonary artery and pulmonary capillaries.

In healthy individuals and patients with compensated heart defects, the cardiac output, as a product of stroke volume times heart rate, stands in direct linear relationship to the exercise up to 70% of the maximal O_2 consumption (Fig. 166b).

The relationship of HR to stroke volume is determined by an individually predominating sympathicotonic or vagotonic regulation (Heiss). Under exercise the sympathicotonic drive causes an increase in HR at only slight increase in volume in the untrained (there is also dependence on bodily posture—Figure 165, and Bühlmann and Gattiker).

The behavior under exercise of the pressures in the pulmonary and systemic circulations is the same. Systolic and average pressures increase distinctly while the diastolic pressure remains almost the same.

The circulatory resistances become reduced.

For assessment of overload insufficiency of the myocardium, the cardiac output, stroke volume, left ventricular filling pressure and contractility are measured. An inadequate increase in cardiac output (tachycardia and reduced stroke volume) and an end diastolic pressure load (elevated filling pressure) indicate myocardial workload insufficiency. In an angina pectoris attack, a left ventricular insufficiency with elevated end systolic volume and elevated end diastolic pressure occurs by way of myocardial ischemia (Fig. 167) (see also McCans and Parker). Because of the good correlation between average pressure in the left atrium, pulmonary capillary pressure and diastolic pressure in the pulmonary artery, the end diastolic pressure in the left ventricle (= diastolic pressure in the pulmonary artery) is relatively easy to measure with a catheter (Stürzenhofecker et al.). On the other hand, the

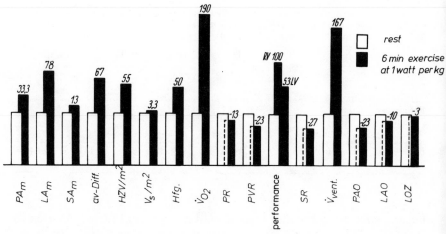

Fig. 166a. Circulatory dynamic factors in those with healthy circulation. Changes in averages in the steady state at a power of 1 watt per kg of body weight as compared with the starting values, in percentages. PA = pulmonary artery, LA = left auricle, SA = systemic artery, m = average pressure, PR = total pulmonary resistance, PVR = pulmonary arteriole resistance, RV = right ventricle, SR = systemic arterial resistance, LV = left ventricle, PAO = circulation times: PAO = PA to ear, LAO = LA to ear, LOZ = time from lung to ear. For absolute values, see Table 51.

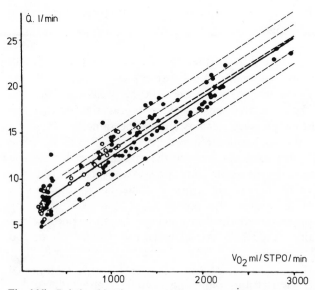

Fig. 166b. Relationships between cardiac output ($\dot{Q}$) and O_2 consumption ($\dot{V}_{O_2}$) at rest and during exercise while reclining in healthy men ♂ and women ♀. Thick line: regression line for all values. Thick broken line: regression line for all exercise levels. Thin broken lines: standard deviation $\pm 1\sigma$ and $\pm 2\sigma$ (after *Ekelund* and *Holmgren*).

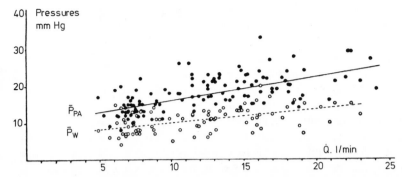

Fig. 166c. Relationships between average pressure in pulmonary artery (P_{PA}), pulmonary capillary pressure (P_W) and cardiac output ($\dot{Q}$) in healthy men and women (symbols same as in Fig. 166b) (after *Ekelund* and *Holmgren*).

ventricular volumes (end systolic and end diastolic volume) can be measured only with great technical dexterity—usually under exercise—by ventriculography, using contrast medium or indicator-washout curves (Kreuzer; Bussmann et al.; Kober et al.; Sharma et al.). The ejection reaction (EF) of the left ventricle (relationship of stroke volume to end diastolic volume):

$$EF = \frac{V_1 - V_2}{V_1} \times 100$$

(V_1 = end diastolic, V_2 = end systolic) is a sensitive yardstick for evaluating the myocardium and the functional condition of the heart (normal 60–90%)

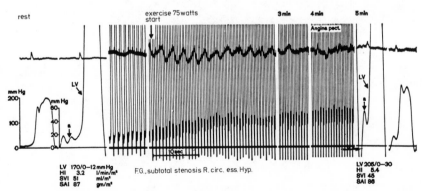

Fig. 167. Relation between abnormal hemodynamics and ischemic pain syndrome. Left: left-ventricular dynamics while at rest. Center and right: hemodynamics immediately upon starting, and 3, 4 and 5 minutes into the exercise. The increase in end diastolic pressure occurs immediately after start of exercise and attains its maximum some minutes before the pain starts. LV = left-ventricular systolic and diastolic pressure; HI = cardiac index; SVI = stroke volume index; SAI stroke-exercise index (after *Lichtelen* in *Schweizerische Rundschau für Medizin, Praxis*, 58, No. 5, 1969, p. 137).

(Schmutzler et al.). The relationship between stroke volume and end diastolic volume is linear with myocardial sufficiency. But if under exercise the
relative stroke volume decreases, there is an insufficiency reaction to exercise (see Roskamm and Reindell).

The same system of regulation is the basis of the correlation of total
cardiac volume (determined by x-ray) with maximal O_2 pulse, as recommended by Roskamm and Reindell.

Among the data on contractility are the speed-based parameters of the
isovolumetric phase (maximal speed of rise in pressure = dp/dt_{max}) and
those of the distribution phase (circumferential speed of abbreviation =
V_{CF}), which stand in close relation with one another (Sonnenblick et al.).

Figures 168 and 169 (by Roskamm, 1) show the close relationships
of dp after dt_{max} or $\dfrac{dp/dt}{p}$ to performance, HR and systolic ventricular pressure. The contractility reserve is a measure of performance reserve. During physical exercise, there comes about a considerable activation of the sympathetic stimulus to the heart and
therewith an increase in contractility (Braunwald et al.). Through

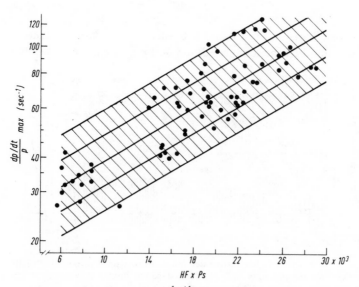

Fig. 168. The relationship between $\dfrac{dp/dt}{p}$ max and HR times P_{RV} in normal individuals aged
19 to 27. The $\pm 2\sigma$ normal range is indicated on semilogarithmic paper. This manner of presentation is best suited for use as a diagram of normal values (after *Roskamm*).

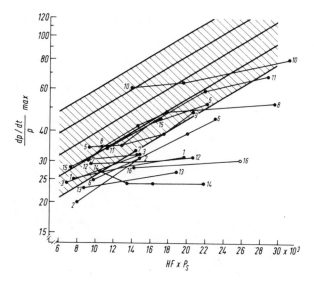

Fig. 169. The relationships between $\dfrac{dp/dt}{p}$ max and HR times P_{RV} while resting and during exercise in patients with primary noncoronary disease of the myocardium. Shaded area: normal range for healthy subjects (after *Roskamm*).

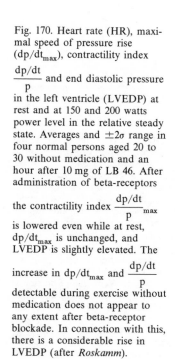

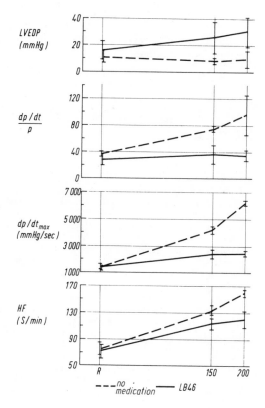

Fig. 170. Heart rate (HR), maximal speed of pressure rise (dp/dt_{max}), contractility index $\dfrac{dp/dt}{p}$ and end diastolic pressure in the left ventricle (LVEDP) at rest and at 150 and 200 watts power level in the relative steady state. Averages and $\pm 2\sigma$ range in four normal persons aged 20 to 30 without medication and an hour after 10 mg of LB 46. After administration of beta-receptors the contractility index $\dfrac{dp/dt}{p}_{max}$ is lowered even while at rest, dp/dt_{max} is unchanged, and LVEDP is slightly elevated. The increase in dp/dt_{max} and $\dfrac{dp/dt}{p}$ detectable during exercise without medication does not appear to any extent after beta-receptor blockade. In connection with this, there is a considerable rise in LVEDP (after *Roskamm*).

beta-receptor blockade, this effect can be largely eliminated (Fig. 170). Normal values for the left ventricle at rest: dp/dt_{max}: 1400 to 2200 mm Hg., $\dfrac{dp/dt}{p}$: 28 to 36 seconds^{-1}, V_{CF}: 1.2 circ/sec. For values at 150 and 200 watts power, see Fig. 170. These figures are obtained as follows: Measure the pressure by means of Tipp manometer (providing the true curve with accuracy of amplitude and frequency). With the aid of a differentiating instrument, the speed of rising pressure dp/dt is continuously recorded. From the partial signals dp/dt and p, the quotient dp/dt over p is continuously calculated with the aid of an electronic analog divider, and is recorded.

IV. Detailed knowledge of central hemodynamics during physical exertion can not be obtained without considerable technology. Of course, noninvasive methods, such as sphygmography or echocardiography, also occupy a prominent place in diagnostic work, but these have only relatively specialized uses, such as continuous observation, as compared with the invasive methods (Gleichmann et al.; Weissler).

An understanding of the physiologic and pathophysiologic regulation of the dynamics of the central circulation is of greatest importance in diagnosis as well as in therapy, not only in cardiology but also in practical sports and performance medicine.

References

Braunwald, E., E. H. Sonnenblick, J. Ross, Jr., G. Glick and S. E. Epstein: An analysis of the cardiac response to exercise. Circulation Res. XX/XXI. Suppl. I-44, 1967.

Bühlmann, A. and H. Gattiker: Herzzeitvolumen, Schlagvolumen und physische Arbeitskapazität. Schw. Med. Wschr. 94, (1964) 443.

Bussmann, W. D., G. Kober, R. Thaler, J. Heeger, R. Hopf, and M. Kaltenbach: Angiographische und hämodynamische Befunde des linken Ventrikels nach Volumenbelastung und körperlicher Arbeit bei Patienten mit koronarer Herzkrankheit Verh. Dtsch. Ges. Kreisl. Forschg. 41, 181 1975.

Donald, K. W.: Exercise studies in heart disease. Med. Conc. Cardiovasc. Dis. XXVIII, (1959) 529.

Ekelund, L.-G. and A. Holmgren: Central hemodynamics during exercise; Central research XX, Suppl. 1-33, 1967.

Gleichmann, U., A. Neitzert, H. M. Mertens, H. Schmidt, U. Sigwart and J. Steiner: Comparison between systolic time intervals and left ventricular pressure and volume changes at rest and during exercise. In: Ventricular Function at Rest and during Exercise, by Roskamm, H. and Hahn, Ch., S. 44-48. Springer, Berlin, 1976.

Heiss, H. W.: Coronary blood flow at rest and during exercise. In: Ventricular Function at Rest and during Exercise, by Roskamm, H. and Hahn, Ch., pp. 17-20. Springer, Berlin, 1976.

Kober, G., W. D. Bussmann, R. Hopf, R. Thaler and M. Kaltenbach: Beurteilung der Ventrikelfunktion aus dem Angiogramm.

Qualitative und quantitative Methoden. Herz/Kreislauf 8/4, p. 180, 1976.

Kreuzer, H.: Ventrikelvolumina und ihre Beziehung zur Herzinsuffizienz. In: Herzinsuffizienz, p. 446, Georg Thieme, Stuttgart 1968.

Kubicek, F.: Bemerkungen zum methodischen Vorgehen beim ergometrischen Arbeitsversuch. Wien. Klin. Wschr. 84, (1972) 522.

McCans, J. L. and J. O. Parker: Left ventricular pressure-volume relationships during myocardial ischemia in man. Circulation XLVIII, 775, 1973.

Roskamm, H. (1): Zur Frage der Indikationen und Kontraindikationen dosierten Trainings in der rehabilitativen Cardiologie. In: Mellerowicz, Rehabilitative Cardiologie, S. Karger, Basel 1974.

Roskamm, H. (2): Hämodynamik und Kontraktilität des gesunden und kranken Herzens bei körperlicher Belastung. Verh. Dtsch. Ges. Kreisl.-Forschg. 37, (1971) 42.

Roskamm, H. and H. Reindell: Belastungsprüfungen in der Cardiologie. Internist 11/8, (1970) 278.

Roskamm, H. and H. Reindell: In: Herzkrankheiten, pp. 321–336. Springer, Berlin-New York 1977.

Schmutzler, H. (1): Methode und Wert ergometrischer Studien während der Herzkatheteruntersuchung. L'ergometrie en Cardiologie. Boehringer (Mannheim), p. 191, 1967.

Schmutzler, H. (2): Die Kreislaufdynamik der Mitralstenose unter konstanter Arbeit. Bibl. Cardiol. 25,4. S. Karger, Basel 1969.

Schmutzler, H., H. Paeprer, H.-W. Liebenschütz (1): Der Wert der Arbeitsbelastung für die quantitative Katheterdiagnostik des kranken Herzens. Verh. Detsch. Ges. Kreisl.-Forschg. 37, (1971) 192.

Schmutzler, H., G. Grosse, W. Rutsch, H. Paeprer, U. Michel and Th. Krais (2): Ventricular function in valvular heart disease before and after prosthetic valve surgery. In: Ventricular Function at Rest and during Exercise, by Roskamm, H. and Hahn, Ch., pp. 125–128. Springer, Berlin, 1976.

Sharma, B., S. Raina, J. F. Goodwin, M. J. Raphael and R. E. Steiner: Raphael and R. E. Steiner: Ventriculography in coronary heart disease. In: Coronary Angiography and Angina Pectoris, pp. 133–151, Symposium of the European Society of Cardiology. Hannover, Georg Thieme, 1975.

Sonnenblick, E. H., E. Braunwald, J. F. Williams and G. Glick: Effects of exercise on myocardial force-velocity relations in intact unanesthetized man. J. clin. Invest. 44, (1965) 12.

Stürzenhofecker, P., K. Schnellbacher and H. Roskamm: Cardiac output and filling pressures at rest and during exercise. In: Ventricular Function at Rest and during Exercise, by Roskamm, H. and Hahn, Ch., pp. 26–30. Springer, Berlin, 1976.

Weissler, A. M.: Systolic time intervals at rest and during exercise. In: Ventricular Function at Rest and during Exercise, by Roskamm, H. and Hahn, Ch., pp. 39–43. Springer, Berlin, 1976.

XV. Additional Performance Functions Applicable to Ergometric Diagnostics

1. Ergometric Oximetry

by Horst Schmutzler

Combining oximetry with ergometry expands the stress test, so important in functional diagnosis of respiration and circulation, by checking the O_2 saturation in the flowing blood (Fig. 171).

By "oximetry" is understood the determination of the oxygen saturation of the blood in percent with the aid of photoelectric methods. The significance of oximetry in ergometry lies less in gaining absolute data on the O_2 saturation, for whose determination the analysis of samples of arterial blood is more precise, than in continuously recording possible changes in the O_2 saturation through bloodless measurement in the tissues themselves.

The possibility of measuring the O_2 saturation of the blood photometrically depends on the following principle: The absorption of light rays is an optical property of hemoglobin that depends on concentration. By measuring the light absorption of a solution of hemoglobin and oxyhemoglobin in the long-wave spectrum range between 600 and 700 mμ it is possible, with the aid of the Lambert-Beer law (linear relationship between the log of the amount of light let through and the O_2 content of the blood), to determine the concentration of the hemoglobin and oxyhemoglobin simultaneously in one and the same blood sample, since the extinction curves of the two forms of hemoglobin behave differently. Kramer confirmed in 1934, by means of a cuvette method in vitro, the applicability of the Lambert-Beer law even to whole blood, and Matthes was the first to apply the photoelectric method to measuring blood in man, in 1935. He demonstrated that measurements

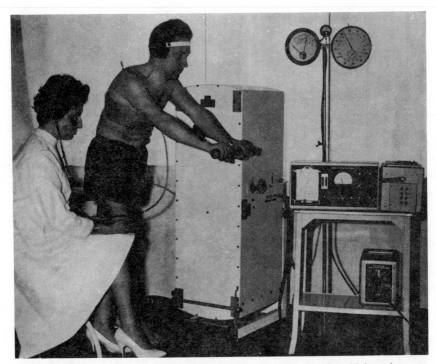

Fig. 171. Oximetric examination during ergometric exercise on the Lauckner Universal ergometer (Lauckner Co., Kurfürstenstr. 7a, Berlin-Mariendorf), using the Atlas oximeter (Atlas-Werke, Bremen, Germany) (ear lobe transmission method), with recording by the Hartmann & Braun (Frankfurt am Main, Germany) Ultra-violet Direktschreiber recorder.

made in a layer of tissue filled with capillaries are subject to the same regularity as a hemoglobin solution in the cuvette. The only requirement is that the blood flow in the area being studied, for example, in the ear lobe, be greatly intensified, by means of histamine-ionophoresis, among other things; then the O_2 delivery becomes so slight in comparison with the intensified blood flow that the O_2 saturation of the venous blood is approximately the same as that of the arterial. Whether these conditions are sufficiently fulfilled for measuring arterial O_2 saturation can be double-checked according to Matthes by altering the pressure of the alveolar O_2. The conditions are optimal as soon as the oximeter reacts to alterations in the alveolar O_2 oxygen pressure with only a lag corresponding to the time taken for circulation from the lungs to the measurement area.

Kramer has recently called attention to the fact that measurement on flowing blood does involve deviations from the Lambert-Beer law, since the linear relationships of the O_2 saturation and the logarithms of the amount of penetrating light are also dependent on the concentration of erythrocytes.

The invasive and bloodless methods in use today both operate on the principles of transmission or reflection of light (Fig. 172), the difference, simply expressed, being that in the transmission procedure the light source and the photocell are on opposite sides of the blood, while in the reflection method light source and photocell are both on the same side of the blood and, of course, of the tissue sample.

The principle of the transmission method consists in the fact that the translucency of the blood in vitro or in vivo is measured in two different wavelength ranges. Since change in blood volume must have an effect on absorption in red light and thus may disguise changes in saturation, it seemed the obvious thing to do to measure the light absorption also in a second infrared wavelength range in which it is dependent only on the hemoglobin content and not on the degree of saturation. Thus with the second photocell the effect of the total pigment concentration on the reading of the first photocell can be eliminated. Since it may happen that the compensation for the changes in blood vessel filling in ergometric exercise is not quite enough (Ulmer), it may be necessary for scientific purposes to record the hemoglobin reading, which varies with the filling of the vessels, by means of absorption in the infrared.

Millikan's oximeter found wide acceptance, although no absolute measurement of O_2 saturation percentages was possible with it, but only the ascertainment of changes in saturation. Wood developed an oximeter in

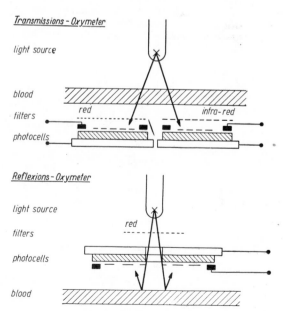

Fig. 172. Principles of the transmission and reflection oximeters (after *Zijlstra*).

1949 by which absolute readings of saturation can be read. Additional, present-day, useful transmission oximeters are the Nilsson and the Atlas (from Atlas-Werke, Bremen, Germany).

In the reflection method light reflected from tissue surfaces—for example, the forehead or finger—is measured to determine the O_2 saturation. This reflection is dependent on O_2 saturation in the same way as is transmitted light. But in this method, also, the total content of hemoglobin and oxyhemoglobin concentration must be taken into consideration. On this reflection principle are based Brinkmann's Hämoreflektor for invasive measurement and the Cyclop for tissue measurement. A further reflective oximeter was constructed in 1951 by Bühlmann in cooperation with Sigrist.

According to Zijlstra, the following advantages are inherent in the reflection principle: First, the amount of light reflected is largely independent of the total concentration of hemoglobin. Therefore, only one spectral band need be measured. In addition, the amount of light reflected is a far greater

Table 53. Normal values for O_2 in healthy men while at rest (sea level) (after *Bartels, Bücherl, Hertz, Rodewald* and *Schwab*).

	Average	$\pm S_x$	$\pm S_{\bar{x}}$	Minimum	Maximum	Number of examinations	Method
Arterial blood Femoral or brachial artery							
O_2 pressure mm Hg	94.2	5.3	1.5	83	102	13	I
	93.0	5.6	0.7	80	104	59	II
O_2 content ml O_2/100 ml blood	19.6	1.2	0.2	17.3	22.3	50	III
	19.1	1.1	0.2	17.6	21.2	31	III
O_2 capacity ml O_2/100 ml	19.6	1.6	0.3	17.0	23.1	29	III
	19.9	1.3	0.2	17.8	21.6	42	III
Percentage O_2 saturation of the blood	95.8	—	—	93	98	154	III
	97.4	1.8	0.4	93.2	101.4	17	III a
	95.6	2.7	0.5	90.5	99.0	31	III b
Mixed venous blood Pulmonary artery (internal jugular vein)							
O_2 pressure mm Hg	39.4	5.76	1.9	29.5	48.5		I
O_2 content ml O_2/100 ml blood	15.0	1.20	0.4	12.6	16.4	9	III
	12.99	1.3	0.2	11.0	16.1	50	III
A-VO$_2\Delta$ ml O_2/100 ml blood	4.2	0.78	0.26	3.2	5.8	9	III
	6.7	0.8	0.1	4.5	8.5	50	III
Percentage O_2 saturation of the blood	76.8	3.85	1.28	70.1	81.9	9	III
	61.8	3.7	0.5	55.3	70.7	50	III

fraction of the light input than is transmitted light. In the reflection methods, a greater part of the light reaches the photocell than in the transmission method. Consequently, weaker light sources and less sensitive galvanometers can be used. With the Hämoreflektor, percentages of O_2 saturation are measured by means of a calibration curve. Individual calibration curves must be set up with two points for fully saturated and for O_2-poor blood, bearing in mind that the calibration curve runs linearly from 0 to 100% oxyhemoglobin. This is also true of the transmission oximeter. According to recent studies by Wood, however, there are no strongly linear relationships in the range of O_2 saturations of 90 to 100%.

Van Slyke's manometric method for calibrating the photometer or oximeter is the one generally used. The surest procedure is to relate the data obtained from analysis of arterial blood to the deviations of the galvanometer as measured at the time. According to Zijlstra, the standard deviation of 36 measurements with a Hämoreflektor, compared with cuvette measurements, amounted to between 38 and 99% of oxyhemoglobin $\pm$ 2.3%. By way of comparison, in 211 comparative manometric analyses using the Wood oximeter, the standard deviation amounted to between 13 and 100% of oxyhemoglobin $\pm$ 2.4%. The precision of oximetric measurement is directly dependent on constancy of blood perfusion at the measurement site.

The O_2 saturation of arterial blood in a healthy person at rest is 97.1 $\pm$ 3.1%, according to Mitschell et al. A survey of the behavior of arterial readings on arterial O_2 in healthy men at sea level is given in Table 53, after Bartels et al. Mitschell et al. found in the brachial and femoral arteries resting readings of 52.6% of O_2 $\pm$ 12.9 and 37.9% of O_2 $\pm$ 16.2, respectively, and after heavy labor 24.9% $\pm$ 7.8 and 19.9% $\pm$ 8.8, respectively.

According to Matthes, the venous O_2 saturation in normal individuals amounts to between 62 and 80% at rest and between 41 and 60% after heavy physical labor.

The O_2 saturation of arterial blood depends on diffusion conditions and O_2 pressure in the alveolae of the lungs, the pH of the blood, CO_2 pressure in the blood and alveolae and blood temperature (Figs. 173a-c). Thus, for example, muscular exercise, through the evolution of acid metabolic products, causes a drop in the O_2 binding curve and thus an increase in O_2 supply to the exercising muscle tissue.

According to Grosse-Brockhoff, the following aberrations are to be regarded as causes of arterial undersaturation with O_2 brought about by a lowering of arterial O_2 pressure:

1. Lowered O_2 content of the inhaled air (as when ascending to great altitudes)
2. Disturbances to the external respiration (by reason of respiratory mechanics, pneumonia, atelectasis, pulmonary edema)

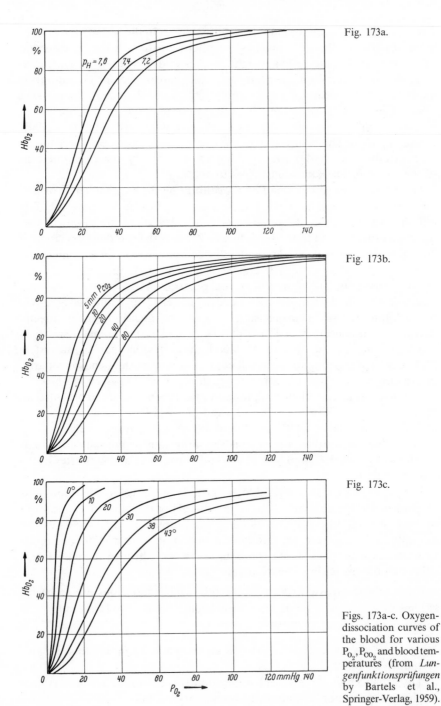

Fig. 173a.

Fig. 173b.

Fig. 173c.

Figs. 173a-c. Oxygen-dissociation curves of the blood for various P_{O_2}, P_{CO_2} and blood temperatures (from *Lungenfunktionsprüfungen* by Bartels et al., Springer-Verlag, 1959).

3. Development of bypasses (right-to-left shunt)
4. Formation of methemoglobin
5. Retarded blood circulation in local or general vascular disturbances.

As the method of choice, Bühlmann suggests that, in a sequence of increasing workload stages of from 10 to 30 watts, it be ascertained at which stage full arterial saturation is just steadily maintained.

Venrath et al. point to the following mechanisms of disturbance of oximetric recording during physical exercise:

1. Relative retardations in blood flow in noninvolved areas are able to appear as arterial undersaturation with greater venous exhaustion during recording.
2. Changes in the hemoglobin content of the blood can exist that can not be controlled at the point of measurement (Knipping, Bolt, Valentin and Venrath).

These influences seem, however, to be of more theoretical than practical importance in standardized ergometric methodology.

It should be emphasized that ergometric oximetry is of great value in routine examinations. More refined studies, which are calculated to afford detailed insight into physiologic and pathologic respiratory processes in physical stress, do not replace it. Such studies can only be performed by means of spirometry and analysis of blood gases, in the course of which CO_2 content, CO_2 pressure and pH are determined. Especially when there is

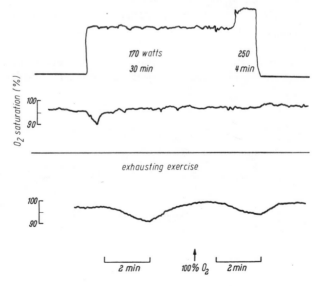

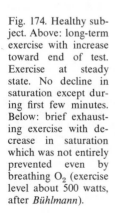

Fig. 174. Healthy subject. Above: long-term exercise with increase toward end of test. Exercise at steady state. No decline in saturation except during first few minutes. Below: brief exhausting exercise with decrease in saturation which was not entirely prevented even by breathing O_2 (exercise level about 500 watts, after *Bühlmann*).

suspicion of disturbances of diffusion, the combination with direct analysis of blood gases is valuable in order to differentiate more clearly the cause of the oximetrically measured drop in O_2 saturation.

There is wide agreement among various authors (Bühlmann; Bühlmann and Schaub; Christensen and Högberg; Comroe; and Walker, among others) that a drop in saturation in the arterial blood of healthy individuals occurring only at very heavy levels of physical exercise is still regarded as normal (Fig. 174). This phenomenon is caused by acidosis arising from heavy exercise and elevation of CO_2 pressure in the blood and resulting displacement of the O_2 binding curve. An increase in the flow of the blood in the pulmonary capillaries above a critical point may also play a role. When a physiologic borderline flow of blood is exceeded, the time spent by the hemoglobin molecules in the alveolar blood may be insufficient for complete saturation with oxygen.

Bühlmann found no drop in O_2 saturation in healthy men exercising at powers up to 200 to 250 watts, except in the first two to three minutes (Fig. 174). This initial drop in saturation is explained through a relative delay in the increase in lung ventilation as compared with O_2 consumption. Doll et al. found neither a significant decline of O_2 saturation nor a drop in arterial O_2 pressure in twenty untrained men at an average maximal power of 212 watts. On the other hand, Friehoff regularly found a drop in arterial O_2 pressure (but not in O_2 saturation) in 45 untrained and trained men at powers of 90 to 200 watts. Trained men capable of high-level performance can very probably perform at still higher levels without significant undersaturation of the blood with O_2. At top powers, O_2 undersaturation does occur even in highly trained individuals (together with hypercapnia and acidosis), which in many instances can not be completely compensated for even through breathing O_2 to heighten alveolar partial O_2 pressure (Fig. 174).

Under pathological conditions of respiratory and cardiac insufficiency of various etiologies (page 193), there can occur considerable reduction of the

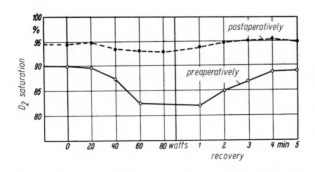

Fig. 175. Graphic representation of the behavior of O_2 saturation under exercise before and after commissurotomy of a mitral stenosis. The decline in saturation is only slight after the operation, whereas it was 7% previously (after *Buhr*).

O_2 saturation, especially during exertion and depending on the magnitude of the exercise.

In disturbances of ventilation as well as of diffusion of various etiologies, including cardiac, the amount of arterial undersaturation corresponds to the extent of functional damage and the magnitude of the exercise. Also, for assessing the effects of heart surgery (Fig. 175) and for determining performance limits both pre- and postoperatively, it is important to check the O_2 saturation in an ergometric test.

In summary, it may be said that ergometric oximetry is a suitable method for determining the limit of cardiopulmonary performance, which is characterized by a significant drop in arterial O_2 saturation. Both the transmission and reflection methods are practically useful if critically and knowledgeably evaluated.

References

Bartels, H., E. S. Bücherl, C. W. Hertz, G. Rodewald and M. Schwab: Lungenfunktionsprüfungen. Berlin-Göttingen-Heidelberg: Springer, 1959.

Brinkmann, R.: in Firma Kipp, Delft/Holland.

Bühlmann, A.: Helv. physiol. pharmacol. acta 9, (1951); Schweiz, med. Wschr. 16, (1951) 374.

Bühlmann, A., F. Schaub and P. Luchsinger: Schweiz, med. Wschr. 11, (1955) 253.

Buhr, G.: Klinische Oxymetrie, in: Kramer, Oxymetrie. Stuttgart: Thieme, 1960.

Christensen, E. H. and P. Högberg: Arbeitsphysiologie 14, (1950) 251.

Comroe, J. H. and P. Walker: Amer. J. Physiol. 152, (1948) 365.

Doll, König and H. Reindell: Pflügers Arch. Physiol. 271, (1960) 283. Pflügers Arch. Physiol. 270, (1960) 431.

Grosse-Brockhoff, F.: Klin. Wschr. 23, (1944) 145.

Knipping, H. W., W. Bolt, H. Valentin and H. Venrath: Untersuchung und Beurteilung des Herzkranken. Stuttgart: Enke, 1959.

Knipping H. W. and H. Valentin: Münchner medizinische Wochenschrift 1, (1961) 11.

Kramer, K.: Oxymetrie. Stuttgart: Thieme, 1960.

Matthes, K.: Kreislaufuntersuchungen am Menschen mit fortlaufenden registrierenden Methoden. Stuttgart: Thieme, 1951.

McIlroy, M. B.: Brit. Heart J. XXI/3, (1959) 293.

Millikan: zit. nach Wood, Oxymetrie, in: Medical Physics, Ed. by Otto Glaser (Chicago) 2, (1950) 644.

Mitchell, J. H., B. J. Sproule and C. B. Chapman: J. Clin. Invest. 37, 4, (1958) 538.

N.J.: Pflügers Arch. Physiol. 262, (1956) 595; 263, (1956) 374.

Ulmer, W. T.: Zschr. Kreisl.-Forschg. 49, (1960) 461.

Venrath, H., H. Valentin and W. Hollmann: Ärztl. Wschr. 526 (1955).

Wood, E. H.: Oxymetrie, in: Medical Physics, Ed. by Otto Glaser (Chicago) 2, (1950) 644.

Zijlstra, W. G.: Fundamentals and application of clinical oxymetry. Assen: Van Gorcum & Comp., 1953.

2. Arterial Blood Gases and Acid-Base Balance in Ergometric Performance

by Fritz A. Schön and Elmar Waterloh

2.1 Methodology of Measurement of Arterial Blood Gases

The development of reliable procedures for microanalysis has contributed essentially to the fact that blood gas analysis today has become an important part of spiroergometric performance studies, chiefly in the area of clinical diagnosis of pulmonary disease and preoperative evaluation of pulmonary function. It has additional applicability in intensive care, in monitoring artificial respiration, cardiac diagnostics and sports medicine.

2.1.1 Obtaining Samples

For blood gas analysis, arterial blood or "arterialized blood" from the ear lobe is used. The capillary blood comes from the arterioles when it flows freely after a puncture of the skin. Squeezing the ear lobe leads to venous admixture and thus to false readings. In order to create a state of local hyperemia, leading to more plentiful bleeding, salves containing nicotinic acid ester are an old standby. It takes only ten minutes to produce complete arterialization in the ear lobe region. Ulmer et al. (1963) succeeded in proving, in the course of comparative studies on subjects free of pulmonary disease, that there are no differences in blood gas and pH readings between arterial blood and capillary blood from the ear lobe. Reichel et al. (1966) were able to confirm these findings in a large population of heart and lung patients.

The correctness and reproducibility of readings depend on the following points:

A. Avoiding contact with air when taking capillary blood. Blood emanating from the ear lobe is caught in heparinized glass capillary tubes about 10 cm long and with a capacity of about 100 μl each. In doing so the tip of the tube should be inserted into the center of the forming drop of blood. To avoid contact with the air and consequent loss of CO_2, Reichel et al. (1966) recommend small plexiglass funnels which can be slipped tightly over the tips of the tubes.

B. Complete prevention of coagulation. Sodium heparinate in a solution of about 0.55 mg per ml of blood serves as anticoagulant. Other anticoagulants such as oxalate, citrate and EDTA are unsuitable since they upset the acid-base parameters.

C. As quick processing as possible. After the blood has been taken, the blood cells, especially the leucocytes, are still metabolically active. Therefore, blood specimens should be analyzed within a few minutes of being taken. If for technical reasons this is impossible, the blood samples must be preserved for analysis in ice water or at refrigerator temperatures of 0 to 4°C. At this temperature range, the glycolytic activity of the blood cells is sufficiently reduced so that changes in the acid-base parameters by acid metabolites may be expected to be delayed for up to two hours.

2.1.2 Measurement of Arterial Partial O_2 Pressure

Structure of the electrode: O_2 partial pressures in fluids and tissues can be measured polarographically with the aid of stabilized all-glass-platinum electrodes. Figure 176 shows the construction of a platinum electrode on the Clark principle.

The measuring and reference electrodes lie together behind a 25-μ teflon membrane that is able to transmit gas but turns back liquids. By this means the electrolyte and the electrode are separated from the analysis fluids and to a great extent protected from soiling and chemical reaction. The platinum

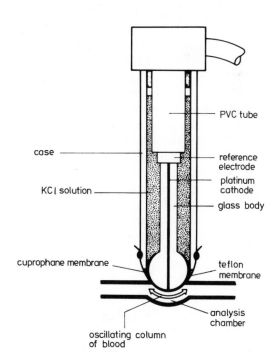

Fig. 176. Schematic construction of a P_{O_2} electrode.

core is embedded free of air bubbles in the glass while the latter is in a molten state. A silver–silver chloride electrode serves as reference electrode and is enclosed in a PVC tube except for its tip, so that the upper surface of the silver dipping into the KCl remains constant even at various filling levels of the electrode housing. The carrier electrolyte is a saturated or phosphate-buffered KCl solution which forms the electrically conducting medium between the platinum and reference electrodes. A piece of cuprophane about 10 μ thick between the platinum tip and the teflon membrane keeps the gap constant. Thus shifts in calibration, caused by mechanical effect on the membrane, are avoided.

Measuring principle: The O_2 diffuses through the membrane and is reduced at the negatively charged platinum tip.

$$O_2 + 4e^- \rightarrow 2\,O^{--}$$

This current flow (reducing current) is dependent on the number of O_2 molecules reaching the tip of the electrode per unit of time. From the magnitude of the reduction current a conclusion can be drawn as to the concentration of O_2 and thus as to the partial O_2 pressure.

2.1.3   Measurement of the Arterial Hydrogen Ion Concentration

Structure of the electrode: For determining the concentration of hydrogen ions in the analysis of blood gases, only glass microelectrodes are used. Figure 177 shows the schematic construction of a chain of glass electrodes.

A glass membrane made of special glass separates the solution being measured from an inner reference solution, which is usually buffered potassium chloride or dilute HCl. Into this reference solution dips a lead-off electrode made of silver and silver chloride. A further important member of the chain of glass electrodes is the reference electrode, which is electrically connected to the solution being measured via an electrolyte bridge. In the illustration is shown a saturated calomel electrode, in which a platinum wire dips into a layer of mercury which forms a precipitate layer with mercurous chloride (calomel). A saturated KCl solution serves as electrolytic bridge. It is either in direct electrical contact with the solution being measured, via a capillary cleft, as shown in Figure 177, or separated from it by a clay or porcelain diaphragm permitting ions to pass through.

Measuring principle: Membranes of glass electrodes are such that when dipped into an aqueous solution they form, through swelling in the border layers, so-called phase-border potentials between the swelled layer and the aqueous solution. Depending on the pH of the solution being measured, differences of concentration develop between the hydrogen and hydroxyl ions of the aqueous solution and those of the swelled layer. The differences

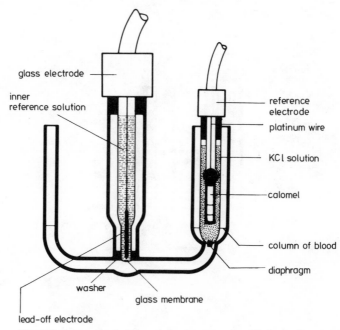

glass electrode

inner
reference solution

reference
electrode

platinum wire

KCl solution

calomel

column of blood

diaphragm

washer

glass membrane

lead-off electrode

Fig. 177. Schematic drawing of the structure of a pH electrode.

in potential that are to be measured are then dependent exclusively on the pH of the solution, since the concentration of hydrogen ions in the inner reference solution is constant.

2.1.4   Measurement of Arterial Partial CO_2 Pressure

Structure of the electrode: The electrode system for direct measurement of the partial CO_2 pressure corresponds essentially to the structure of a glass electrode chain. Figure 178 shows the schematic structure for measuring P_{CO_2}.

The gas electrode is in a millimolar solution of $NaHCO_3$ and is separated by a 12-μ teflon membrane from the solution actually being measured. This membrane lets CO_2 through but is impervious to ions which could alter the pH of the bicarbonate solution. An intermediate layer of nylon cloth serves to stabilize the electrode, keeping the fluid cleft between the teflon and glass membranes. A saturated calomel electrode is used as a reference electrode and is housed in a separate vessel, being in communication, through a diaphragm, with the bicarbonate solution of the glass electrode. A further possibility is the use of silver and silver chloride as a reference electrode, in the

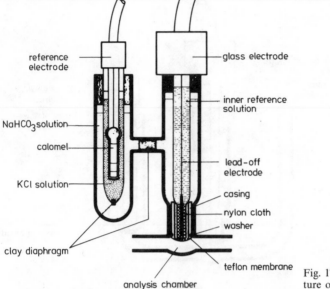

reference electrode

glass electrode

inner reference solution

NaHCO₃solution

calomel

KCl solution

lead-off electrode

casing

nylon cloth

washer

clay diaphragm

teflon membrane

analysis chamber

Fig. 178. Schematic structure of a P_{CO_2} electrode.

form of the single measuring chain for P_{CO_2} housed in the same vessel as the glass electrode. A disadvantage of this, as compared with the calomel electrode, is the somewhat lower stability, since silver electrodes show drift phenomena if the chloride coating is not uniform.

Measuring principle: CO_2 diffuses through the teflon membrane into the bicarbonate solution until both media are of the same CO_2 pressure. The CO_2 is first hydrated to H_2CO_3 and then dissociates into H^+ and HCO_3^- ions. The increase in H^+ ions alters the pH of the bicarbonate solution, which the glass electrode finally shows as a difference in potential. From the Henderson-Hasselbalch equation (for further details see Siggaard-Andersen, 1974), it is seen that the pH is a linear function of the decade logarithm of the arterial carbon dioxide partial pressure divided by the hydrogen concentration.

2.1.5 Measuring Device for the Combined Determination of the Arterial P_{O_2}, P_{CO_2} and pH

Instrument manufacturers in Germany and other countries today offer a number of blood gas analyzers that are very competent and easy to use. In structure and function of the electrode system, there are no basic differences among the several instrument types. On the basis of the restricted size of the analysis chambers and the special arrangement of the electrodes, the simultaneous measurement of the arterial P_{O_2}, P_{CO_2} and pH is possible only in blood samples 100 to 200 μl in volume. Since all readings are highly dependent on temperature, constancy of temperature in both the blood phase and the gas phase is of primary importance. The same is true of the full saturation of the calibrating gases with water vapor. All measurements are made at a temperature of 37 °C. To temper the electrodes, analysis chambers and gas lines, water bath thermostats with sufficient pumping effects and a range of regulation of only $\pm$ 0.05 °C are generally used. Figure 179 shows the Combi-Analysator MT supplied by the firm of Eschweiler, in Kiel, Germany.

In the left half is located all the electronic gear of the measuring devices, in the right is the water-tempered glass triple-measuring unit, affording a convenient visual check on the electrodes and the analysis chamber. The water bath thermostat, suction device and the entire gas feed system are in the right side of the housing. Cleaning and calibration are, as in most such instruments, largely mechanized, making for ease of operation and handling. The fully automatic blood gas analyzers represent the latest developments in specialized technology and are well adapted for use by the majority

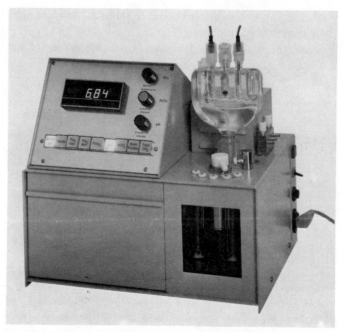

Fig. 179. Combi-Analysator from the firm of Eschweiler, Kiel, Germany.

of users or for intensive around-the-clock operation. They are known as the ABL 1 (from Hillerkus, Uerdinger Str. 463, D-415 Krefeld), AVL 940 (from AVL GmbH, Dietigheimer Str. 3, D-6830 Bad Homburg), IL 613 (from Instrumentation Laboratory Boskamp GmbH, Klein-Str. 14, D-5303 Hersel) and Technicon BG (From Technicon GmbH, Im Rosengarten 11, D-6368 Bad Vilbel 1), all from Germany.

2.1.6   Calibration and Quality Control

As a rule for calibration of the P_{O_2} and P_{CO_2} electrodes, two calibrating gases are used whose upper calibrating value should lie in the neighborhood of the expected readings. Calibration of the pH unit is done by means of two phosphate buffer mixtures.

To ensure quality operation in analysis of blood gases, control solutions are available that cover both the normal and pathological ranges. The solutions are stable for one to two years at room temperature in their glass ampules. Once opened, the contents must under no circumstances be exposed to the air for longer than a single moment, since changes in the concentrations of the dissolved gases occur very rapidly. The following relative standard deviations are at present regarded as acceptable and may be used to calculate the warning and checking limits: pH: $\pm 0.2\%$, P_{O_2} and P_{CO_2}: $\pm 5\%$.

According to the International System of Measurement Units (SI), pressure is measured in pascals (Pa). To make it easier to get oriented in the new system, the following conversion factors are given for mm Hg.:

Old Unit	Conversion Factor	SI Unit
mm Hg	$\xrightarrow{0.1333}$ $\xleftarrow{7.5020}$	kPa

2.2   Parameters of Arterial Blood Gas Analysis and Acid-Base Balance

2.2.1   Arterial O_2 Partial Pressure

In older textbooks on physiology of the lungs, a normal value of 12.0 kPa (90 mm Hg) is usually given as the normal value for arterial O_2 partial pressure. Studies on the behavior of P_{O_2} in conjunction with age and sex, such as those by Loew and Thews (1962), Ulmer et al. (1963), Lange and Hertle (1968), and others, show a distinct age-dependency, as will be seen from Figure 180.

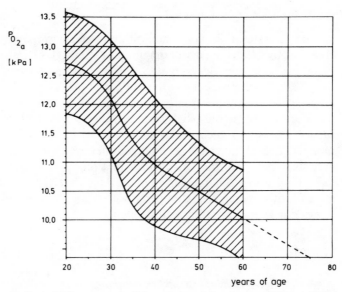

Fig. 180. Dependence of arterial P_{O_2} on age in 390 employees (after *Loew* and *Thews*, 1962).

Below are the regression formulas of Ulmer et al. (1970), obtained from the P_{O_2} readings on 1200 men and 741 women, all with sound lungs and of various ages:

$$P_{O_2}\,(\male) = 109.4 - 0.26 \cdot \text{age in years} - 0.098 \cdot \text{Broca index} \; (\pm\,14.14;\; p < 0.05)$$
$$P_{O_2}\,(\female) = 108.86 - 0.26 \cdot \text{age in years} - 0.073 \cdot \text{Broca index} \; (\pm\,15.11;\; p < 0.05)$$

$$\text{Broca index} = \frac{\text{body weight}}{\text{height} - 100} \cdot 100$$
$$= \frac{\text{kg}}{\text{cm} - 100} \cdot 100$$

With equal Broca index and equal age, the arterial P_{O_2} in women is about 0.2 kPa above the figure for men.

Circulatory, restrictive and also less severe obstructive distribution anomalies are named as the main causes of the age-linked decrease in oxygen partial pressure. Body posture is also a significant influence.

Ulmer et al. (1963) succeeded in demonstrating that resting P_{O_2} is, on the average, 0.5 kPa lower when sitting than when reclining. In addition, there are considerable individual variations in the arterial P_{O_2} while resting, which according to Geisler and Rost (1971) can amount to 0.8–1.3 kPa, and can in individual instances be as much as 2.7 kPa.

Corrected diurnal variations could not be verified.

2.2.2   Arterial O_2 Saturation

Arterial O_2 saturation is obtained within the framework of blood gas analysis either by means of curve nomograms (Thews, 1967), with the aid of the blood gas slide rule (Severinghaus, 1966) or by special computer programs (Fig. 181). It is dependent on arterial P_{O_2} and pH. The O_2 dissociation curves on page 286 present this clearly. As can be seen from the way the curves run, O_2 saturation varies only slightly in the range of arterial pressure because of the flat nature of the curve. Here the arterial P_{O_2} is the more sensitive parameter. The relation changes if we consider the lower (venous) ranges. The very steep nature of this curve shows that the O_2 saturation figures change more than do the O_2 pressure figures. This time the O_2 saturation is the more sensitive parameter. Compared with the arterial P_{O_2}, the normal range of arterial O_2 saturation is well defined.

Normal range: 94-98%

2.2.3   Parameters of the Acid-Base Balance

The acid-base parameters can be arranged in three different components, as shown in Table 54, below.

Table 54. Components of the acid-base balance.

Component for hydrogen ion concentration	Respiratory component	Metabolic component
pH (Balance value for respiratory and metabolic processes)	PCO_2	Active bicarbonate Standard bicarbonate Buffer bases Base deviation

Arterial pH: Arterial hydrogen ion concentration shows no age dependency. While the subject is at rest the concentration lies within relatively narrow limits. To be sure, the averages differ in women by +0.007 pH units as compared with men, but in practice it has proved to be desirable and sufficient to consider the normal range for both sexes as being the same.

Normal range: pH 7.36 to 7.44

Arterial CO_2 partial pressure: An age-dependent relationship could not be shown for the arterial P_{CO_2} either. There are mean differences of 0.4 kPa for women, but in practice it is again sufficient to consider the normal range for both sexes to be the same.

Normal range: 4.8-5.9 Pa

```
                                    BLUTGASANALYSE

NAME        MAY MICHAEL                                        SOLL        IST
BERUF       BEAMTER
GEB-DAT        1. 2.52           HAEMOGLOBIN        G/L    140 - 180      160
GROESSE   CM    178              ERYTHROZYTEN       BILL/L  4.6 - 6.2      5.4
GEWICHT   KG     68              M C H              PG     27  -  36       31
ALTER     J      25              HAEMATOKRIT              0.42-0.54      0.48
GESCHLECHT  MAENNLICH
RAUCHEN     NICHTRAUCHER         PCO2 ALV.          KPA           5.3      5.5
SPORT       LANGSTRECKE          PCO2 ART.-ALV.     KPA    0.0 - 0.8      0.2


                          RUHE    BELASTUNG                                        ERHOLUNG
LEISTUNG    WATT                   30    70   110   150   190   230   270   310     0     0     0
DAUER       MINUTEN  SOLL IST       3     3     3     3     3     3     3     3     4     7    10
PO2  ART    KPA   10.7 12.4       12.7  12.9  12.8  13.1  12.8  12.5  12.1  11.6  14.9  13.1  12.7
PCO2 ART    KPA 4.8 - 5.9 5.5      5.6   5.5   5.3   5.3   5.1   4.9   4.8   4.8   4.1   4.4   4.5
PH   ART    7.36-7.44 7.42        7.42  7.40  7.39  7.38  7.36  7.30  7.24  7.22  7.18  7.22  7.33

SO2         PROZ  94 - 98 96.9    97.1  97.1  96.9  96.9  96.5  95.5  94.0  92.8  95.7  94.6  96.0
HCO2AKT MMOL/L PLASMA 20.5 - 27 25.7  26.3  24.5  23.4  22.9  20.7  17.6  14.3  14.2  11.2  13.1  17.3
CO2 TOT MMOL/L PLASMA 21.5 - 28 26.9  27.6  25.8  24.6  24.1  21.9  18.7  16.0  15.3  12.1  14.0  18.3
BASENABW    MMOL/L B/ 0 +- 2.5 1.7  2.1   0.3  -0.9  -1.6  -3.7  -7.9 -11.7 -12.6 -16.5 -13.8  -7.3
BASENABW OX MMOL/L BL 0 +- 2.5 1.5  2.0   0.1  -1.0  -1.7  -3.9  -8.1 -12.0 -13.2 -16.7 -14.1  -7.5
PUFFERBASEN MMOL/L BL  45 - 50 50.2 50.7  48.8  47.6  47.0  44.8  40.6  36.7  35.5  32.0  34.6  41.2
STAND-HCO3 MMOL/L PL      24 25.4  25.8  24.3  23.3  22.8  21.1  18.1  15.6  14.8  12.8  14.3  18.5
STAND-PH             7.40 7.43   7.43  7.41  7.39  7.38  7.35  7.28  7.21  7.19  7.13  7.18  7.29
BEREICH                 1    1      1     1     1     1     1     8     9     9     9    17    17    17


 1 NORMBEREICH
 8 LEICHTE METABOLISCHE ACIDOSE
 9 METABOLISCHE ACIDOSE
17 TEILWEISE KOMPENSIERTE METABOLISCHE ACIDOSE
```

Fig. 181. Alpha-numeric readout of gas analysis and acid-base balance from the fast printer of a large computer setup (after *Schön*, *Rittel* and *Waterloh*).

Actual bicarbonate: This parameter is calculated, as are all those below, in the framework of the blood gas analysis, and is not measured. Nevertheless, this figure is the actual concentration of HCO_3 at any given moment in the plasma of anaerobically obtained blood. The bicarbonate at the given moment, however, does not exclusively represent the metabolic component, since there is a strong dependency on the P_{CO_2} through reciprocal reactions between carbonic acid and nonbicarbonate buffers.

Normal range: 20.7 to 27 mmol/liter of plasma

Standard bicarbonate: This figure is defined as bicarbonate concentration in the plasma after establishing equilibrium in the blood sample with a P_{CO_2} of 5.3 kPa and full O_2 saturation. The respiratory influence of the P_{CO_2} is here cancelled out.

Normal value: 24 mmol/liter of plasma

Buffer bases: The buffer bases represent the sum of all buffer ions (e.g., hemoglobin, organic and inorganic phosphates, and plasma proteins) in 1 liter of whole blood. There is no influence on the part of possibly predominating carbonic acid partial pressure, but instead a strong dependency on the hemoglobin concentration, which contributes an essential part to the buffer capacity of the blood.

Normal range: 45 to 50 mmol/liter of blood

Base deviation: The base deviation is influenced neither by the carbonic acid partial pressure nor by the hemoglobin concentration in the blood. The figure permits a direct statement as to the lack or excess of base in 1 liter of blood. Because it is altered primarily by exercise it is the most interesting item in considering physiological matters having to do with performance.

Normal range: ±2.5 mmol/liter of blood

2.2.4   Calculation Possibilities

Raw parameters obtained in blood gas analysis and acid-base balance are P_{O_2}, P_{CO_2}, pH and hemoglobin concentration. From these figures all the other parameters can be obtained by various methods. One way that the data can be derived is from various nomograms, such as the acid-base nomogram according to Thews (1967). Another tool for calculating blood gas is the slide rule of Severinghaus (1966). Further, blood gas analyzers of the latest generation comprise inherent circuited automatic calculators for the most important acid-base parameters.

A particularly convenient way of calculating and documenting is offered by computer programs which can read all the parameters of blood gas analysis and acid-base balance and present them in plain language. Such programs are described by Maas et al. (1972), Heck and Hollmann (1974) and Schön, Rittel and Waterloh (1976). Figure 181 shows a readout sheet from blood gas analysis produced by a CD 6400 calculator at the TH Computer Center in Aachen, Germany.

2.2.5   Disturbances in the Acid-Base Balance

Disturbances in the acid-base balance that accompany a rise in pH are called alkalosis; when pH declines it is called acidosis. Such disturbances may originate in pulmonary gas exchange or in altered metabolic processes. If the alterations in the acid-base balance are of respiratory as well as metabolic nature, we speak of combined disturbances. From Table 55, which shows the four most important disturbances, it is evident that in purely respiratory disturbances the values of the metabolic components lie within the normal range, while in purely metabolic ones the arterial CO_2 partial pressure is normal. The organism is trying to compensate either partially or completely for any disturbance in the acid-base equilibrium. Thus, respira-

Table 55. Primary disturbances of the acid-base balance.

Disturbance	PCO$_2$ (kPa)	pH	Base deviation (mmol/l)
Respiratory alkalosis	< 4.7	> 7.44	(+2.5)-(−2.5)
Acidosis	> 6.0	< 7.36	(−2.5)-(+2.5)
Metabolic alkalosis	4.8–5.9	> 7.44	> +2.5
Acidosis	4.8–5.9	< 7.36	< −2.5

tory disturbances are compensated metabolically; metabolic disturbances are compensated respiratorily.

In metabolic acidosis, for example, compensatory hyperventilation causes a drop in the arterial P_{CO_2}, bringing about a lesser shift in pH toward the "acid side."

2.3 Arterial Blood Gases and Acid-Base Balance in Ergometric Performance

Arterial O_2 partial pressure: No simple data are available in the literature on behavior of the P_{O_2} under exercise. There is merely mention of an in-

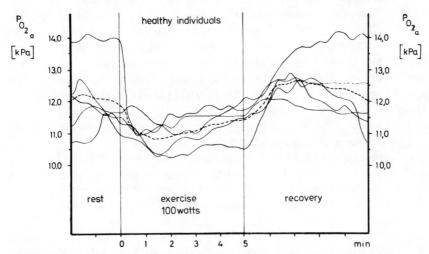

Fig. 182. Behavior of arterial P_{O_2} at rest, during exercise and recovery in five subjects with healthy lungs as determined through continuous measurement of O_2 pressure (after *Fabel*, 1968).

crease, a constancy or a drop during exercise. These contradictory statements are in part explained by the varying rest values at the start of the exercise (the sharpest drop occurs when the resting rate is already elevated) and also by the various types of exercise and various intensities (in submaximal exercise, no steady drop in P_{O_2} occurs).

Fabel (1968) succeeded in carrying out continuous readings of O_2 pressure with the aid of a quick-reading platinum electrode (lag time 2 to 3 seconds) and a special measuring unit. A special two-way cannula in the brachial artery permitted blood to be taken continuously over the course of hours. Figure 182 presents the behavior of the arterial O_2 partial pressure during rest, exercise and recovery on the part of five subjects with sound lungs.

Worthy of note is the great individual variation in the values for the resting and recovery phases, while the individual readings during exercise are grouped closely about the average level. During exercise, there is noted without exception, as has already been briefly alluded to, an increase in arterial O_2 pressure after an initial decline. At a power of 100 watts for five minutes, the arterial O_2 pressure is generally not affected by the blood temperature. However, Holmgren et al. (1964) pointed out that an increase in blood temperature of one degree Celsius, as is often noted during extremely intense exercise, makes it necessary to correct the arterial O_2 pressure reading by about $+0.8$ kPa, the P_{CO_2} by $+0.2$ kPa and the arterial pH by -0.014. Accordingly, for example, a drop of 0.8 kPa in arterial P_{O_2} caused by exercise could be traceable solely to the absence of temperature correction. This aspect should always be borne in mind in a critical consideration. Even taking this factor into account, a significant drop in arterial O_2 pressure has been confirmed in highly trained athletes in instances of top exercise intensity ranges (Eckoldt et al., 1968). Doll et al. (1966), who obtained both in teenage and adult athletes under vita maxima conditions an average P_{O_2} decline of about 1.5 kPa, made no correction for temperature. Figure 183 presents the relationships for arterial O_2 and CO_2 partial pressure in normal individuals and athletes.

The causes of the decline in O_2 pressure accompanying exercise in athletes are unknown. Since athletes' regulation capacity of the pulmonary circulation can hardly be inferior to that of normal individuals, in whom such a decline is not found even at like exercise intensities, the cause has been supposed rather to lie in an inequality in ventilation and perfusion. Trained persons breathe more economically during exercise, that is, more slowly and deeply. It is therefore conceivable that in individual areas of the lungs there exists relatively lower ventilation with increased perfusion. In the border area of exercise loading, not available to the untrained, the shortening of contact time might play a role in the further decline in the arterial O_2 partial pressure.

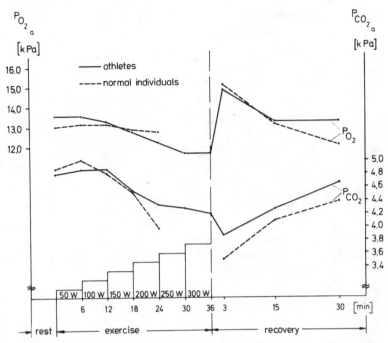

Fig. 183. The behavior of the arterial P_{O_2} and P_{CO_2} while at rest, during exercise and recovery on the part of normal individuals and athletes.

Reports of the behavior of arterial P_{O_2} during recovery all note a sharp increase immediately after interruption of the exercise. The O_2 partial pressures generally reach their starting values ten to fifteen minutes after the conclusion of the exercise.

Arterial O_2 saturation: On the basis of the flat curve for O_2 dissociation at higher pressure ranges, the arterial O_2 saturation generally remains in the normal range even with a decline in P_{O_2} caused by exercise. The normal range is, however, usually exceeded if the pH falls below 7.25 through metabolic influences (shift of the dissociation curve to the right; see Fig. 173a). For example, even under extreme physiological conditions of intense exercise, in which a P_{O_2} of 11.3 kPa and a pH of 7.00 were recorded, the arterial O_2 saturation still read 87.5%. In this instance the pH decline (starting values, P_{O_2} = 12.7 kPa and pH = 7.40) led to a drop of only 7.5% in O_2 saturation.

It can therefore be said that a drop in arterial O_2 saturation due to exercise, accompanied by unchanging or slightly lowered P_{O_2}, is to be traced chiefly to a sharp drop in pH.

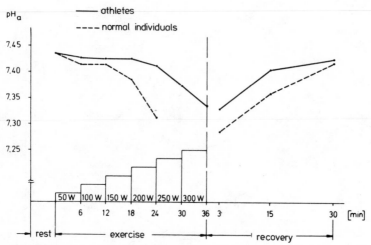

Fig. 184. The behavior of the arterial pH at rest, during exercise and during recovery in the normal individual and athletes. (after *Doll et al.*, 1968.)

Arterial CO_2 partial pressure: The arterial CO_2 partial pressure changes very little up to a power of 100 watts in trained and untrained individuals. Compared with athletes, normal individuals as a rule show a sharper drop in P_{CO_2} at high exercise intensities because of relative hyerventilation.

Immediately after the conclusion of an exercise, there occurs in both trained and untrained individuals a long-lasting reduction in arterial CO_2 partial pressure, reaching about 4.0 kPa during the third to tenth minute of the recovery phase. Even as late as thirty minutes into the recovery phase, the resting values are not regained, depending of course on the intensity of the foregoing exercise. The reduction in arterial CO_2 partial pressure in the recovery period constitues an important mechanism in the compensation for the metabolic processes. As can be easily seen in the behavior of the standard pH (pH at a P_{CO_2} of 5.3 kPa) from Figure 181, the pH shift would become still more serious without the influence of the respiratory component in the first minutes of recovery.

Arterial hydrogen-ion concentration: Exercise intensities above the endurance limit of performance lead to a steady increase in hydrogen-ion concentration. Together with this, as exercise gets greater, the anaerobic portion of the gain in energy increases. Untrained individuals show a more pronounced pH shift toward the "acid side" at the same intensity of exercise than do the trained. The reason lies in an earlier and sharper rise on the part of the fixed acids (mainly lactate).

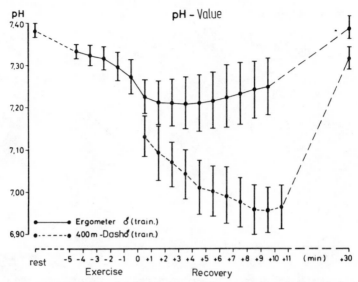

Fig. 185. The behavior of arterial pH in eight highly trained 400-meter runners during and after an exhausting ergometer exercise and after a 400-meter dash under world championship conditions (after *Metzner et al.*, 1968).

Figure 184 shows the behavior of the arterial pH in normal individuals and athletes during step-by-step exercise loading and in the recovery phase. It is worthy of note that the lowest pH in the trained as well as in the untrained is found in about the fourth minute of recovery, although the intensified production of CO_2 in this phase has a compensatory effect on the pH shift. The cause of the further drop in pH after exercise lies in the fact that lactate and pyruvate reach their peak at this time and at the same time the free fatty acids increase abruptly. The lowest pH levels were measured (Meitzner et al., 1968) in highly trained 400-meter runners under world championship conditions. Figure 185 shows the behavior of the pH on the bicycle ergometer (Venrath and Hollmann's method) and after a 400-meter dash in which times of 47 to 48 seconds were achieved.

In comparison with the ergometer loading to endurance load with maximal exercise intensity in the final exercise phase, the 400-meter run represents a brief exercise at highest intensity. The pH changes are correspondingly clear. Thus, highly trained athletes had blood pH readings as low as 6.885 after a 400-meter race (Metzner et al., 1968). These figures, obtained under world championship conditions, strengthen the assumption that trained individuals achieve and tolerate lower pH than untrained.

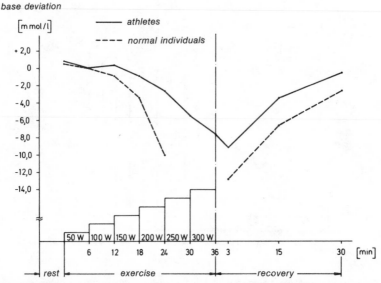

Fig. 186. The behavior of the base deviation at rest, during exercise and in the recovery phase in normal individuals and athletes (after *Doll et al.*, 1966).

Base deviations: This parameter represents the most important part of the metabolic component of the acid-base balance for the physiological consideration of performance, since it is affected primarily by exercise. In contrast to the current pH value, which reflects both the respiratory and metabolic situations, this parameter represents exclusively the metabolic side of the picture. Even so, the behavior patterns of both parameters resemble one another under ergometric exercise, since the pH shifts are essentially metabolically caused. Here too the sharpest deviations are found in the fourth minute of recovery. At that point the extent of the shift is greater than in the current pH, since the latter is respiratorily influenced at this point. The duration of the deviation is remarkable; it frequently has not been entirely compensated for until 30 minutes after the conclusion of the exercise, depending on the intensity of the exercise. Figure 186 shows the behavior of the base deviation in normal individuals and athletes during and after step-by-step increasing ergometer exercise.

To characterize briefly the acid-base situation during ergometer exercise, it might be said that with increasing intensity of exercise there arises a situation of acidosis which is more or less compensated respiratorily during the ensuing recovery phase (see Fig. 181).

2.4   The Arterial Blood Gases Under Pathological Conditions During Ergometric Performance

Sufficient O_2 consumption and exhalation of CO_2 at rest and during physical exercise are determined by ventilation, diffusion and perfusion.

The relationship of the various individual parameters to one another determines the effect of the external respiration. Any change in this relationship necessarily leads to changes in the arterial blood gases.

Disturbances in the pulmonary gas exchange may have their causes in increased venous contaminations, in disturbances in distribution, disturbances in diffusion or in a general alveolar hypoventilation.

Practical experience shows again and again that disturbances in gas exchange can be detected only after considerable alteration in the air passages and the lung tissues, since the lungs possess great functional reserves. At the start of disturbances in gas exchange, the arterial O_2 partial pressure is the first thing to be affected. Thanks to the considerably better diffusion properties of CO_2, changes in CO_2 partial pressure are not to be expected until ventilation is disturbed to a high degree. Table 56 gives an overview of the behavior of the arterial P_{O_2} and P_{CO_2} in various disturbances of the respiratory function.

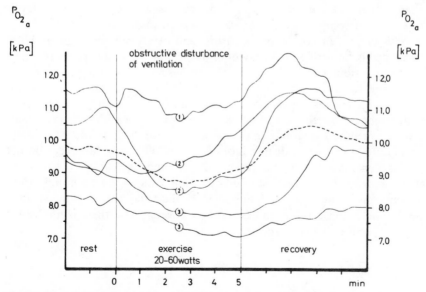

Fig. 187. The behavior of arterial P_{O_2} at rest, during exercise and recovery for five patients with obstructive emphysema of varying degrees of severity, as examples of continuous measurement of O_2 pressure (after *Fabel,* 1968).

Table 56. Disturbances of the respiratory functions.

Disturbance		Rest	Exercise	Hyperoxia
Anatomic shunt (increased venous contamination)	PO_2	lowered	drops	lowered
Functional shunt (disturbed distribution)	PO_2	lowered	rises	normal
Disturbance in diffusion	PO_2	lowered	drops	normal
Alveolar hypoventilation	PO_2	lowered	drops	normal
	PCO_2	elevated	rises	elevated

During O_2 breathing, the arterial O_2 pressure values are normalized provided there is no venous contamination. If there is, the arterial P_{O_2} remains low even under conditions of hyperoxia.

In contrast to the physiology of highly trained athletes, a pathological steady decline in arterial O_2 partial pressure under exercise is an indication of respiratory insufficiency, especially if the value is already low while at rest. The causes of this decline in P_{O_2} resulting from exercise are either insufficient ventilation reserves, increased venous contamination or insufficient increase in diffusion capacity. In advanced disturbances of gas exchange, there is an increase in P_{CO_2} under exercise with corresponding development of a compensated or noncompensated respiratory acidosis.

With the aid of continuous measurement of O_2 pressure, Fabel (1968) succeeded in depicting the behavior of the arterial P_{O_2} in five patients suffering from various stages of obstructive emphysema of the lungs. Figure 187 shows the various O_2 pressure profiles during rest, exercise and recovery.

In this illustration, curve 1 corresponds to the P_{O_2} behavior in one patient with minor obstructive emphysema of old age. It resembles the curve pattern of a healthy individual. In two patients (curve 2), there was moderately pronounced obstructive disturbance of ventilation which, however, did not infringe on the performance reserve of the lungs, as can be seen by the increase in P_{O_2} under exercise. Finally, curve 3 shows the extent of an obstructive disturbance of ventilation in which the arterial P_{O_2} declines steadily during the exercise and even during the recovery phase there is no distinct rise in pressure despite hyperventilation.

References

Clark, L. C., R. Wolf, D. Granger and Z. Taylor: Continuous recording of blood oxygen tension by polarography, J. appl. Physiol. **6** (1953), 189–193.

Doll, E., J. Keul, Chr. Maiwald and H. Reindell: Das Verhalten von Sauerstoffdruck, Kohlensäuredruck, pH, Standardbicarbonat und base excess im arteriellen Blut bei verschiedenen Belastungsformen. Int. Z. angew. Physiol. einschl. Arbeitsphysiol. **22** (1966), 327–355.

Eckoldt, K., W. Roth, E. Thiele and W. Thiele: Blutgasanalytische und spiroergometrische Messungen bei Normalpersonen und Sportlern, Medizin u. Sport, **8** (1968), 102–107.

Fabel, H.: Die fortlaufende Messung des arteriellen Sauerstoffdruckes beim Menschen, Arch. Kreisl.forschg. **57** (1968), 145–189.

Geisler, L. and H.-D. Rost: Zur Problematik eines „Normwertes" für den arteriellen Sauerstoffdruck, Med. Welt **22** (1971), 49–52.

Gleichmann, U. and D. W. Lübbers: Die Messung des Kohlensäuredruckes in Gasen und Flüssigkeiten mit der pCO2-Elektrode unter besonderer Berücksichtigung der gleichzeitigen Messung von pO2, pCO2 und pH im Blut. Pflügers Arch. ges. Physiol. **271** (1960), 456–472.

Heck, H. and W. Hollmann: Berechnung der Werte des Säure-Basen-Status im Blut mit Hilfe eines Tischcomputers, Sportarzt u. Sportmed. **25** (1974), 154–159.

Holmgren, A. and M. B. McIlroy: Effect of temperature on arterial blood gas tensions and pH during exercise, J. appl. Physiol. **19** (1964), 243–245.

Lange, H. J. and F. H. Hertle: Zum Problem der Normalwerte. In: Hertz, C. W.: Begutachtung von Lungenfunktionsstörungen, Thieme (1968), 44–64.

Loew, P. G. and G. Thews: Die Altersabhängigkeit des arteriellen Sauerstoffdruckes bei der berufstätigen Bevölkerung, Klin. Wschr. **40** (1962), 1093–1098.

Maas, A. H., J. A. Kreuger, A. J. Hoelen and B. F. Visser: A computer program for calculating the acid-base parameters in samples of blood using a mini-computer, Pflügers Arch. **334** (1972), 264–275.

Metzner, A., J. Willmann and E. Gadermann: Säurebasengleichgewicht nach Maximalbelastung am Fahrradergometer und nach sportlichem Wettkampf, Med. Welt **19** (1968), 2161–2167.

Reichel, G., E. Schürmeyer, and E. W. Bartelheimer: Untersuchungen über die arterielle Blutgasanalyse im Capillarblut des hyperämisierten Ohrläppchens bei Herz- und Lungenkranken. Klin. Wschr. **44** (1966), 386–388.

Schön, F.-A., H.-F. Rittel and E. Waterloh: Analyse des gaz du sang avec calcul, par ordinateur, de l'equilibre acid-base. Broncho-Pneumologie **26** (1976), 124–132.

Severinghaus, J. W.: Blood gas calculator. J. appl. Physiol. **21** (1966), 1108–1116.

Siggaard-Andersen: The Acid-Base-Status of the Blood Munksgaard, Copenhagen 1974.

Thews, G.: Ein Nomogramm Für die O2-Abhängigkeit des Säure-Basen-Status im menschlichen Blut. Pflügers Arch. ges. Physiol. **296** (1967), 212–221.

Ulmer, W. T., G. Berta and G. Reichel: Sauerstoff- und Kohlensäurepartialdruckmessung im arteriellen und Ohrläppchenkapillarblut mit stabilisierten Mikroelektroden. Med. thorac. **20** (1963), 235–249.

Ulmer, W. T., G. Reichel and D. Nolte: Die Lungenfunktion, Thieme, Stuttgart 1970.

3. The Mechanical Duration of Systole During Ergometric Performance

The mechanical duration of systole (measured from Q until the start of the second heart sound) becomes shorter during ergometric performance in regular relationship to the magnitude of the exertion. Only in ergometric exercise while reclining, when the ergometric exercise is interrupted for a few seconds, can it be measured perfectly.

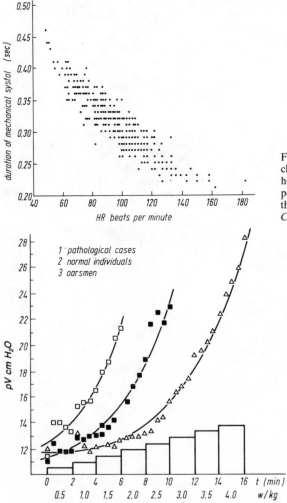

Fig. 188. The duration of mechanical systole in relation to heart rate during ergometric pedaling in 30 healthy men in their 20s through their 40s (after *Cardus* and *Vera*).

Fig. 189. Venous pressure in the cubital vein in mm H_2O (pV) (after *Moritz* and *Tabora*) in ergometric cycling while reclining (in watts per kg) in 27 normal individuals, 13 patients with cardiac insufficiency and 12 top-flight oarsmen (after *E. Kaempfe*).

From a knowledge of the normal range of variation of the mechanical duration of systole in absolutely and relatively equal exercise intensities in certain age and sex groups, we can expect to distinguish pathological changes in cardiac insufficiency (Fig. 188). Under resting conditions there occurs at first a prolongation as cardiac insufficiency progresses, but later with very advanced insufficiency there comes a shortening of the mechanical duration of systole, as was demonstrated by Blumenberger; Echte and others. The pathological changes in mechanical duration of systole as ergometric exercise is increased can make possible a determination of cardiac performance capacity and the extent of the performance insufficiency in pathological conditions of the heart. A prerequisite for this is the knowledge of the average duration of systole and its standard deviations as ergometric performance intensifies.

4. Venous Pressure During Ergometric Performance

Venous pressure increases slightly in healthy individuals during exercise in regular relationship to the magnitude of the exercise (Fig. 190) (Barger et al.; König; Lotvin; Porojkova). Measuring the pressure in the right atrium in six healthy individuals during ergometric power of 100 watts, however, showed no elevation of the performance pressure compared with the tests while at rest (Reindell et al.). After the exercise, it drops in the course of a few seconds or minutes (depending on the magnitude of the exercise), returning to the resting level (Fig. 191).

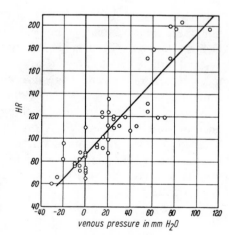

Fig. 190. Venous pressure in the cubital vein (in mm H$_2$O; 1 mm Hg = 13.6 mm H$_2$O) in relation to HR during increasing treadmill exercise (after *Barger, Greenwood, Dipalma, Stokes* and *Smith*).

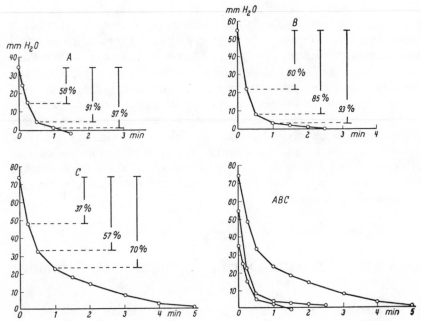

Fig. 191. Average drop in pressure after exercise of clinically distinct groups—Ordinate: pressure increase above resting level. Abscissa: time since exercise. Group A: patients without right-heart insufficiency; Group B: patients with questionable signs of right-heart insufficiency; Group C: patients with right-heart insufficiency; ABC shows the differences in venous pressure in the three groups after approximately equal pedaling exercise while reclining to be about three times the resting O_2 consumption. (The curves are based on a total of 200 measurements on 96 patients by König.)

In right-heart insufficiency, with increasing stasis in the systemic circulation, there comes about a pathological rise in venous pressure (Budelmann, Delius, Hultgren, Schott and Szekely, cited by König) (Fig. 189), and a delayed drop in venous pressure after exertion (König) (Fig. 191). From the measurement of the venous pressure with slowly increasing ergometric performance, a right-side insufficiency can be detected and determined quantitatively from the occurrence of pathological pressure readings at performance of various magnitudes. A prerequisite for this, however, is a more detailed knowledge of normal venous pressure as ergometric performance levels increase. The diagram in Figure 190, showing the relations between venous pressure and performance HR in healthy individuals, affords an approximate basis.

The venous pressure can be measured during ergometric exercise while reclining with the simple method used by Moritz and Tabora. A saline or dextrose infusion into a cubital vein is performed at the level of the right atrium and connected with a calibrated standing tube by way of a three-way cock. By switching the cock to the standing tube, the pressure can be read at brief intervals.

References

Barger, A. C., W. F. Greenwood, J. R. Dipalma, J. Stokes and L. H. Smith: J. Appl. Physiol. 81, (1949) 2.

Blumberger, K.: Klin. Wschr. 3, (1943) 55; proceedings of Dtsch. Ges. Kreisl.-Forschg. Frankfurt/Main 15, (1949) 118; Proceedings of Dtsch. Ges. Kreisl.-Forschg. Darmstadt 16, (1950) 121; Ärztl. Forsch. 1958, Nr. 8/9, 477.

Budelmann, Delius, Hultgren, Schott and Szekely: after König, Dtsch. med. Wschr. 140, (1958) 4.

Cardus, D. and L. Vera: Cardiology 59, (1974) 133.

Echte, W.: Zschr. Kreisl.-Forschg. 49, (1960) 559.

Kaempfe, E.: Dissertation Med. Hochschule Lübeck 1978.

König, E.: Dtsch. med. Wschr. 140, (1958) 4.

Lotvin, V. B.: Terap. arch. (Moskva) 4, (1954) 37.

Minx, W. and H. Mellerowicz: Zschr. Kreisl.-Forschg. 54, (1964) 448.

Porojkava, G. D.: Sovet. med. 6, (1955) 41.

Reindell, H. et al.: Herz, Kreislauf und Sport. München: Barth, 1960.

XVI. Physiological Criteria of Physical, Cardiac and Pulmonary Performance Limits

1. The Subjective Maximal Physical Performance

The subjective maximal physical performance is achieved with the subjectively greatest exercise of will power. The "competitive situation," especially in the presence of an audience, is the one most likely to bring the performer closest to the limit of his individual performance, but the ability to completely exhaust one's performance reserves varies very much with the individual. It is determined chiefly by the personal, trainable ability to resist the physical and mental stresses due to increasing metabolic changes resulting from fatigue.

Using the application of maximal will power, especially in the actual or supposed competitive situation, the subjective maximal power under these conditions and under definite duration (of for example three, six or nine minutes) leads to a completely possible estimation of physical performance. These conditions can in general not be taken for granted in the situation of compensation evaluations. The subjective maximal values measured in these cases can only be used in comparative consideration with the objective criteria of the limits of physical performance.

2. HR at Maximal Endurance Performance

At maximal physical power, maximal HR is attained. It is conditioned by age, sex, constitutional factors and environmental conditions, and to a lesser

315

extent by the duration of the performance. Knowledge of the maximal ranges for HR is an important prerequisite in identifying a maximal ergo-metric power. Passing beyond the $+2\sigma$ limit for the maximal HR in particu-lar age and sex brackets is an essential criterion of the physical and cardiac maximal performance.

Figures 46 and 47 in Chapter V show the maximal ranges for HR in a three or six minute maximal performance on the hand crank ergometer in 100 untrained, healthy males aged 20 to 30. At maximal pedaling perform-ance while reclining, the HR is about ten to fifteen fewer beats per minute than in pedaling while seated and hand cranking while standing (after Galle and Mellerowicz).

The average HRs of 160 untrained male teenagers aged 12 to 19 in a maximal ergometric performance on the hand crank ergometer are shown in Figure 43 in Chapter V. They are about five to ten heart beats higher than those of the 20 to 30 year olds.

The maximal frequencies in the older age groups are lower than those of the younger ones. A rough survey of their behavior is presented in Figure 192 and Table 57. There we see a regular decrease in maximal HR with advancing years.

According to our knowledge at the present time (Mellerowicz and Lerche; Dransfeld and Mellerowicz; S. Robinson and P. Åstrand, Christensen, Bengtsson, and others), the average maximal HR in the individual age level is:

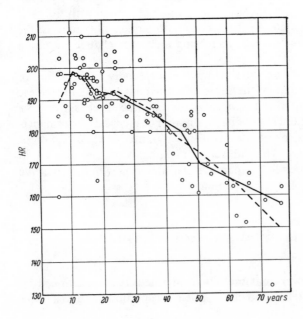

Fig. 192. The highest HR in healthy male individuals aged 6 to 75 at maximal ex-ercise on the treadmill (after *Robinson*).

Table 57. The maximal HR in various age levels at hand cranking (after *Hollmann*).

Age levels Normal persons	Number	HR	± 2σ
12 and 13	55	198	± 26
14 and 15	51	192	± 22
16 and 17	38	187	± 16
18 and 19	43	181	± 12
20 to 40	80	176	± 16
41 to 50	36	173	± 18
51 to 60	42	169	± 12
61 to 70	18	160	± 14
71 to 80	11	138	± 14
Athletes 20 to 40	127	178	± 12

Years	10–20	20–30	30–40	40–50	50–60	60–80
HR per min	≈200	≈190	≈180	≈170	≈160	≈150

The lower limit ($\approx -2\sigma$) of the maximal range is about 10 to 20 per minute below these values (Fig. 193). If the HR as measured exceeds these values during ergometric performance, then it can be assumed that this is indeed a maximal power.

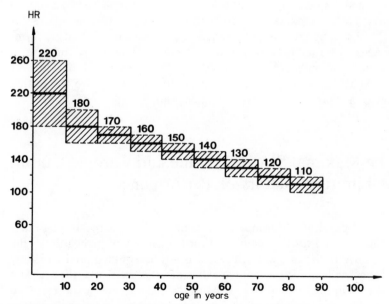

Fig. 193. Schematic representation of the lower limits of the maximal range of the HR ($\approx -2\sigma$) in relation to age.

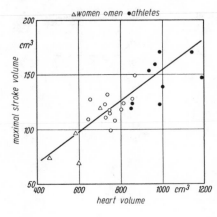

Fig. 194. The heart volume in relation to stroke volume at maximal exercise (pedaling while reclining) (after *Musshoff, Reindell* and *Klepzig,* 1959).

The HR for women at maximal power levels seems not to diverge essentially from that of men. Düntsch found, in 80 healthy women aged 20 to 30, an average HR of 178 per minute (s = 11.4) at the conclusion of a ten-minute maximal performance on the hand crank ergometer. Metheny, Brouha, Johnson and Forbes have measured an average maximal HR of 197 per minute in women after exhausting running performance. Åstrand's studies found an average HR of 198 per minute (σ = 9.9) at maximal exercise on the pedaling ergometer. Additional studies seem to be necessary on the behavior of the maximal HR in healthy women of various age levels.

E. A. Müller designates as "endurance-performance limit" that performance which can be maintained for several hours without any increase in pulse rate and without any increase in the total recovery HR. It lies, according to E. A. Müller and Karrasch, about 30 to 40 beats above the resting rate, that is, at about 100 to 120 beats per minute.

3. The Maximal Stroke Volume and Cardiac Output as Limiting Factors of Performance

The maximal physical endurance performance is limited by, among other factors, the maximal stroke volume and cardiac output of the healthy or the damaged heart. In the case of healthy hearts it is determined predominately by the size of the heart. While people with small ("office-workers") hearts of a volume amounting to about 700 to 900 cm³ maximal cardiac output reach from 20 to 25 liters per minute, athletes with hearts of great performance capability with volumes of about 1000 to 1200 cm³ are capable of pumping from 30 to 35 liters per minute (with an A-VO₂Δ of about 12 to 15 volume percent and a maximal O₂ consumption of about 3000 to 6000 cm³). Maximal stroke volumes have been observed in ergometric catheter examinations of trained individuals by Musshoff, Reindell and Klepzig at about 70% of the top performance, with HRs of 120 to 150 per minute. The approximately linear relation between maximal stroke volume and heart volume is shown in Figure 194. Higher cardiac outputs and performances can be attained through a further increase in HR. A decrease in the stroke volume in the range of the highest HR in conjunction with a drop below a critical duration of diastole, which still just permits filling with a maximal stroke volume, is to be assumed, though it is not definitely proven.

4. The Maximal O₂ Pulse

The maximal O₂ pulse is attained, according to studies by P. Åstrand, approximately in the range of the maximal HR, but the maximal stroke volume at a HR of about 120 to 150 (Musshoff, Reindell, Klepzig). A further increase in the O₂ pulse at higher HR can therefore be caused only by a further increase in the A-VO₂Δ. The behavior of the average maximal O₂ pulse in ten men aged 20 to 40, in ergometer exercise increased to the point

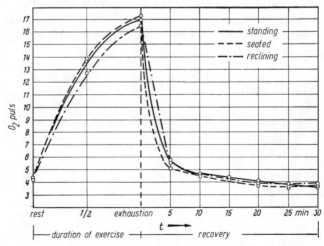

Fig. 195. The O₂ pulse in the course of an ergometric exercise increasing to the level of exhaustion in 10 untrained male subjects aged 20 to 40 while standing ———, sitting — — — and reclining —·—·— (under standard conditions, after *Galle* and *Mellerowicz*).

Table 58. The maximal O_2 pulse at various age levels at hand cranking (after *Hollmann*).

Age levels Normal persons	Number	O_2 Pulse	$\pm 3\sigma$
12 and 13	55	9.1	± 2.4
14 and 15	51	12.4	± 3.8
16 and 17	38	14.6	± 3.2
18 and 19	43	17.1	± 3.5
20 to 40	80	16.8	± 3.3
41 to 50	36	15.6	± 2.9
51 to 60	42	13.0	± 3.8
61 to 70	18	11.1	± 2.0
71 to 80	11	11.0	± 3.1
Athletes 20 to 40	127	21.6	± 3.4

of exhaustion, is shown in Figure 195 after Galle and Mellerowicz. A maximal performance may be assumed when the O_2 pulse no longer increases in the course of an examination with steadily increased performance stages. Table 58 shows the maximal O_2 pulse at various age levels during hand cranking.

5. The Maximal O_2 Consumption

The maximal O_2 consumption is the most important conditioning factor and most reliable criterion for the maximal (aerobic) physical performance. But it must be borne in mind that additional exercise can be performed by accruing an O_2 debt of about 5 to 15 liters. With slowly increasing exercise,

Table 59. The maximal O_2 consumption at various age levels with hand cranking exercise (after *Hollmann*).

Age levels Normal persons	Number	Maximal O_2 consumption in cm^3	$\pm 3\sigma$
12 and 13	55	1810	± 220
14 and 15	51	2390	± 310
16 and 17	38	2730	± 284
18 and 19	43	3100	± 290
20 to 40	80	2970	± 305
41 to 50	36	2680	± 331
51 to 60	42	2220	± 326
61 to 70	18	1790	± 263
71 to 80	11	1520	± 325
Athletes 20 to 40	127	3848	± 402

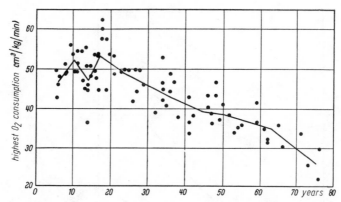

Fig. 196. Highest O_2 consumption per minute per kg of body weight on the part of male subjects aged 6 to 75 at maximal exercise on the treadmill (after *Robinson*).

O_2 consumption reaches its maximal level (Fig. 197), while the physical performance can rise still higher with greater O_2 debt. The maximal physical performance is determined more by the maximal O_2 consumption as the duration increases. The maximal O_2 consumption in individuals aged from 10 to 80 is shown in Figure 115, Table 21, Table 59, and Figure 196.

The maximal steady-state performance is the endurance performance with the highest O_2 consumption without mounting O_2 debt. This "limit of O_2 endurance performance" (after Hollmann) lies above the "limit of pulse endurance performance" (after E. A. Müller). According to E. A. Müller's definition, an exercise lies below the limit of O_2 endurance performance if as much O_2 is taken up by respiration as is needed for the exercise. The exercise lies below the limit of pulse endurance performance, however, if the exercising muscles take up as much O_2 as they need for the exercise.

6.   The Rise in the Respiratory Equivalent

The relationship of the respiratory time-volume to the O_2 consumption, the so-called respiratory equivalent

$$\frac{\text{respiratory time-volume in cm}^3 \text{ [BTPS]}}{O_2 \text{ consumption in cm}^3/\text{min [STPD]}}$$

at first declines to a minimum at increasing submaximal performances (Figs. 197 and 198). As the performance steadily increases, the quotient rises; the respiratory time-volume increases relatively more than the O_2 consumption

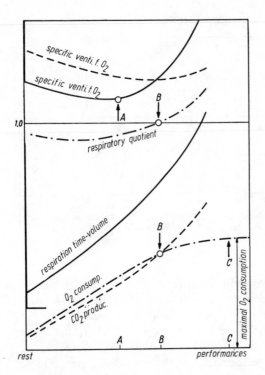

Fig. 197. Respiratory equivalent (specific ventilation for O_2), respiratory quotient, O_2 consumption, CO_2 production and respiratory time-volume during increasing ergometric performances up to the maximal range in healthy individuals. A = lowest value of the respiratory equivalent, B = respiratory quotient = 1.0, C = maximal O_2 consumption (after *Joss*).

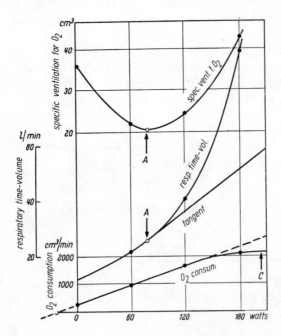

Fig. 198. Determination of the minimal respiratory equivalent and its increase with increasing ergometric performances (after *Joss*).

for an individually different magnitude of performance, and an "excessive" increase in respiratory equivalent comes about. At this cardiopulmonary performance level, the respiratory economy starts to decline. Greater respiratory volumes are required for the consumption of the same quantity of O_2.

This increase in the respiratory equivalent, occurring long before the attainment of the maximal HR, is a characteristic point (performance point A in Figs. 197 and 198). It characterizes performance at optimal respiratory economy. Since, however, the respiratory time-volume depends also on subjective factors, the accurate ascertainment of this point, especially in compensation cases, is not always possible.

7. The Respiratory Quotient at Limits of Physical Performance

When resting values of the respiratory quotient are as low as 0.8, the quotient rises gradually as (endurance) performance increases and reaches a value of about 1.0 at the maximal HR and maximal (endurance) performance (see Figs. 106, 197 and 199). With simultaneous recording of O_2 and CO_2, there is a further criterion for a maximal physical endurance performance (performance point 8, according to Joss).

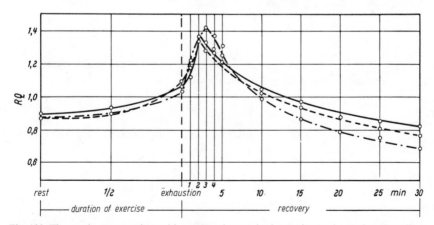

Fig. 199. The respiratory quotient with ergometric exercise increasing to the performance limit and in the recovery phase: hand cranking while standing (————), pedaling while seated (—— ——) and reclining (—·—·—) in 10 untrained male subjects aged 20 to 40 under standard conditions (after *Galle* and *Mellerowicz*).

8. The Respiratory Time-Volume, Tidal Volume and Respiration Rate at Maximal Physical (Endurance) Performance and Their Relationship to Vital Capacity and Maximal Ventilatory Capacity

During endurance performances, the values of the respiratory time-volume, the tidal volume, and the respiratory frequency in healthy respiratory systems are considerably lower than their limit values during a brief, maximal exertion of six to ten seconds (Table 25). They depend on age, sex, constitutional factors and also on the nature and duration of the performance. Knowledge of their age- and sex-related averages, as well as their standard deviations, makes possible a comparative evaluation of these values in individual cases.

Maximal values for the respiratory time-volume in male and female subjects aged 7 to 33 are shown in Figure 200.

Fourteen of Balke's subjects attained a maximal respiratory time-volume of 80 liters after thirty minutes of slowly increasing exercise on the treadmill. Robinson found, at maximal treadmill exercise in men aged 16 to 38, an average respiratory time-volume of 120 liters. With advancing years, the figures become lower. The average maximal figures for 40-to-50 year olds was 98 liters; for those 60 to 70 it was 81 liters (Table 60). The not inconsiderable divergences in the results of various investigators are traceable to differences in the populations being studied, nature and duration of the

Table 60. Respiratory time-volume, respiration rate and tidal volume at maximal treadmill exercise in male subjects aged 6 to 75 (after *Robinson*).

Age group	No. of subjects	Avg. age	Avg. wt. in kg	Respiration rate per min		Respiration time-volume	
				Avg.	Extremes	Avg.	Extremes
I	4	6.1	21.0	62	58–68	33.3	28– 43
II	9	10.4	30.0	57	48–68	53.4	41– 68
III	8	14.1	57.5	50	40–64	92.2	71–121
IV	6	18.0	67.8	46	40–56	121.0	103–143
V	9	25.3	72.4	43	32–56	118.2	104–135
VI	10	35.1	79.3	43	32–48	122.4	103–147
VII	9	44.3	74.1	39	28–48	97.6	72–133
VIII	6	50.7	68.6	38	28–58	86.8	57–114
IX	7	62.7	69.3	35	26–44	80.8	62–106
X	3	75.0	67.4	29	26–34	47.7	45– 50

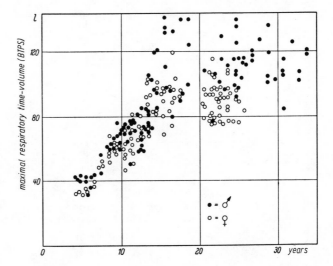

Fig. 200. Maximal values for respiratory time-volume in male and female subjects aged 7 to 33 (after Åstrand).

exercise and also to the equipment being used (differences in impedance to breathing, among other factors) and methodology in taking readings.

The tidal volume at maximal exercise usually amounts to about 50% of vital capacity in ergometric pedaling in men and women (Fig. 138). According to Nielson, respiration at about 50% of vital capacity is very economical in relation to amount of exercise and amount of absorbed O_2. The respiratory frequency at maximal (treadmill) exercise in men aged 20 to 33 amounted to 40 ± 1.3 and in women aged 20 to 25 amounted to 46.0 ± 1.0

Table 60, continued.

RMV per kg		Tidal volume		Tidal volume · 100 vital capacity	
Avg.	Extremes	Avg.	Extremes	Avg.	Extremes
1.59	1.49–1.65	0.54	0.41–0.68	45.5	34–69
1.78	1.56–2.11	0.92	0.73–1.12	43.5	31–52
1.60	1.51–1.84	1.88	1.48–2.34	52.0	40–63
1.60	1.39–2.10	2.66	2.27–2.91	55.8	52–59
1.64	1.40–1.95	2.93	1.86–4.13	56.0	44–77
1.55	1.37–1.86	2.88	2.33–3.59	59.4	55–69
1.32	1.02–1.72	2.53	1.71–3.14	56.3	45–68
1.26	0.91–1.52	2.34	2.02–2.55	53.0	42–69
1.16	0.93–1.47	2.33	1.89–2.82	59.6	55–72
0.71	0.67–0.73	1.64	1.40–1.93	50.8	43–58

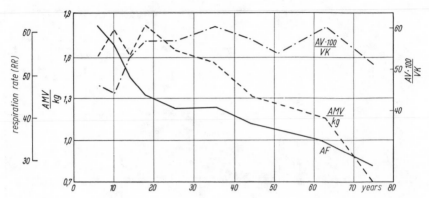

Fig. 201. Respiration rate (RR), respiratory time-volume per kg of body weight and volume in % of vital capacity during maximal treadmill exercise in males aged 6 to 75 (after *Robinson*).

Table 61. Breathing rate at maximal exercise (after *Åstrand*).

Years	4–6	7–9	10–11	12–13	14–15	16–17	♂20–33 ♀20–25
♂	70.4 ± 2.5	67.0 ± 2.7	57.5 ± 2.9	54.1 ± 2.5	52.9 ± 3.2	44.7 ± 3.9	39.9 ± 1.3
♀	66.4 ± 3.9	67.1 ± 3.0	61.3 ± 2.7	54.4 ± 3.3	51.6 ± 2.7	51.2 ± 1.8	46.0 ± 1.0

(according to Åstrand). The maximal breathing rates in children and teen-agers were considerably higher (Table 61).

In Robinson's older subjects, the maximal respiratory frequency showed a decline with advancing years (Table 62 and Fig. 201).

Depending on the constitution of the subject, the maximal respiratory minute-volume in healthy (not obese) individuals generally shows regular relationships to body weight, stature and body surface area, as shown by Åstrand's studies (Fig. 202). These results, although obtained on a not entirely random sampling, make it possible to decide, on the basis of body weight, whether a subject has attained maximal respiratory time-volume. The maximal respiratory time-volume in relation to body weight declines with advancing age (Fig. 201).

Table 62. Breathing rate at maximal physical exercise in untrained males aged 6 to 75 (after *Robinson*).

Years of age	6	11	14	17	25	35	45	52	63	75
Number of subjects	8	10	11	12	11	10	10	9	8	3
Maximal respiration rate	62	57	50	46	43	43	39	38	35	29

The maximal respiratory time-volume is also dependent on the type of exercise being performed. Thus, ten male subjects reached an average maximal respiratory time-volume of 82.4 ± 10.7 liters at hand cranking, of 80.0 ± 9.2 liters at pedaling while seated and of 73.0 ± 11.2 liters at pedaling while reclining (after Galle and Mellerowicz). At pedaling while reclining, it is thus possible to achieve only about 90% of the maximal respiratory time-volume.

If the respiratory apparatus is healthy, an approximate calculation of the maximal respiratory time-volume can be obtained based on vital capacity. At maximal performance, the subject breathes at about 50% of his vital capacity (Åstrand). The maximal respiration rate in men and women of average age is about 30 to 40 per minute. Therefore the following approximate relationships may be assumed:

$$RMV_{max} = \frac{VC}{2} \times 35$$

(RMV = respiratory time-volume and VC = vital capacity.)
That is, for example,

$$RMV_{max} = \frac{51}{2} \times 35 = \approx 90 \text{ liters.}$$

The respiratory time-volume is only about 60% of the maximal voluntary ventilation (according to Heine, Benesch and Hertz). For example, with a maximal voluntary ventilation of 120 liters, we must reckon with a maximal respiratory time-volume of about 70 liters.

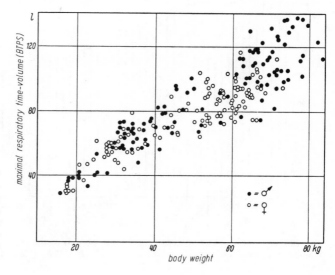

Fig. 202. Respiratory time-volume at maximal pedaling exercise while sitting, in relation to body weight in male and female subjects aged 7 to 33 (after Åstrand).

9. The Maximal O_2 Debt

In maximal physical exercise of a particular duration, a maximal O_2 debt that has a limiting effect on performance is reached either with steady exercise or else during its final phase. According to studies by Helbing and Mellerowicz, this amounted on the average to 6300 ± 1050 cm³ in the case of maximal hand-cranking work in 32 untrained men aged 20 to 40 (Fig. 203). In highly trained middle- and long-distance performers, Fandrey and Nowacki found values of about 10 to 20 liters of O_2 debt after maximal ergometric pedaling while seated. The measurement of maximal O_2 debt on a sufficiently large representative population of various age and sex groups is needed. Exceeding the -2σ threshold of the average maximal O_2 debt may be assumed to be the criterion of maximal exercise for a performance of a certain magnitude and duration. The O_2 debt is recovered by approximately 55% of trained and untrained individuals in five minutes of rest, and by 70–75% in ten minutes (Fandrey and Nowacki).

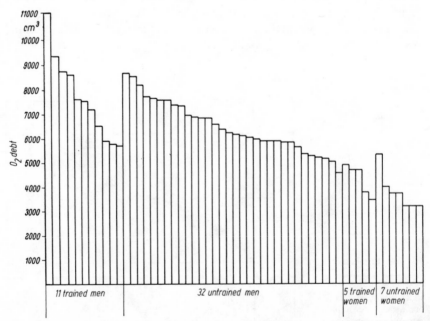

Fig. 203. O_2 debt at maximal hand cranking on the part of trained and untrained men and women of average age under standard conditions (after *Helbing* and *Mellerowicz*).

10. Decrease in O_2 Saturation of the Blood and the Spirographic O_2 Debt

In the range of maximal physical exercise, arterial undersaturation with O_2 is an important performance-limiting factor, under both normal and pathological conditions of heart and lungs. This can be detected bloodlessly by oximetric means. As a consequence of and in quantitative connection with this arterial undersaturation and other factors, a spirographic O_2 debt can be detected, if it is great enough.

References

Åstrand, P.: Experimental studies of physical working capacity in relation to sex and age. Kopenhagen: Munksgaard, 1952.

Balke, B.: Arbeitsphysiologie 15, (1954) 311.

Dransfeld, B. and H. Mellerowicz: Internat. Zschr. angew. Physiol. einschl. Arbeitsphysiol. 17, (1958) 207.

Düntsch, G.: Diss. FU Berlin 1960.

Galle, L. and H. Mellerowicz: Der Sportarzt 10, (1962) 332.

Heine, Benesch and Hertz: Zschr. Tbk. 102, (1953) 273.

Helbing, G.: Dissertation FU Berlin 1966.

Hollmann, W.: Proceedings of Tagg. der dtsch. Hochschulsportärzte Münster 1960.

Hollmann, W.: Kriterien der körperlichen, kardialen und pulmonalen Leistungsgrenzen. In: 1. Internationales Seminar für Ergometrie. Berlin: Ergon-Verlag, 1965.

Hollmann, W. and Th. Hettinger: Sportmedizin—Arbeits- und Trainingsgrundlagen. Schattauer, Stuttgart-New York 1976.

Joss, E.: Helvet. med. acta 24, (1959) 26.

Mellerowicz, H. and D. Lerche: Internat. Zschr. angew. Physiol. einschl. Arbeitsphysiol. 17, (1959) 459.

Messin, R.: The practice and limitation factors of ergometric tests. In: 1. Internationales Seminar für Ergometrie. Berlin: Ergon-Verlag, 1965.

Metheny, E., R. Brouha, R. Johnson and W. Forbes: Amer. J. Physiol. 137, (1942) 318.

Müller, E. A.: Arbeitsphysiologie 14, (1950) 271.

Müller, E. A. and K. Karrasch: Zbl. Arbeitsmed. 2, (1953) 37.

Musshoff, K., H. Reindell, H. Klepzig and H. W. Kirchhoff: Cardiologica 31, (1957) 359.

Musshoff, K., H. Reindell and H. Klepzig: Acta Cardiol. (Bruxleles) 14, (1959) 427.

Nielson, M.: Skand. Arch. Physiol. 74, (1936) 299.

Robinson, S.: Arbeitsphysiologie 10, (1938) 251.

XVII. Computerized Ergometry

by Elmar Waterloh and
Hans-Friedmund Rittel

1. Basic Concepts in Electronic Data Processing

In electronic data processing (EDP), information processing systems are used. Recently, microcomputers have gained in importance. There are two types of electronic computers: analog calculators, which function with physical variables (analog-electric voltages), and digital calculators, which use discrete individual quantities (numbers). Programmed digital calculators are especially well suited for calculating individual spiroergometric functional quanta. The basic digital calculator consist of an input-output unit, a storage unit, a calculator, and controls.

1.1 Input-Output Unit

Keyboards, teletypes, punch-card or punch-strip readers and magnetic-card, magnetic-band or magnetic-plate readers serve as input units. For data output are employed numerical paper strips (numeral output), alphanumeric printers and high-speed printers (numeral and text output) or projection screen devices (video terminals, displays). Output data can be transferred via punch-card and punch-strip stampers to the corresponding data carriers or to magnetic cards, magnetic tapes or magnetic plates. With the aid of cathode ray tubes and cameras, data storage on microfilm is also possible. Graphic output of data is possible with graphomats or plotters (automatic drawing devices).

1.2   Storage Unit, Calculator, Controls

The central computer is made up of storage unit, calculator and controls. Internal and external storage units serve to store commands or alphanumeric data. Core storage units, consisting of magnetic cores or monolithic circuit coils and, more recently, integrated semiconductor storage units, are used as internal (central) storage units. Extend storage units are magnetic cores, magnetic tapes, or magnetic disks. The actual processing of data takes place in the calculator in connection with the controls, which regulate the proper sequence of calculating operations.

1.3   Programming

A computer program sees to it that storage unit, calculator and controls operate in coordination with one another. A program represents the definite sequence of commands by which directives can be given to the computer. Programs must be couched in computer language, distinguishing between machine-oriented and problem-oriented languages. Machine-programming means the direct input of a command in machine language to a particular

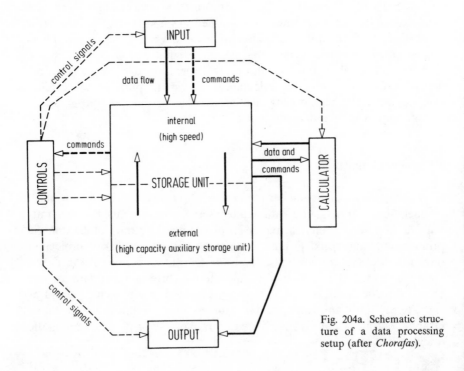

Fig. 204a. Schematic structure of a data processing setup (after *Chorafas*).

computer. Smaller table model computers demand special programming languages intended specifically for them. Higher level programming languages are independent of particular systems and can be used for many different data-processing setups. A compiler (translation program) can be used to translate into a specialized machine language.

1.4   Hardware-Software

All the mechanical parts of the data processing setup (input-output units, computers with storage, calculating and control units) are called "hardware." The "software" comprises calculating and control programs and the know-how for operation of the computer.

1.5   Off-Line and On-Line Processing

Data input may be "off-line" or "on-line." We speak of off-line processing when the primary data are fed into the computer manually by way of an input system. In on-line operation, the data of the study unit are picked up

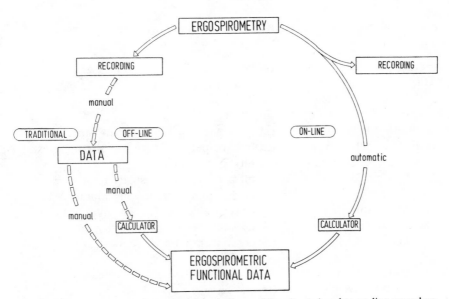

Fig. 204b. Data flow in a traditional (extreme left), an off-line (center) and an on-line procedure (right) for obtaining spiroergometric functional data (*Rittel*). Broken arrows: manual data transfer, solid arrows: automatic data transfer.

electronically from the start and transmitted to the data-processing setup. For this purpose, data which are already analog-electrically available must be digested for the computer's needs by means of a suitable adapter unit (interface).

2. Spiroergometric Testing of Performance

In spiroergometry (spirometric ergometry), the reactions of respiration, HR and blood pressure are measured against a prescribed amount of work. To record respiration, open and closed systems for measurement of the functions are used. HR is best determined from electrocardiographs. They furnish by means of electronic integrators an analog-electrical voltage for the HR for data processing. Blood pressure data obtained pneumatically from Korotkoff's sounds are likewise available as analog-electric voltages. In electrically braked bicycle ergometers, a corresponding recording voltage can be obtained for any set number of watts.

2.1 Measured and Calculated Data

In ergometric functional studies, the following parameters are customarily recorded:

wattage	(in watts)
HR	(in beats per minute)
systolic blood pressure	(in Torr)
diastolic blood pressure	(in Torr)
respiratory time-volume	(in liters per unit time, usually minutes)
respiration rate	(in breaths per unit time, usually minutes)
tidal volume	(in ml)
O_2 consumption	(in ml per unit time, usually minutes)
CO_2 production	(in ml per unit time, usually minutes)
respiratory quotient	$(= CO_2 \text{ production}/O_2 \text{ consumption})$
respiratory equivalent	$(= O_2 \text{ consumption/respiratory time-volume})$
O_2 pulse	$(= O_2 \text{ consumption/heart beat,}$ in ml/heart beat)
O_2 consumption per kg of body weight	(in ml/kg)

This list includes units of measurement and calculation. In calculations, the following must be taken into consideration: corrections for BTPS (body temperature and pressure, saturated) and STPD (standard temperature and pressure, dry), the nitrogen correction in open systems and the quotients as listed. Ideal values in spiroergometry must be determined according to age, sex, stature and weight of the subject.

2.2 Calculation by Electronic Data Processing

The traditional calculation was done with calculating recorders, conventional calculators and by use of tables or guide nomograms. The multiplicity of routinely occurring data demands a great waste of time in calculation and filling out blanks and record sheets. The use of data-processing machines (computers) affords the following advantages:

1. relieves the researcher of much time-consuming calculation
2. reduces human sources of error
3. increases the pace of research
4. reduces the expense of long-term procedures
5. increases the volume of information per study
6. provides quick availability of test results through automatic printout of results
7. facilitates comparisons by repetition
8. provides automatic comparison with norms
9. provides automatic storage of study results
10. allows ready access to data from archives for statistical formulations.

3. Off-Line Procedure

3.1 Programmable Table Model Computers

A simple and rapid evaluation of spiroergometric functional data using a programmable table model computer (Programma 102 from Olivetti) is described by Löllgren (Fig. 205).

The computer programs are fed in via magnetic cards and the experimental data are typed in on the keyboard. All calculations, including the determination of mean spirometric resting values and their deviations, are performed and the result turned out in numeric form on paper tapes. The programming language and handling of the computer are easy to learn. Setting up the program is simple and thus adaptable to various machines and methods. An especial advantage is to be seen in the low cost of the computer. A disadvantage is the fact that the printout of results on tape is

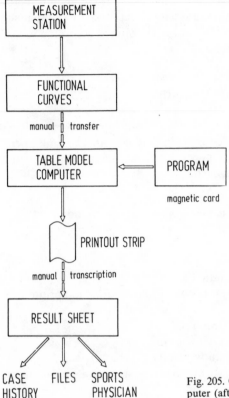

CASE   FILES   SPORTS
HISTORY   PHYSICIAN

Fig. 205. Off-line procedure using table model computer (after *Löllgren*).

not readily readable in tabular or chart form, and must be copied out in presentable shape. No immediate storage of data is provided.

3.2 Small Computers Coupled with Teletype

A table model computer with greater storage capacity (Wang 720) combined with a teletype has been used since 1972 by Heck and Hollmann. The working and computing program is here fed into the computer via magnetic tape cassettes. All the customary calculations and determination of certain additional calculation data are carried out (Fig. 206).

The decisive advantage of this procedure lies in the printout of a result sheet containing all data on the spiroergometric performance with clear text remarks, all immediately available for analysis and use. In addition, the data on the result sheet can simultaneously be punched out on tape and thus filed away, all in a single operation.

```
          INSTITUT FUER KREISLAUFFORSCHUNG UND SPORTMEDIZIN
                 DEUTSCHE SPORTHOCHSCHULE KOELN


NAME    :
VORNAME:
BERUF   :    STUDENT
ADRESSE:     5 KOELN 60 TURMSTRASSE 12


U.-DATUM :      9.  11.  73                ARCH.-VR:       538
GEB-DAT. :     12.  12.  52                TEST-VR. :    16301
GROESSE  :    183 CM                       GEWICHT  :   71.0 KG
ALTER    :     20                          GSCHL.   :       1
ARZT     :     11                          MTA      :       3
TEMP.    :     21.5 C                      L.-DRUCK:    757 TORR
L= 16.6 CM     B= 12.5 CM    TMAX= 10.8 CM  HERZVOL.:    873 ML
BLUTVOL. :     5600 ML                      HAEMOGL.:   15.2 G%


                            SPIROMETRIE


VK:     5.90 L             AGW:    218 L          TIFF.-WERT:      %


                          SPIROERGOMETRIE
                 (STANDARDTEST NACH HOLLMANN UND VENRATH)

MKP/                     AMV/                            RR     RR
SEK     O2-A     AMV     O2-A    AF      PF     O2-P    SYST   DIAST

RUHE     341    10.9     31.9    10      56     6.1     120     85
  3      674    18.5     27.5    15      76     8.8     130     80
  7     1079    24.0     22.2    21      92    11.7     140     75
 11     1529    33.9     22.1    24     108    14.1     155     70
 15     1799    40.4     22.4    26     120    14.9     190     65
 19     2249    56.8     25.2    30     144    15.6     205     65
 23     2609    74.3     28.5    35     160    16.3     215     60
 27     2969    82.0     27.6    36     172    17.2     225     60
 31     3374   108.2     32.0    41     180    18.7     230     55
 35


MAX.O2-AUFN.(ASTRAND):      3519 ML           REL.MAXO2A:     49.5 ML/KG
MAX. O2-PULS( 195)   :      18.0 ML           O2-A.(170):     2968 ML
AUSDAUERGRENZE( 130 ):      2002 ML           O2-P.(170):     17.4 ML

HERZVOL.:    873 ML         HV/KG:    12.3 ML          HVAE:      48.4
BLUTVOL.:   5600 ML         BV/KG:    78.8 ML
HAEMOGL.:   15.2 G%         GES.-HB:    851 G          GES.-HB/KG:   11.9 G
```

Fig. 206. Alphanumeric output of the off-line procedure using a table model computer with attached teletype (*Heck* and *Hollemann*).

3.3 Large Computers

A convenient possibility in data processing in the off-line procedure is opened up with the availability of a full-size computer. Waterloh and Rittel have been processing spiroergometric data since 1966 on a full size CD 6400 computer in the computation center of the Aachen Technical (see Fig. 207).

In this procedure, the primary data are transferred from a protocol sheet to punch cards and made available to the computer by means of a punch-card scanner. In addition to the usual spiroergometric calculations, cardiac volume and quotients determinable therefrom are determined.

The advantages of this procedure consist of the extensive amount of data possible per patient and the convenient presentation, along with clear text, on 11-3/4″ × 15-3/4″ sheets, copies of which can be supplied in any desired number from the high-speed printer. In addition, direct documentation of data on punch cards and/or magnetic tape is available. The disadvantage that some might find in the data being punched out just as produced by the data processing is made up for through the advantage gained from the direct documentation of all the data. The only unavoidable disadvantage is the time consumed in waiting.

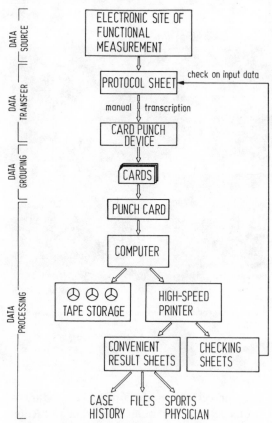

Fig. 207. Off-line procedure with a full-size computer using punch cards (*Waterloh* and *Rittel*).

Fig. 208. Convenient alphanumeric output from the high-speed printer of a full-size computer bank (*Waterloh* and *Rittel*).

SPIROERGOMETRISCHE FUNKTIONSUNTERSUCHUNG

1

NAME	KRAFTFAHRE
BERUF	4. 7.20
GEB.-DAT.	178
GROESSE	80
GEWICHT	55
ALTER	MAENNL.
GESCHLECHT	210
RAUCHEN	

2

ARCHNR.	200704.2
TESTNR.	5.1
NATION	
UNI.-DAT.	27. 2.75
UHRZEIT	9
RAUMTEMP.	23
FEUCHTE	36
LUFTDRUCK	775

3

```
I HOCHSCHULAERZILICHES INSTITUT I
I (LEITER DR.E.WATERLOH)        I
I TECHNISCHE HOCHSCHULE         I
I                               I
I 51  A A C H E N               I
I ROERFONDERSTR. 7              I
```

	SOLL	IST
HAEMOGLOBIN	14 - 18	15.1
ERYTHROZYTEN	4.6-6.2	4.86
M C H	27 - 36	31.1
HAEMATOKRIT	42 - 54	0
HERZVOLUMEN		408.0
-LAENGE		12.3
-BREITE		9.7
-TIEFE		9.5
KOERPEROBF.		1.980
HERZVOL./KG.		0.0
HERZVOL./GE.		0.0
SOLLGRUNDUMSATZ		1688
VO2 MAX(ASTRAND)		0

4

VOLUMINA

		SOLL	IST
ATEMVOLUMEN	CCM	532	759
INSP.RESERVEVOLUMEN	CCM	2578	2339
INSPIRATIONSKAPAZITAET	CCM	3110	3098
EXP.RESERVEVOLUMEN	CCM	1037	1366
INTRATHORAK.GASVOLUMEN	CCM	2750	3229
RESIDUALVOLUMEN	CCM	1713	1862
RESIDUAL./TOTALK.	PROZ	29	29
VITALKAPAZITAET	CCM	4147	4465
TOTALKAPAZITAET	CCM	5860	6327

ABWEICHUNG VOM SOLL

VITALKAPAZITAET	PROZ		8
ATEMGRENZWERT	PROZ		0
TOTALKAPAZITAET	PROZ		6

5

ATEMDYNAMIK

		SOLL	IST
ATEMZEITQUOTIENT		1/1-1.5	1/1.18
APNOE INSP.	SEC	50 - 60	64
APNOE EXP.	SEC	30 - 40	40
ABSOL.SEC.KAP.	CCM	2903	3615
RELAT.SEC.KAP.	PROZ/VK	70	81
MAX.ATEMSTOSSGESCHW.	LIR/SEC		0.00
MAX.ATEMSTROMGESCHW.	LIR/SEC		0.00
ATEMGRENZWERT	LIR/MIN	114.8	114.8
ATEMRESERVE		1/1.4.4	1/8.4.4

ATEMMECHANIK

INSP.RESISTANCE	CM H2O/L/S	BIS 3.5	2.15
EXP.RESISTANCE	CM H2O/L/S	BIS 3.5	1.99
MITTLERE RESIST.	CM H2O/L/S	BIS 3.5	1.95

6

```
                           RUHE    BELAST.                                ERHOLG.
LEISTUNG        WATT       SOLL  IST   50   50   75   75  100  100     4    7   10
DAUER           MINUTEN                                                 4    7   10
BLUTDRUCK SYST. MM HG       120  160  160  165  170  170  180  185    115  105  110
BLUTDRUCK DIAST.MM HG        80   80   75   70   70   70   70   70     70   70   70
PULSFREQUENZ    P.MIN        84  112  113  129  128  139  145  145    103  102  100
ATEMFREQUENZ    P.MIN        17   23   30   23   28   31   32   22     24   23   22
ATEMVOLUMEN     CCM         759 1465 1463 1510 1632 1819 1969  677    846  761  677
ATEMMINUTENVOL. L/MIN      12.9 33.7 34.1 45.3 45.7 63.0 20.3 14.9   20.3 17.5 14.9
O2-AUFNAHME  PROZ.ANV       4.1  4.7  4.6  3.8  4.1  3.7  3.7  4.1    3.6  3.7  4.1
CO2-ABGABE   PROZ.ANV       3.4  3.9  4.6  3.5  3.5  3.5  3.5  3.3    3.6  3.3  3.3
O2-AUFNAHME  CCM/MIN        437 1309 1306 1412 1548 1724 1926  505    604  535  505
CO2-ABGABE   CCM/MIN        362 1086 1099 1310 1359 1631 1822  406    621  477  406
RESPIRAT. QUOTIENT    .82-.86  .83  .85  .92  .88  .95  .95  .80   1.03  .89  .80
ATEMEQUIVALENT        20-35  25.8 26.3 31.9 29.5 32.7 32.7 29.5   33.6 32.7 29.5
SAUERSTOFF-PULS             5.2 11.7 11.5 11.0 12.1 12.4 13.3  5.0    5.9  5.2  5.0
O2-AUFN./GEWICHT CCM        5.5 16.4 16.2 17.8 19.4 21.6 24.1  6.3    7.5  6.7  6.3
```

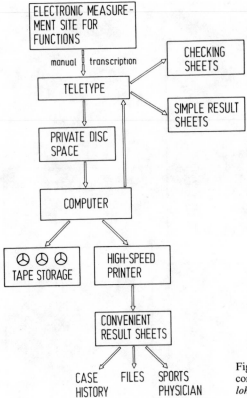

Fig. 209. Off-line procedure with teletype connected to a full-size computer (*Waterloh* and *Rittel*).

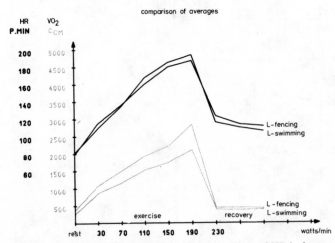

Fig. 210. Comparison of averages for O_2 consumption and HR in fencers and swimmers drawn by a graphomat (original in full color) (*Waterloh* and *Rittel*).

3.4   Teletype Attachment to the Full-Size Computer

An off-line procedure that eliminates the disadvantage of time wasted in waiting is the coupling of a teletype to the full-size computer.

The primary data are transmitted via a Siemens teletype (physician's terminal) to the full-size computer (computer terminal). There the program, stored in a "private disc space," is summoned up for computations. The resultant data are transmitted back again to the teletype at the physician's terminal. The printout then is made in alphanumeric form in clear text on 8-1/2" × 11" sheets. 11-3/4" × 15-3/4" sheets can be prepared at the same time by the high-speed printer in the full-size computer setup in any desired number of copies. All data are stored away on magnetic tapes at the computer station (Fig. 209).

3.5   Possibilities of a Full-Size Computer Setup

The particular advantage of storage on magnetic tape lies in the practically unlimited storage capacity, in space-saving along with instant retrievability, and in the possibility of processing data electronically from the most varied points of view. Thus, alphabetic name lists can be obtained from choronologically filed blocks of data and be sorted for age levels, clinical findings, different sports and according to certain attained workload levels or other aspects. For statistical inquiries, correlation and regression analyses of blocks of data of certain groups can be carried out with corresponding programs, as well as calculations of averages, standard deviations and t-values.

Moreover, the full-size computer setup offers the possibility of converting all results expressed numerically to graphic presentations by means of graphomats or plotters and printing them out that way. The functional parameters which are to be presented are transferred to punch strips under automatic control of a preset program. The punch strip also contains preprogrammed data on the desired dimensions, typeface, type size and format of the axial distribution (Figs. 210 and 211a).

The digital plotter receives its commands and data via a magnetic tape. For lettering the drawings, there is available a symbol-printer with 48 symbols, making it possible to print rapidly in typewriter quality. In this way a great deal of software and computer time can be saved as compared to the graphomat.

3.6   Microfilm Storage by Means of a Full-Size Computer

A new filing procedure, called COM (computer on microfilm), affords the possibility of transferring data from magnetic tape to microfiches. On each

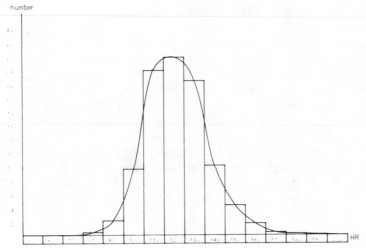

Fig. 211a. Frequency distribution of HR at 70 watts in subjects aged 20 to 30, N = 1004, drawn by a plotter (*Waterloh* and *Rittel*).

microfiche (Fig. 211b) it is possible to place in up to 104 miniaturized blocks the data from the same number of typewritten pages, which can be projected in enlarged form on a projection screen for retrieval reading, and if desirable recopied on a larger 11-3/4" × 15-3/4" sheet. Microfilm cards afford a space-saving filing system for data and diagrams. They are handy and readily scannable, so that even with a huge amount of stored material a quick survey of all the patient data is quite possible.

Before being transcribed on microfilm cards, the blocks of data filed chronologically on magnetic tape are sorted alphabetically by patient name by the computer every quarter or every year. The top line of each microfiche, corresponding to eight frames, has a title information written by the calculator in large, easily readable letters. On the last part of the frame, the calculator writes the contents for the microfiche. This way, it is easy to find the desired microfilm cards and all other individual data on the microfiche.

4.   On-Line Procedure

The chief disadvantage of all off-line procedures lies in the manual input of data. This can give rise to data errors which are avoidable in the on-line procedure.

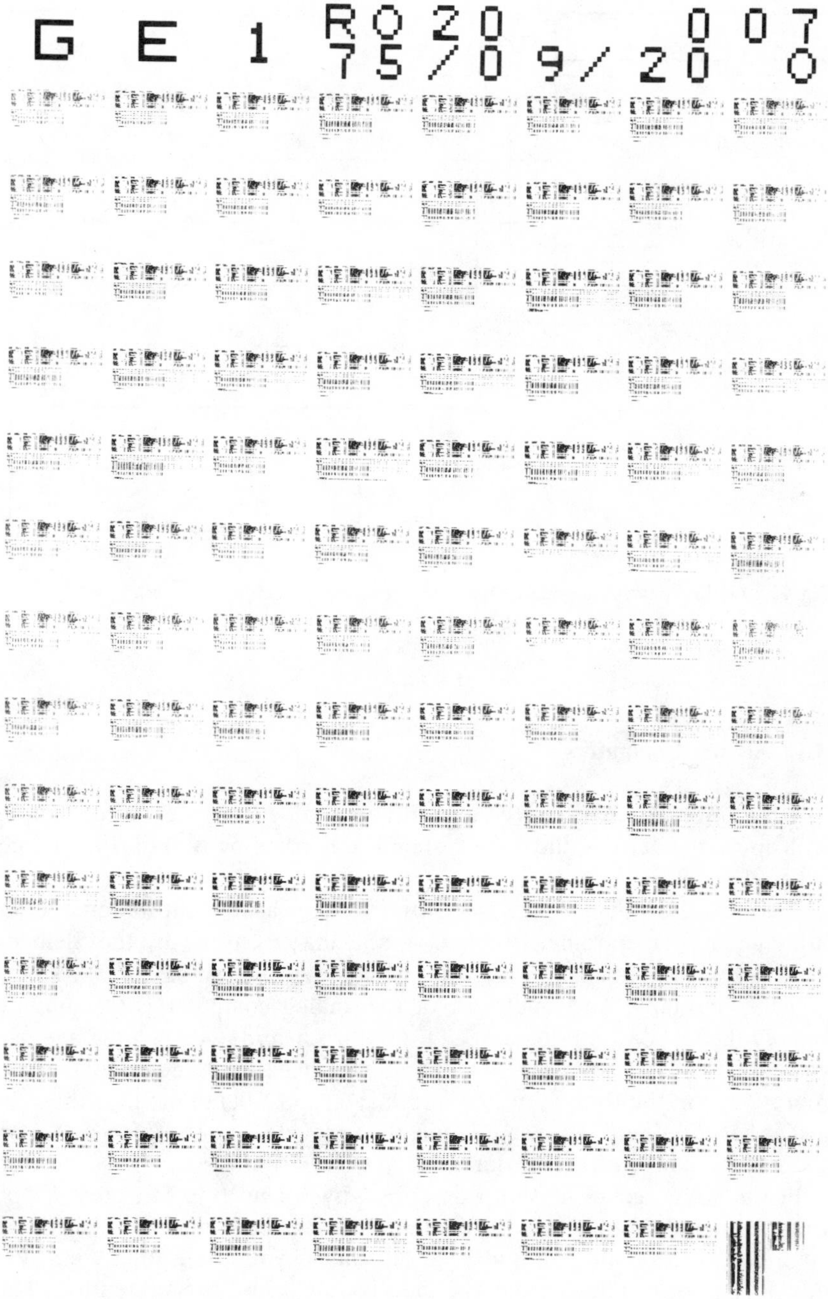

Fig. 211b. Microfiche (microfilm card) with 14 × 8 = 112 frames (size of the original: 94 × 78 mm). The last frame at lower right is the table of contents for the microfiche.

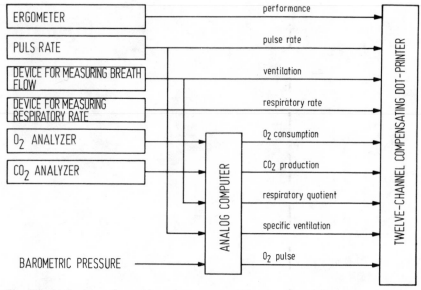

Fig. 212. On-line procedure with analog computer (after *Brandt* and *Bünau*).

4.1 Analog Computers

The use of on-line data processing with an analog computer in connection with spiroergometry in the open system is described by Brandt, Bünau and Flügel (Fig. 212).

Brandt and Brünau use the Siregnost FD 78 measurement station operating on the open spirometric principle and manufactured by the Siemens Company, Department of Medical Technology, Henkestrasse 127, 852 Erlangen, Germany. The chief task of the analog computer is to compute rapidly the O_2 consumption and CO_2 production and to correct the average gas flows to STPD conditions. The parameters measured and calculated are represented in the form of curves and make it possible to monitor the subject as he works out. At the same time, they provide synoptic information on the interplay of the various data.

In the spiroergometric setup described by Flügel (the Siregnost FD88 from Siemens; see Fig. 213), the computations are performed by two analog computers. One analog computer, A, calculates by multiplication the STPD and BTPS corrections for the O_2 and CO_2 data and the ventilation. The other analog computer, B, calculates the quotients—respiratory equivalent, respiratory quotient and O_2 pulse.

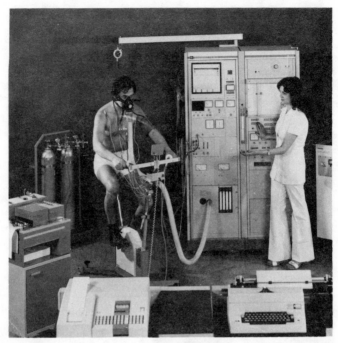

Fig. 213. Siregnost FD 88 S measurement station with analog computer and data output on a multicolor dot-printer, tape printout and/or electric typewriter, 1977 (Photo: Siemens Co.).

In cyclic sequence, the individual data are called for and are printed out by means of two-second series of dots during the exercise examination on a multicolor dot-printer in a so-called "synoptic ergospirogram" which contains all the customary data. These data can be processed with alphanumeric output of the functional parameters by means of an Olivetti computer bank (Programma P 652) in connection with the Olivetti Editor 4 ST.

In the Pulmosport spiroergometric measuring station, product of the firm of Dr. Fenyves and Gut, Leonhardstrasse 26, CH 4051 Basel, Switzerland, an analogous depiction of six to twelve parameters is possible in different colors on a dot-printer. For the digital output, a recording printer is available, which periodically prints out as many as ten parameters in succession every one, two or five minutes. Likewise, numeric values for the same parameters can be provided every minute.

4.2 Digital Computers

Howald and Schönholzer describe on-line data processing using a programmable Olivetti table model computer (Programma 102) in spiroergometry with the Pneumotest open-spirometer system from the firm of Erich Jaeger, Roentgenring 5, 87 Wurzburg, Germany. In addition to the analog recording of spirogram, respiratory minute-volume (BTPS) and CO_2 and O_2 content of the exhaled air on a multichannel direct printer, an analog-digital transformer makes it possible to process the fresh data as it appears. Before the start of the examination the programming is done by means of magnetic cards. The BTPS-STPD correction factor for the barometric and temperature conditions of the moment is keyed in manually. Every 30 seconds during the examination, the functional parameters and calculated quotients are reproduced numerically on the output tape. After storage of the data in the computer, averages for respiratory time-volume, O_2 consumption, O_2 pulse, respiratory equivalent and RQ can be calculated in any desired number of the 32 available cycles and printed out on record tapes. The authors see the advantage of this procedure in the considerably easier processing, as compared with the traditional manual evaluation and calculation. A disadvantage would be that the numeric printout on tape lacks overall ready visibility due to the fact that the data are printed out in the order in which they are received.

By expanding this setup with a larger table model computer (Olivetti's Programma 602), a magnetic tape unit (Olivetti's MLU 600) and an electric typewriter provide a more comprehensive programming capacity, data storage and more readable printout of data in typewriter paper format (Howald).

A digital data gathering system was conceived for the Magna-Test spirometer system type 710 from Meditron (formerly Dargatz), Lange Strasse 51, 2111 Kakenstorf, Germany, which can be used in addition to the conventional analog recording. This gathering system prints out as many as 10 parameters in numerical form on a tape printer at intervals of 30 or 60 seconds.

This same firm (Meditron) has supplied open-system spirometric equipment for several years, in addition to their closed-system devices. Here the measurement of volume is done by means of Fleisch's pneumotachograph. The analysis of the respiratory gases for O_2 is done with the quick-registering Oxytest-S (paramagnetic principle, from the firm of Hartmann and Braun) and for CO_2 with the URAS (infrared principle, from the same firm). Computers H99 or H100 are used for electronic processing in the latest model. This is based on the commercially available Hewlett-Packard table model computers 9815 and 9825. The computers are equipped with a cassette unit and a tape printer which prints out data in alphanumeric form and allows for direct dialog between computer and operator. The programs required for carrying out the examination and for the EDP are prepared on a cassette. The interface developed for collecting data makes it possible to search the various individual measurement channels and provides analog-digital changeover and coded transmittal of the individual signals to the computer.

After all calculations have been carried out, the resulting data are printed out on a tape printer with alphanumeric elucidation or in a synoptic readable result report in typewriter paper format.

Since 1976–77 a compact, mobile system for metabolic measurements with on-line data processing has been available commercially from Beckman Instruments, Advanced Technologic Operations, Anaheim, CA, USA. The device was developed in the USA by Beckman (1976, 1977a, b) in consultation with Wilmore et al. (1974, 1976). A turbine collector with a linear measuring range of from 3 to 250 liters per minute and precise determination of respiratory frequency up to 60 breaths per minute was developed for measuring ventilation. For respiratory gas analysis the O_2 Monitor OM-11 (polarographic principle) and the LB-2 CO_2 analyzer (infrared method) are being used, which have a reaction time of 0.1 second for 90% of the data. The built-in programmable table model computer, which controls the collection of data after input from a magnetic card, prints out the resulting data on a paper tape at preselected time intervals.

Schindl uses a larger table model computer (Olivetti's Programma 602) with magnetic tape unit, tape-punch stamper and scanner and electric typewriter in the on-line connection to Erich Jaeger's Pneumotest spirometer measurement station mentioned above. In more extensive study programs, the data can be stored on magnetic tape. The calculation of norms, comparison of norms with observed values and output of data and diagnostic suggestions in clear text via an electric typewriter on standard-size typewriter paper take place after the conclusion of the examination. After the printout the data from the examination are stored on punch tapes. After a large accumulation of data, the punch tapes can be further processed by means of a larger and faster computer (this is known as computer hierarchy).

In the Erich Jaeger Pneumotest system, referred to above, Olivetti's P603 and P652 computers, as well as their P102 and P602, can be used. A software package for standard programs in spiroergometry is available for each of the expansion stages of the measurement station. In the latest development of spiroergometry equipment with electronic data processing, the analog data collection unit has been newly conceived by the Erich Jaeger firm. A computer system in four expansion stages is provided for on-line data processing. The connecting element between the analog-operated measurement station and the digital computer consists of a universal-patterned laboratory interface. The expansion stages differ chiefly in convenience of operation,

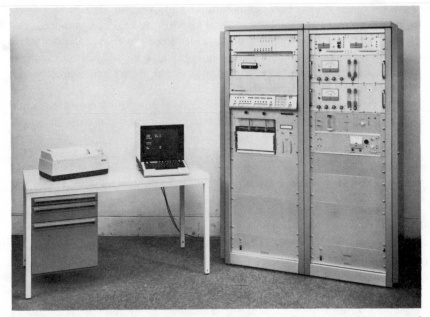

Fig. 214. Spiroergometric measurement station with on-line data processing by means of a process computer (LSI 2/20) from Computer Automation Inc. (CAI). At left is a noiseless printer (Teleprinter, series AH 30 CPS from Extel Corp.) and beside it is a video terminal (Display, model 1440 from TEC Inc., Photo: Fenyves and Gut).

data output (tape output in abbreviated text, typewriter, visual projection screen, high-speed printer and digital plotter) and the manner of storing and filing data. In all four computer systems, the same measurement programs are used and all four put out the customary computation data (see Fig. 215 and also the following subsection on processing computers).

4.3 Processing Computers

Processing computers are able to collect analog and digital values and process them in "real time." They are used in combination with measurement stations of the open and closed systems. High-speed data turnover permits of a quasi-instantaneous signal delivery and monitoring of the data output. In addition to conventional spiroergometric uses, these properties make it possible to analyze each individual breath, provided the measuring devices being employed afford sufficiently high speed of indication.

Among the latest developments in measurement stations for spiroergo-metry with electronic data processing, the firms of Dr. Fenyves and Gut,

Jaeger and Meditron, all referred to above, have introduced processing computers for their full-size installations. Dr. Fenyves and Gut employ a processing computer with a storage capacity of 8, 16 or 24 K, as desired. The possibility is provided for direct access to the central storage for rapid data transmitters such as magnetic tapes or magnetic plates as well as rapid interfaces. The interface is equipped with universal input and output possibilities which make it possible to couple in various peripheral devices for data input and output. The communication with the computer takes place via a video terminal with typewriter keyboard. During the examination the data appear on the screen of the video terminal. For data output there is also, in addition to the display, an alphanumeric matrix-printer for the preparation of 8-1/2″ × 11″ result sheets (Fig. 214).

The Jaeger people use series PDP 11 processing computers from Digital Equipment, with a storage capacity of up to 32 K and floppy discs or changeable record discs, for their larger spiroergometry systems. As an input-output medium, a typewriter can be used as well as a picture projection terminal in connection with a high-speed printer for preparation of up to five copies of a result sheet (Fig. 215).

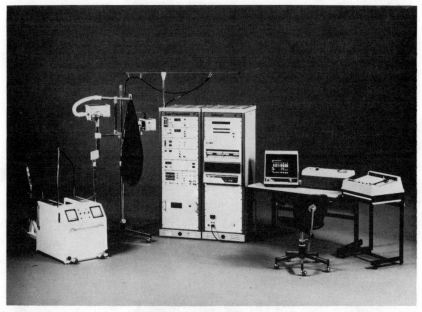

Fig. 215. Pneumotest measurement station with the Dataspir data processing system. Results are put out via visual projection screen, high-speed printer and/or digital plotter 1977 (Photo: E Jaeger).

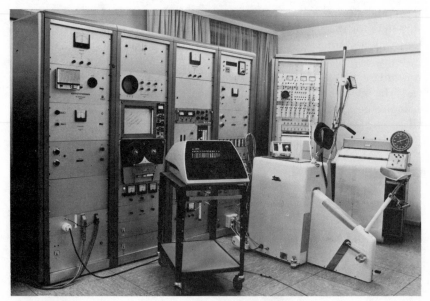

Fig. 216a.

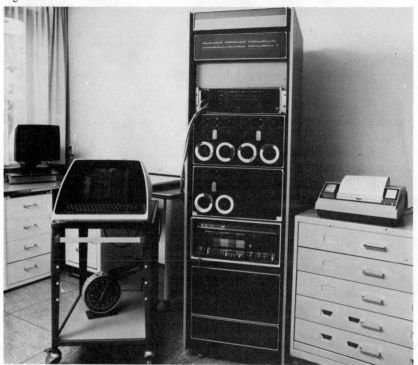

Fig. 216b.

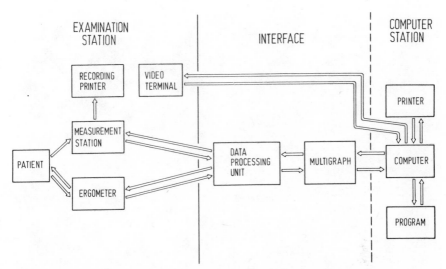

Fig. 217. Functional units of the on-line examination system (*Waterloh* and *Rittel*).

Waterloh and Rittel use the processing computer PDP 8/E (from Digital Equipment) with a storage capacity of 16 K, a magnetic tape unit, a video terminal and a thermo-printer in combination with an open, valveless, electronically operated measurement station for lung function (from Dr. Fenyves and Gut, Leonhardsstrasse 26, CH-4051 Basel, Switzerland), an eddy-current bicycle ergometer that is independent of speed of revolution, and electrocardiogram and a blood pressure cuff. In on-line operation, three functional units are distinguished: examination station, interface and computer station (Figs. 217 and 218). Before the start of each examination, the special control commands for that particular examination procedure are given the computer via the video terminal. Given in addition are data on the patient, the storage code, and the figures for room temperature, humidity and barometric pressure for calculating the standard corrections.

For the on-line processing of the ergometric readings, an interface and a control unit have been developed that introduce the incoming readings to the computer in suitable form. The wattage of exercise is controlled by the

Fig. 216a. Spiroergometry set: Pulmonary function equipment, electrocardiograph (cardiopan), Achtfach recorder, bicycle ergometer (next to blood pressure apparatus), video-terminal (Foto H.-F. Rittel).

Fig. 216b. Computer station: processing computer PDP 8/E with a storage capacity of 16 K and three magnetic tape units plus built-in interface; at the right stands a "Silent 700" printer; at the left is the mobile video terminal; in the background is the scanning device for microfiches (Photo: H.F. Rittel).

```
NAME                              ARCHNR           250429.1
BERUF      HAUMEISTER             TESTNR                5.0
GEB-DAT    28. 4.25               NATION                  1
GROESSE    159                    UNT-DAT          20. 5.77
GEWICHT    66                     UHRZEIT                 8
ALTER      52                     RAUMTEMP               23
GESCHL     MAENNL                 FEUCHTE                45
RAUCHEN    25                     LUFTDR                761


HERZVOLUMEN                       0.
KOERPEROBF                        1.681
HERZVOL/KO                        0.0
HERZVOL/GW                        0.0
SOLLGRUNDUMSATZ                   1418.
VO2 MAX (ASTRAND)                 0.
```

ERGO - SPIROGRAPHIE

WAT	MN	RRS	RRD	PF	AF	AV CCM	AMV L/MN	O2 %	CO2 %	O2 CCM	CO2 CCM	RQ	AE	O2-P CCM	O2/G
SOLL					15	447.	6.7	3.0	2.5	203.	166.	0.82	27.0		
0	6	95	65	70	22	387.	8.5	3.1	2.5	219.	176.	0.80	38.9	3.1	3.3
25	4	120	65	99	27	796.	21.5	4.3	3.5	771.	621.	0.81	27.8	7.8	11.7
25	6	120	70	96	30	754.	22.6	4.3	3.5	812.	654.	0.81	27.8	8.5	12.3
50	4	140	70	108	26	1074.	27.9	4.5	3.8	1043.	876.	0.84	26.8	9.7	15.8
50	6	135	65	110	29	934.	27.1	4.3	3.7	963.	828.	0.86	28.1	8.8	14.6
75	4	155	70	124	30	1141.	34.2	4.4	3.9	1240.	1103.	0.89	27.6	10.0	18.8
75	6	165	70	148	34	1373.	46.7	4.4	4.6	1681.	1775.	1.06	27.8	11.4	25.5
0	4	105	70	91	24	502.	12.0	3.4	3.0	335.	298.	0.89	36.0	3.7	5.1
0	7	90	60	90	23	474.	10.9	3.5	3.0	314.	270.	0.86	34.7	3.5	4.8
0	10	100	60	85	21	499.	10.5	3.7	3.0	323.	260.	0.80	32.4	3.8	4.9

Fig. 218a. Output of the "Silent 700" thermoprinter for a performance test in on-line operation (*Waterloh* and *Rittel*).

WAT	= watt	$O_2\%$	= O_2 consumption in % of RTV
MN	= Exercise time	$CO_2\%$	= CO_2 production in % of RTV
RRS	= Systolic BP	O_2 CCM	= $V_{O_2}/cm^3/min$
RRD	= Diastolic BP	CO_2 CCM	= CO_2 production/cm^3/min
PF	= HR/min	RQ	= RQ
AF	= RR/min	AE	= AEg
AV	= Tidal Volume (cm^3)	O_2P	= O_2 pulse
AMV	= RTV/l	O_2G	= V_{O_2} cm^3/kg

computer by way of a control voltage, is altered at prescribed times in accordance with the preset program, and the wattage at any given time is indicated on the video terminal. Blood pressure readings are taken semi-automatically and are available in the form of analog-electric voltages. The signals for determination of the HR are obtained from an electrocardiograph. From two successive R-peaks the prevailing average is calculated so that systemic stress can be detected early on. HR, respiration rate and respiratory minute-volume are counted according to definition during a full minute.

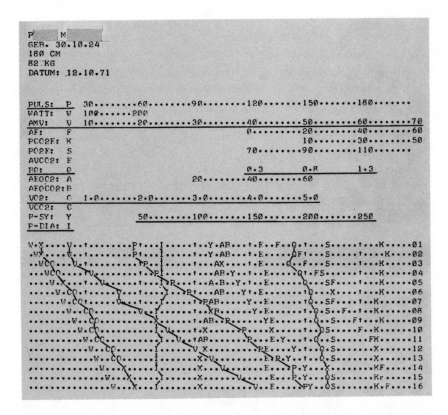

Fig. 218b. Output with quasi-graphic presentation of the functional parameters as furnished every minute. In the upper part of the picture the measurement scales are reproduced. Each calculated value is indicated by a letter. If a line lacks a scale, then the numerals of the previous line apply. The lower half of the illustration shows in 16 lines the calculated values for each minute at the locations which are to be projected to the scales above. If two or more letters fall on the same location an X is printed. The increase in the respiratory time-volume (V) is recognized, for example, or the constancy of the diastolic blood pressure (*Smidt* and *Finkenzeller*).

Pulse rate	—PULS	per minute
exercise	—WATT	in watts
respiratory minute-volume	—AMV	in liters STPD
respiratory rate	—AF	per minute
end-expiratory P_{CO_2}	—PCO2E	in Torr BTPS
end-expiratory P_{O_2}	—PO2E	in Torr BTPS
alveolar ventilation for CO_2	—AVCO2	%
respiratory quotient	—RQ	in ml/ml
respiratory equivalent for O_2	—AEQO2	in ml/ml
respiratory equivalent for CO_2	—AEQCO2	in ml/ml
O_2 consumption	—VO2	in liters STPD
CO_2 production	—VCO2	in liters STPD
systolic blood pressure	—P-SY	in Torr
diastolic blood pressure	—P-DIA	in Torr

For the analysis of the respiratory gases, the concentrations of O_2 and CO_2 in the expired air are analyzed for each successive breath. Previously received signals, such as respiration rate and tidal volume, are temporarily stored until the corresponding O_2 and CO_2 readings, arriving later because of time elapsed during transit, are in. From the primary data of tidal volume, O_2 consumption and CO_2 production are calculated the respiratory equivalent, respiratory quotient and O_2 pulse. The processing computer has the capability to break into the course of the examination. The work on the ergometer can be interrupted if a critical HR is exceeded. The rpm of the eddy-current ergometer are monitored to give warning if they fall below a certain minimum; this will automatically alter the program.

All resulting data are shown minute by minute on the video terminal of the examination station. In this way synoptic digital indications of all parameters measured and calculated are always available to the investigator after a given recording interval is completed. All data are first stored on magnetic tape. After the conclusion of the examination, the recording intervals relevant to the evaluation are printed out by the thermoprinter (Fig. 219).

A program system was developed in 1977 by Rössmann and Waterloh which automatically puts out a brief report of findings in clear text, based on the data obtained. The procedure falls naturally into two phases. First, the parameters relevant to the diagnosis are evaluated in an algorithm of computation and decision composed of three elementary types of functions. Next, a formulating algorithm converts the information obtained into clear text. In this step simple sentence structures are produced by a syntactical program, with the aid of a context-free grammar, and this is then filled in with the facts by means of a semantic program. The necessary textual constants are stored in the form of tree-like structures in order to avoid redundancies. It is, of course, obvious that this computer knowledge must be evaluated only in connection with other diagnostic criteria. The assessment of the validity of the various readings on which the computer knowledge is based can naturally not be done by the computer; this is the task of the experienced physician, and interactions with other organic systems must always be taken into consideration (Ulmer 1977).

As early as 1972, Smidt described breath-by-breath analysis with on-line processing using the pneumotachogram, with O_2 and CO_2 partial pressures in the breathed air determined by mass spectrometry on a continuous basis. In addition to these input data, the HR, blood pressure and wattage setting of the ergometer can be obtained on-line. A PDP-12 from Digital Equipment is used as the computer, having a basic storage facility of 8 K, two magnetic tape units, a real-time clock, a projection screen and a teletype. The primary signals, pneumotachogram and P_{O_2} and P_{CO_2} readings, both inspiration and expiration, appear as a standing picture on the screen of the video terminal. The time lag between the appearance of the pneumotacho-gram and the P_{O_2} and P_{CO_2} readings, arising from the transit time of the gases being analyzed, is set manually on a potentiometer. The pneumotacho-gram is always stored in the computer for a corresponding period of time. By multiplication of the P_{O_2} and P_{CO_2} readings by the corrected simultaneous reading of the strength of the breath flow and subsequent integration of the product obtained, the computer calculates the O_2 consumption and the CO_2 production.

Scales for all parameters to be measured or calculated are printed out on a teletype before the start of the actual examination. Each parameter gets a letter-assignment to earmark it, and at the end of each minute the teletype puts out a line with the earmark letters of the parameters measured and

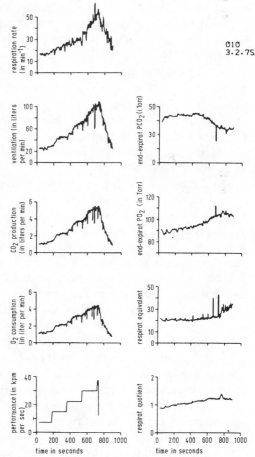

Fig. 219. Recording of spiroergometric parameters obtained in a vita maxima test by the breath-by-breath method using online procedures. The output of analog curves takes place after the conclusion of the examination and is done by means of an incremental plotter.

Commentary:
Abscissa:
   time in seconds
Ordinates:
   respiration rate (in min⁻¹)
   ventilation (in liters per min)
   CO_2 production (in liters per min)
   O_2 consumption (in liters per min)
   performance (in kpm per sec)
   end-expiration P_{CO_2} (in Torr)
   end-expiration P_{O_2} (in Torr)
   respiratory equivalent
   respiratory quotient
   (*Stegemann*).

calculated. At the end of several minutes of examination with the patient at rest and under exercise, there is available a quasi-graphic representation of all parameters, which can in addition also be put out in numerical form. The minute-by-minute output of data permits monitoring of all the readings as they are taken in the course of the actual examination. This affords a check on the functioning of the equipment and also the pathophysiological reactions of the subject. All data are continuously stored on tape and can be retrieved again at any time (see Figs. 216a and b). Of course a purely digital output of all parameters is also possible and they can be expressed either on a breath-by-breath basis (involving a huge mass of data) or minute by minute, as is customary in conventional spiroergometry.

The advantages of this procedure are the large content of information possible, its immediate availability, the relatively clear quasi-graphic presentation and the direct storability. Among the disadvantages must be mentioned the high cost of computers and connected paraphernalia.

The most elegant system known to us for breath-by-breath analysis in on-line procedure with a processing computer was described in 1976 by Stegemann. He uses Fleisch's pneumotachograph for measuring the strength of the breath flow. To analyze the respiratory gases he uses, as does Smidt, the M3 (Varian-MAT) mass spectrometer and determines the O_2, CO_2 and N_2 concentrations on a continuous basis. He uses the PDP 12 digital processing computer from Digital Equipment, which works with real numbers and offers, in conjunction with a video display, the possibility of analog and digital output of data and also permits graphic presentations to be prepared on an X-Y printer.

The continuous analog voltages are program-controlled by way of an analog-digital converter and digitalized at a pace supplied by a programmable quartz clock. The two analog signals for the pneumotachogram and for gas analysis, arriving one after the other at the input of the analog-digital converter, are synchronized as follows: The analog curves for gas concentration drop back in sudden jumps to their inhalation levels at the start of each inhalation. This sudden backtrack is pinned down as the time for the start of an inhalation. The transit of the pneumotachogram for the respective breath must be adapted to this zero line. Since the zero transit of the pneumotachogram has already previously taken place, the time interval between this zero transit and the previously mentioned sudden reversion of the gas concentration curve must be determined at the inhalation level. This done by storing the readings on the strength of the breath flow for a definite but adjustable delay time and retrieving it according to program for further use. The program developed by Stegemann corrects possible changes in the delay time automatically during the course of the examination.

All examination results can be put out either in digital or analog form. The numeric output can be performed during the examination itself by printing out on a breath-by-breath basis the parameters obtained on a line printer. Immediately at the conclusion of the examination the results can also be drawn in the form of a curve with lettered abscissa and ordinate by means of an incremental plotter (Fig. 219).

5. EDP Procedures Available Published in English

The application of EDP in studies of pulmonary function has been reported on by numerous authors in English-language publications. A detailed reference to all these articles is not within the scope of the present work. We will proceed to present here below a brief summary of the procedures of the leading specialists.

5.1 Off-Line Procedure

Predicted spirometric data and actual values at rest were processed by Ellis et al. (1975) on a programmable computer, and on the basis of a comparison between ideal and actual figures an interpretation was printed out by the computer according to clinically customary criteria.

The off-line collection and processing of general data (on the individual, barometric pressure, temperature, etc.), readings on ventilation, diffusion and gas exchange while at rest as well as data on blood gas analysis at rest and with exercise were described by the investigating teams of Rosner et al. (1966, 1967, 1971) and Ayers et al. (1969). In their system, the raw data can be passed on to the computer center by mail or telephone and transmitted via a teleprinter connection direct to the digital computer (Control Data Corp. 160 A) after preparing a punch tape. All customary computations including the determination of predicted values and comparison of predicted and actual values for the parameters while at rest are carried out by the computer. Functional data falling outside the normal range (an upper and lower limit for the normal range are given) are marked with an asterisk. These starred values are processed separately in a subroutine and a descriptive term or association with a physiological dysfunction is appended to these in clear text.

The off-line processing on the CDC 1700 computer (32 K 16-bit words) of the Control Data Corporation was described in 1973 by Protti et al. As early as 1968, a program in Fortran was developed at a computer center for the electronic processing of data on pulmonary functions and was simplified and improved after three years' experience with it.

In the procedure described in 1973 by Protti et al., the patient's personal data, transfer diagnosis, clinical data and the barometric pressure are noted on the first page of the three-page input blank. On the second page are entered the raw data from the spirometric tests and on the third the figures for gas exchange and arterial blood gases. The raw data from repetitions of the test (for example, after administration of bronchial dilators) can be filled in on the appropriate page. In addition there is space reserved for remarks from the investigator (or technicians) about the course of the examination (cooperativeness of the patient, devices used in the examination, etc.), so that the examining or directing physician of the hospital can judge the relevance of the examination results.

Each evening all the filled-in blanks are brought to the computer department, punched on cards, checked and processed. The structure of the program, because of its modular conception with fifteen subroutines and the properties of the computer (overlaying capabilities), requires only 4 K stored words. Through this program all input data are checked: they must lie between tabularly filed minimal and maximal limits. If data are correct even though they lie beyond the set limits (for instance, a patient who weighs more than 175 kg), this fact is emphasized by special notation. Erroneous input data (for example, punching errors) are corrected at the computer center and the whole batch of data is reprocessed.

Two subroutines calculate ideal values for nine parameters based on age and height. In the comparison of actual and ideal figures it is ascertained whether the actual reading lies below the 80% limit of the appropriate regression grades. If this happens the actual reading is regarded as "abnormal" and marked with an asterisk. The results are printed out on two sheets of typewriter paper.

The first of these two pages contains the personal data, transfer diagnosis, actual and ideal values for static and dynamic volumes (with indication of the percentage of deviation, if any, marked with an asterisk), completed with the determination of the diffusion capacity. Results of a re-test (for example, after administration of a broncho-dilator) are inserted in a separate column. A verbal interpretation, based on the above comparison of actual and ideal figures, is printed out under the columns of figures. The second page contains, in addition to the data on the patient, the readings and some ideal figures for the investigation of ventilation, gas exchange and blood gas analysis at rest and, in certain cases, under exercise.

This article (Protti et al., 1973) expressed the intention of further developing the technique to include graphic data output as well as on-line collection and processing of the functional data. The authors felt that an important requirement for this was a shift from the previously used full-size IBM 360/65 computer, with twenty terminals in various departments of the hospital, to the smaller CDC 1700 computer, which serves only a few users.

In a cost-value analysis, Protti et al. (1973) achieved a saving of about 100 minutes (235 minutes compared to 134.5 per patient) compared to manual processing. This estimate covers the entire study of pulmonary function: evaluation, calculation of ideal values, interpretation of the results, and preparation of a typewritten result sheet.

5.2   On-Line Procedure

Wilmore and Costill (1974) and Wilmore et al. (1976) describe the on-line processing of ventilation and gas analysis readings with a programmable computer (Hewlett-Packard 9810). This team, in conjunction with the Beckman Co., developed the "Metabolic Measurement Chart" (MMC). The developments leading to this system of measurement, by way of the Douglas-bag method with automatic gas analysis and data processing (Wilmore and Costill, 1974), as well as the comparative studies on the precision of measurement attained with the MMC (a comparison with two independent systems of ergospirometry), and described by Wilmore et al. (1976).

Turney et al. (1972) and Blumenfeld et al. (1973) report on an automatic monitoring system for parallel monitoring of the respiratory gases over a long period in the case of twelve patients in an intensive care station. Each patient is connected to the sampling line by means of a three-way valve, through which the gas samples are fed into a mass spectrometer. A computer controls the opening and closing of the valves in programmed sequence. The analysis readings from the mass spectrometer for inspiration and expiration are digitalized and put out at once (real-time) numerically, including the peaks for O_2 and CO_2 concentration and the minimal O_2 concentration. Average values are computed for a fixed interval (36 seconds), giving $\dot{V}_{O_2}$, $\dot{V}_{CO_2}$, and RQ. There are two protocols: In the first place, every hour the readings for all occupied beds (maximum: twelve patients) are automatically recorded. In the second place, the personnel of the intensive-care station are able to monitor the readings obtained for a selected patient at intervals of one minute.

Neely et al. (1971) also measured bedside spirometric parameters, mainly mechanical ones related to breathing, which were then processed by means of a small analog computer.

5.3   Breath-by-Breath Analyses

Beaver, Whipp, and Wasserman (1972, 1973) use in their on-line procedure for breath-by-breath analysis a Fleisch pneumotachograph (model 3) to which the patient is connected via an Otis-MacKerrow two-way valve (W. E.

Collings, Cambridge, MA), which itself is connected on the exhalation side with a differential pressure manometer (Statham, Model PM 97). The linearity of this pneumotachograph system runs up to 600 liters per minute at the respiratory frequencies usually met with during exercise. Fine hoses (PE 90) lead from the mouthpiece to a high-speed O_2 analyzer (Westinghouse Model 211) and CO_2 analyzer (Beckman Model LB-1).

The electric signals for the expiration breath flow when there is a difference in concentration of O_2 and CO_2, and those for the HR are connected to the input of an oscillographic recorder (Beckman Type RM Dynograph). The analog output channels of the oscillograph recorder are connected via a multiplexer and an analog-digital converter to the input of the computer. The computer (Varian 620/i) has a central storage facility for 12 K 16-bit words. It simultaneously processes (by time-sharing) on-line data of a second pulmonary function lab with which it is connected. The computer possesses sixteen analog input channels, only four of which are used in the on-line analysis here described: for the signals of exhalational flow, O_2 concentration difference, CO_2 concentration difference and HR.

The data are collected in each sampling interval and retained in storage until the delay in some signals can be compensated for. The computer results can be recorded on digital magnetic tape and at the same time be transmitted via digital-analog output channels for recording in the oscillograph recorder (detailed description also in Wasserman et al., 1973, and Whipp and Wasserman, 1972).

Similar procedures for breath-by-breath analysis are reported by Osborn et al. (1969), Cardus and Newton (1970), Elliot et al. (1970), Domizi and Earle (1970), and Linnarsson and Lindborg (1974), although there are differences in the method of precise determination of the zero point of the pneumotachogram, the detection of delay, the gas analyzers and the preparation of the primary data for electronic processing. For the most part, they use digital computers (Linnarsson and Lindborg use an analog computer) and the functional data are shown in analog or digital form on a projection screen during the course of the examination. The final output of results corresponds to the formulation of the questions by the individual teams.

The articles referred to above represent the present state of EDP use in spirometric and ergospirometric studies, according to the documentation in the literature covered up until July of 1977 (DIMDI—Deutsches Institut für medizinische Dokumentation and Hoechst Documentation of Literature).

References

Albers, C.: Nomogramme zur Berechnung des Sauerstoffverbrauchs mit dem offenen System. Int. Z. angew. Physiol. einschl. Arbeitsphysiol. 25, (1968) 80–88.

Beaver, W. L., B. J. Whipp and K. Wasserman: On-line computer analysis and graphical display of exercise function tests. Manuskript der Fa. Varian MAT, Bremen, 1972.

Beaver, W. L., K. Wasserman and B. J. Whipp: On-line computer analyses and breath-by-breath graphical display of exercise function tests. J. Appl. Physiol. 34, (1973) 128–132.

Beckman: Metabolic Measurement Cart. Beckman Instruments, Bulletin 5115, Illinois/USA 1976.

Beckman: Metabolic Measurement Cart: The bedside program—operating instructions. Beckman Instruments, Program Instructions No. 675502. California/USA 1977a.

Beckman: Metabolic Measurement Cart: The exercise program—operating instructions. Beckman Instruments, Program Instructions No. 675502, California/USA 1977b.

Blumenfeld, W., S. Wolf, Ch. McCluggage, R. Denman and S. Turney: On-line respiratory gas monitoring, Computers and Biomedical Research 6 (1973) 139–149.

Brandt, A.-J. and H. von Bünau: Meßwertverarbeitung durch Analogrechner zur Sofortdarstellung standardisierter Zeitmittelwerte in der Spiroergometrie. Pneumologie (Berl.) 143, (1970) 61–77.

Buchheim, F. W.: Erfassung, Verarbeitung und Dokumentation atemphysiologischer Kenngrößen in Ruhe und unter Belastung. Technik in der Medizin (1973) 1–8.

Buchheim, W. and H.-P. Heynen: Fortschritte in der Sportmedizin mit neuen Meß- und Überwachungsgeräten. Siemens-Zeitschrift 46 (1972) 599–603.

Cardus, D. and L. Newton: Development of a computer technique for the on-line processing of respiratory variables. Comput. Biol. Med. 1 (1970) 125–131.

Chorafas, D. N.: Computer in der Medizin. de Gruyter, Berlin-New York 1973.

Dargatz (Medizin-Elektronik): Hausmitteilungen Nr. 5/1971.

Dargatz (Medizin-Elektronik): MagnaTest-Typ 710. Firmenprospekt.

Domizi, D. B. and R. H. Earle: On-line pulmonary function analysis: program design. Decus Proceedings, Fall 1970 19–22.

Elliott, S. E., Ch. W. Miller, W. T. Armstrong and J. J. Osborn: The use of the digital computer in the study of patients during exercise-induced stress. Am. Heart J. 79 (1970) 215–222.

Ellis, J. H., S. P. Perera and D. C. Levin: A computer program for calculation and interpretation of pulmonary function studies. Chest 68 (1975) 209–213.

Fenyves, F. and W. Gut: Beschreibung unserer Computer-Anlage. Manuskript, Basel 1976.

Fenyves, F. and W. Gut: Personal Communication 1977.

Fleisch, A.: Neue Methoden zum Studium des Gasaustausches und der Lungenfunktion. Edition Leipzig 1964.

Flügel, E.: Die apparative Einrichtung für die ergospirometrische Belastungsuntersuchung. Elektromedica (1972) 84–89.

Flügel, E.: Personal Communication 1977.

Griffith, P. H. and W. L. Beaver: Real time analysis of pulmonary function data. Varian Associates, Palo Alto/California.

Heck, H. and W. Hollmann: Personal Communication, Köln 1973 and 1977.

Hollmann, W.: Höchst- und Dauerleistungsfähigkeit des Sportlers. Barth, München 1963.

Howald, H.: Eine Ergospirometrie-Anlage mit on-line-Datenverarbeitung durch Mikrocomputer. Med.-Markt/Acta medicotechnica 21 (1973) 115–120.

Howald, H. and G. Schönholzer: Erfahrungen bei der Ergospirometrie in einem offenen System mit direkter elektronischer Datenverarbeitung. In: Stucke, K.: Deutscher Sportärztebund, Verhandlungen 24. Tagung, Würzburg 1971, Demeter, Gräfelfing 1973.

Hüllemann, K.-D. and D. Matthes: Spiroergometrie mit elektronisch arbeitenden Geräten. Medizinische Technik 95 (1975) 69–73.

Jaeger, E.: "Dataspir-Systeme" für Datenverarbeitung in der Medizin. Würzburg 1973.

Jaeger, E.: Moderne Lungenfunktionsdiagnostik. Firmenprospekt Würzb. 1973.

Jaeger, E. and F. Hampl: Personal Communication Würzburg 1976, 1977.

Köhler, R.: Prozeßrechner. Online 11 (1973) 676–687 and 775–783.

Kummer, F.: Die Dokumentation von Lungenfunktionsdaten mit Hilfe eines Computers. In: Fellinger, K.: Computer in der Medizin. Hollinek, Wien 1968.

Linnarsson, D. and B. Lindborg: Breath-by-breath measurement of respiratory gas exchange using on-line analog computation. Scand., J. clin. Lab. Invest. 34 (1974) 219–224.

Löllgren, H.: Die Auswertung spirometrischer, atemmechanischer und exspirationsgasanalytischer Untersuchungen mit einem programmierbaren Tischrechner. Prax. Pneumol. 26 (1972) 701–709.

Meditron (Anlagen zur Funktionsanalytik): Personal Communication. Hamburg 1973.

Neely, W. A., W. T. Robinson, J. D. Hardy and W. O. Bobo: A computer analysis of pulmonary function in surgical patients. Ann. Thorac. Surg. 11, (1971) 565–569.

Neely, W. A., W. T. Robinson, G. H. Holloman and M. H. McMullan: An inexpensive bedside analogue computer for measuring respiratory work and certain other parameters. Surgery, St. Louis, Mo. 69, (1971) 309–313.

Osborn, J. J., S. E. Elliott, F. J. Segger and F. Gerbode: Continuous Measurement of lung mechanics and gas exchange in the critically ill. Medical Research Engineering (1969) 19–32.

Pirtkien, R.: Computereinsatz in der Medizin. Thieme, Stuttgart 1971.

Protti, D. J., N. Craven, A. Naimark and R. M. Cherniack: Computer assistance in the clinical investigation of pulmonary function studies. Meth. Inform. Med. 12, (1973) 102–107.

Rittel, H.-F. and E. Waterloh: Entstehung, Erfassung und elektronische Verarbeitung von Signalen für die Atmung. Prax. Pneumol. 27, (1973) 27–35.

Rittel, H.-F., G. Biener, H. Blackert, H. Lueg and E. Waterloh: On-line-Datenverarbeitung beim spiroergometrischen Leistungstest. Leistungssport 3, (1973) 190–193.

Rittel, H.-F.: On-line-Datenverarbeitung bei leistungsmedizinischen Untersuchungen. Physiotherapie 66, (1975), S. 89–91 and S. 156–158.

Rittel, H.-F. and E. Waterloh: Utilisation d'un petit calculateur dans l'ergospiromé-trie. Broncho-Pneumologie 26, (1976) 114 bis 123.

Rittel, H.-F., E. Waterloh, K. Rössmann and F. A. Schön: Klein- und Großrechner-Einsatz bei Lungenfunktionsuntersuchungen. Prax. Pneumol. 31, (1977) 1–24.

Rittel, H.-F. and E. Waterloh: Computers in lung function tests. In: Shoemaker, W., Brenildo Tavares: Proceedings 6th International Symposium on acute care "Current topics in critical care medicine," vol. 4, Karger, Basel 1977.

Rittel, H.-F.: Elektronische Datenverarbeitung bei der Ergospirometrie. Thieme, Stuttgart 1979.

Rössmann, K., H.-F. Rittel and E. Waterloh: Mikrofilm-Archivierung von Lungenfunktionsdaten. Biomed. Techn. 20, (1975), Supplementary Volume 245–246.

Rössmann, K., H.-F. Rittel and E. Waterloh: Mémorisation parallèle de données sur microfilm et bandes magnétiques. Broncho-Pneumologie 26, (1976) 142.

Rössmann, K. and E. Waterloh: Rechnergestützte Diagnose-Hilfe bei Lungenfunktionsuntersuchungen mit Klartextausgabe des Befundes. Biomed. Techn. 22, (1977), supplementary volume.

Rosner, S. W., A. Palmer and C. A. Caceres: A computer program for computation and interpretation of pulmonary function data. Computers and Biomedical Research 4, (1971), 141–156.

Schindl, R.: Elektronische Datenverarbeitung atemphysiologischer Meßgrößen. Prax. Pneumol. 27, (1973) 365–374.

Schindl, R.: Elektronische Datenverarbeitung in der Pneumologie. Pneumologie 150, (1974) 327–336.

Schindl, R. and R. Mach: Persönliche Mitteilung. Linz, 1973.

Schindl, R., K. Mayer and K. Aigner: Praktische EDV-Erfahrung und Weiterentwicklung im Atemfunktionslabor. Med. Klin. 70, (1975) 1815–1820.

Schön, F. A., H.-F. Rittel and E. Waterloh: Analyse des gaz du sang avec calcul, par ordinateur, de l'equilibre acide-base. Broncho-Pneumologie 26, (1976), 124–132.

Schönholzer, G., G. Bieler and H. Howald: Ergometrische Methoden zur Messung der aeroben und anaeroben Kapazität. In: Hansen, G., H. Mellerowicz: 3. Internationales Seminar für Ergometrie 84–97, Ergon, Berlin 1973.

Shonfeld, E. M., J. Kerekes, C. A. Rademacher, A. L. Weihrer, S. Abraham, H. Silver and C. A. Caceres: Methodology for computer measurement of pulmonary function curves. Dis. Chest 46, (1964) 427 ff.

Siemens: "Meßplätze für die cardiopulmonale Funktionsanalyse." Brochure.

Smidt, U.: A computer program for ergometry. Bull. Physio.-path. resp. 8, (1972) 73–84.

Smidt, U.: On-line Datenverarbeitung in der Lungenfunktionsdiagnostik. Biomed. Techn. 21, (1976) 138–140.

Smidt, U. and P. Finkenzeller: Ein Computerprogramm für die Ergometrie. Pneumonologie (Berl.) 147, (1972) 245–250.

Smidt, U., K. Muysers and G. v. Nieding: Nichtlineare Formeln zur Berechnung spirometrischer Sollwerte. Pneumonologie (Berl.) 144, (1971) 52–58.

Smidt, U., K. Casper, H. J. Schilling and G. Worth: Computer-Einsatz in der modernen Pulmonologie. Münch. med. Wschr. 116, (1974) 169–173.

Stegemann, J.: Rechnergesteuerte Spiroergometrie nach der Methode der Einzelatemzuganalyse. Sportarzt u. Sportmed. 27, (1976) 1–7.

Turney, S. Z., C. McCluggage, W. Blumenfeld, T. C. McAslan and R. A. Cowley: Automatic respiratory gas monitoring, Ann. Thorac. Surg. 14, (1972) 159–171.

Ulmer, W. T.: Lungenfunktionsdiagnostik als Grundlage computeranalytischer Beurteilung. Die Berufsgenossenschaft (1977) 313–314.

Wald, A., D. Jason, T. W. Murphy and V. D. B. Mazzia: A computer system for respiratory parameters. Computers and Biomedical Research 2, (1969) 411–429.

Wasserman, K., B. J. Whipp, S. N. Koyal and W. L. Beaver: Anaerobic threshold and respiratory gas exchange during exercise. J. Appl. Physiol. 35, (1973) 236–243.

Wasserman, K., B. J. Whipp and S. N. Koyal: Quantitative exercise testing procedure manual. Medical Instruments Perkin-Elmer Corporation, Pomona, California 91767.

Waterloh, E., H.-F. Rittel and E. Leide: Elektronische Datenverarbeitung bei spiroergometrischen Leistungsuntersuchungen. Med. Welt 22, (1971) 926–931.

Waterloh, E., H. Lueg, H.-F. Rittel and G. Biener: Ergospirographische Funktionsanalyse im vollautomatisch gesteuerten Untersuchungsgang mit direkter elektronischer Datenverarbeitung. Biomed. Technik 16, (1971) 142–145.

Waterloh, E. and H.-F. Rittel: Anwendung der elektronischen Datenverarbeitung im Lungenfunktionslabor. Wehrmed. 10, (1972) 35–40.

Waterloh, E., G. Biener, H. Lueg and H.-F. Rittel: Computer-Einsatz in der Ergometrie. In: Hansen, G., H. Mellerowicz: 3. Internat. Seminar für Ergometrie, Ergon, Berlin 1973.

Waterloh, E. and H.-F. Rittel: Computereinsatz bei der spiroergometrischen Leistungsüberwachung jugendlicher Sportler, in: Stucke, K.: Deutscher Sportärztebund, Verhandlungen 24. Tagung, Würzburg 1971, Demeter, Gräfelfing 1973.

Waterloh, E., H.-F. Rittel and K. Rössmann: Utilisation d'un ordinateur dans l'exploration fonctionelle du poumon. Broncho-Pneumologie 26, (1976) 133–141.

Whipp, B. J. and K. Wasserman: Oxygen uptake kinetics for various intensities of constant-load work. J. Appl. Physiol. 33, (1972) 351–356.

Wilmore, J. H. and D. L. Costill: Semiautomated systems approach to the assessment of oxygen uptake during exercise. J. Appl. Physiol. 36, (1974) 618–620.

Wilmore, J. H., J. A. Davis and A. C. Norton: An automated system for assessing metabolic and respiratory function during exercise. J. Appl. Physiol. 40, (1976) 619–624.

XVIII. Ergometric Diagnostics in Preventive and Rehabilitative Cardiology

In the framework of preventive cardiology, early diagnosis, the recognition of already premorbid conditions, is of decisive importance in order for measures to be taken at the proper time. The requirement here is a regular preventive cardiological examination performed at least once a year and preferably every three or six months, and this especially in high-risk population groups.

Health and the performance of the cardiovascular system naturally go hand in hand. A progressive reduction in performance of the heart and vascular system is almost surely an early symptom of degenerative cardiac and circulatory diseases. This symptom can be detected by ergometric methods.

1. The simplest and most reliable method is to measure the HR under physical stress at submaximal, relatively (or even absolutely) equal power levels of 1 or 2 watts per kg of body weight, lasting three to six minutes by the stopwatch. If, in several successive examinations, a steady increase in the HR under physical stress lying outside the narrow range of standard deviation for this method crops up, there is an indication of increasing deficiency in physical and cardiac performance. Tachycardial behavior is closely related to a reduction in coronary and cardiac reserves. It usually arises from morphological and vegetative changes in the vascular and other organic systems. Its persistence can gradually lead to degenerative organic disease. There must of course be no delay in turning to thorough qualitative diagnostic measures and consideration of other possible causes on the basis of differential diagnosis.

2. A steady increase in arterial blood pressure during and after equal ergometric exercise may likewise be an indication of mounting loss of economy in the vascular system. It is also to be thought of as a source of increased mechanical wear and tear in the arterial system.

3. A steady decrease in maximal O_2 consumption and maximal physical power may also be caused by a progressive reduction in cardiac performance. It is important with reference to preventive diagnosis only if it exceeds by a considerable margin the natural degree of reduction in performance expected with advancing years.

4. With progressive reduction in performance on the part of the vascular system, the O_2 pulse also decreases under equal ergometric performance. This indicates uneconomic HR work with decreasing volume work and possible reduced peripheral capillarization with reduction in the A-$VO_2\Delta$. With progressive reduction in the cardiac performance reserves, the maximal O_2 pulse also decreases. If this reduction in cardiac performance is caused by degenerative or even inflammatory changes in the myocardium or the valves, the quotient of cardiac volume over maximal O_2 pulse, the so-called cardiac performance quotient, increases steadily. This is a rather sure sign of a faulty relationship between the size and performance of the heart, which can be detected early on by repeated comparative examinations.

5. A considerable increase in ST-depression and T-wave flattening during and after ergometric work in equal, successive preventive electrocardiographic examinations is likewise to be regarded as an indication of changes in O_2 supply, metabolism and vegetative regulation of the heart.

6. In addition, oximetric and spirographic methods can be used to detect arterial undersaturations and spirographic deficits in ergometric exercise.

Through regular and comprehensive application of ergometric methods in cardiologic diagnostic work, preventive measures can be instituted in time. Ergometry is thus a very useful tool in preventive cardiology, and can help save much suffering and expense.

1. What is the Significance of Ergometry in Rehabilitative Cardiology?

In the presence of functional changes and damage in the heart and the vascular system, cardiac and general physical borderline performances can be determined by ergometric methods; with these in mind the proper amounts of rehabilitative training can be established. Moreover, success in rehabilitative training can be objectively verified by ergometric methods.

Prerequisite to this is ergometric measurement and ascertainment of physical or organic borderlines of performance.

2. Determination of Cardio-Physical Borderlines of Performance by Ergometric and Electrocardiographic Means (the Ergo-EKG)

Methodology: The measurements are to be carried out with pedaling while reclining or seated.

Leads: V_1 to V_6 or V_2, V_4, V_6 and/or Nehb.

Stages: 10 watts for one minute
                           or   (depending on results)
            25 watts for two minutes

Start with 25, 30 or 50 watts.

Greater duration in the individual stages provides no differentiation in results (Zerdick, 1979). Monitor continuously on an oscilloscope and record EKG during the last ten seconds of each minute.

Evaluation: Upper borderline performance is reached:
a) On the appearance of EKG changes such as ST-depression (horizontal or descending), extrasystoles or disturbances in stimulus-transmission such as blocks, etc.
b) On the arrival at the age-appropriate maximal range for HR, corresponding to the recommendations of the Rehabilitation Council of the International Society of Cardiology:

Age	Maximal HR
<20	180
20–30	170
30–40	160
40–50	150
50–60	140
60–70	130

c) On arriving at the age-appropriate maximal range for systolic pressure of about 200 to 250 mm Hg. The older (biologically) and more sclerotic the patient is, the lower the indicated maximal systolic pressures.
d) At a respiratory quotient of about 1
e) Upon appearance of subjective difficulties on the patient's part, such as stenocardia (usually preceded by ST-depression), dyspnea (with high respiratory quotient, >30 ml), pain in the calves of the legs, etc.

Rehabilitative training must be programmed to remain about 10–30% below maximal performance as determined ergometrically. The increase in HR during each successive training period should amount to about 30 to 60 beats per minute. The training is best carried out on the ergometer, since this permits an accurate dosage.

At intervals of about three weeks, under exercise of 1 watt/kg of body weight, determinations should be made of HR, arterial O_2 pressure, O_2 pulse and perhaps cardiac performance quotient. If rehabilitative training succeeds, the HR under work stress will be reduced, the O_2 pulse will increase and the cardiac performance quotient will become smaller. ST depression will not occur until ergometric performance becomes greater, or may not occur at all.

References

Brunner, D.: Ergometrische Untersuchungen an Patienten nach Myocardinfarkt. In: Ergebnisse der Ergometrie. Berlin, Ergon Verlag, 1974.

Mellerowicz, H., H. Weidener and E. Jokl: Rehabilitive Cardiologie. Karger: Basel-Freiburg-New York 1974.

Messin, R., S. Degre, P. Vandermoten, and H. Denolin: Ergometry in Cardiology. In: Ergebnisse der Ergometrie. Berlin, Ergon Verlag, 1974.

Zerdick, J.: Diss. FU Berlin 1970.

XIX. Ergometry in Compensation Case Evaluation

by Hans Zapfe

In the majority of compensation case examinations, the estimation of physical power plays a leading role. It is almost always a matter of evaluation of pathological conditions. This means that there must be a qualitative diagnosis before any quantitative measurement of performance is undertaken. This diagnosis is often of paramount importance, since it is required in advance for purposes of proper interpretation of the measurements that will be forthcoming. It also affords a highly significant prognostic evaluation, which in compensation work modifies the final result of any other expert opinion received.

Physical power in a broad sense is affected by numerous factors. Almost all acute organic diseases do this, as do also the majority of chronic infirmities, such as those of the cardiovascular, endocrine or metabolic systems. In the final analysis, of course, normal performance capacity depends on the free transport of blood gases, and therefore on oxygen consumption and carbon-dioxide production via the lungs, the delivery capabilities of the heart muscles and a normal hemoglobin content. This assumption is correct provided no further changes are present which could set a limit on performance; for instance, changes in the use of skeletal muscles or locomotion. If we leave significant anemias out of consideration for the moment, then, in addition to the varied forms of circulatory deficiencies, diseases of the heart and lungs are the ones that most decisively affect general physical performance. A quantitative evaluation of cardiovascular deficiencies, especially, is in very many instances best achieved through ergometric tests. This is said in full realization of what we have said above, under the proviso that acute or chronic infirmities of other sorts (in compensation cases they are generally chronic) are not present.

Thus, it would seem pointless in the case of an individual with polyarthritis and resultant impaired locomotion and movement of the joints, plus muscular atrophy, to undertake an ergometric test simply because heart damage is also present.

1. Compensation Problems and Physical Requirements in Insurance Policies

If a thorough examination gives reason for suspicion of some malfunction in the cardiovascular or pulmonary systems, then before an exercise stress test is done it must be made clear:

a) Whether performance measurement is necessary in order to shed light on medical matters or whether there are contraindications against this for medical reasons

b) Whether a full work load will be required; that is, whether there is any need to measure maximal power or whether submaximal power will be adequate

c) What data are needed to answer the particular questions being raised and how much objectivity a performance test would offer in the certification context, where the subject's goodwill and readiness to cooperate can generally not be relied on in the way it could in a sports-medicine context.

With regard to a) above, it may be said that certification examinations usually have to do with social insurance. Here it is important to distinguish among the several fields of insurance based on their several purposes, which raise different questions about the same infirmities and thus call for different methods of examination.

In workmen's compensation insurance, the examiner has to decide, according to the new German regulatory laws concerning compensation and annuities in effect since February 1957, whether from a medical standpoint the infirmity diagnosed leads more frequently or less so to inability to work at a particular job category as compared with the requirements of the general labor market. According to Paragraph 1246, Section 2, of the RVOY of Germany, an insured is unfit for work if his ability to earn a living has, as a result of illness or other physical or mental infirmity or weakness, fallen below half that of a physically and mentally healthy person of the same education and skill. According to the same paragraph, an insured is not incapable of working until he can no longer perform his gainful duties with a certain degree of regularity for an unpredictable length of time or cannot earn more than a meager amount of income. Type of work, working hours and place of employment (standing, sitting, necessary breaks, confined quarters, etc.) must be taken into consideration.

Therefore in compensation insurance the ability to perform has to be judged in the closest of connections with the work loads to be encountered in the place of employment. For example, if an above-knee amputee is employed in a job done in a sitting position, he does not necessarily suffer any limitation worth mentioning with regard to his ability to earn a living, even as compared with a perfectly healthy person.

In the case of war victims, accident insurance and damage suits, however, the medical expert is far less often asked about the extent of reduction in earning power independently of working conditions. The damage to health has then to be estimated only for confirmation of its causation and solely as to the mere fact of its having occurred, or, under certain circumstances, the fact that it is growing worse. Very often an organ or system has a pathological condition that is supposed to be paid for, but which is not in fact due to the event blamed for it. There is no need here to go into the dubiousness of a percentage estimation of damage to health in itself, nor into the question of an alleged reduction in earning power which has nothing to do with actually earning money, but is of importance rather as a loss of integrity.

In workmen's insurance cases, the most precise possible knowledge of the physical and mental requirements of a day's work on the job in question is absolutely necessary in order to evaluate an applicant for compensation. For instance, the examiner must know:

a) The external conditions under which the job is performed, namely, peculiar or varying working hours, abnormal environmental temperatures, noise, enforced speed-up, etc.
b) Nature of the movements involved and difficulty of the work, whether performed while seated or standing, or in bent-over posture, whether static or dynamic
c) The length of time during which continuous labor of a certain degree of difficulty must routinely be performed and details about any brief peak loads.

Beyond any doubt, a question of long-term performance capability is thus posed that represents something quite different from and is distinctly lower than a maximal performance ergometrically attainable for one or several minutes. These differences have been elucidated very clearly by E. A. Müller by means of long-term work tests with observation of concomitant behavior of the HR. The latter, as the expression of an equilibrium between O_2 consumption by the muscles and O_2 absorption, even over a period of two hours, remains unchanged.

Table 63. Energy requirements for labor of various degrees of difficulty (Basal metabolism $\approx$ 1 kcal per minute $\approx$ 200 ml of O_2 per minute). Easy and medium-difficult jobs as long-term performance for more than 30 minutes (after *G. Lehman*).

	Working kcal per minute:	Total O_2 consumption per minute:	Watts, seated on bicycle
Light	<3	<800 ml $\approx$600 ml	$\approx$30
Moderate	$\approx$3–4	<1000 ml $\approx$800	$\approx$50
Heavy	4	$\approx$1000 ml or more	$\approx$70

In the majority of jobs in this age of automation and conveyor belts, the physical work load is amazingly low. In addition to the data reported by G. Lehmann, the tables by Spitzer and Hettinger reveal the energy requirements for the various physical activities and movements various jobs involve. To readings based solely on calories of work must be added the worker's basic energy consumption. The total oxidative energy turnover is measured ergometrically by O_2 consumption. This is to be taken as corresponding to the average energy equivalent of one liter of $O_2 = 5$ kcal. The basic turnover amounts to about 1.0 to 1.5 kcal, corresponding to 200–300 ml of O_2 per minute. Table 63 shows energy consumption for activities of various degrees of difficulty after the manner of Lehmann.

Tables 64 and 65 show the actual physical work loads for activities of everyday life. The medical pronouncement of unfitness for work in classes of jobs involving only light physical labor or none at all, some of them performed while seated, others while standing, is almost never possible without ergometric testing except on the basis of other proofs of illness such as examination findings, anamnesis, x-ray, EKG, blood-pressure and pulmonary tests. Under urban conditions, the majority of female compensation applicants fall into this group. These days only major health problems preclude such low work loads.

Table 64. Energy-consumption in housework tasks (after *Spitzer* and *Hettinger*).

	kcal/min		kcal/min
General housecleaning	1.9	Dusting	3.1
Making beds	4.1	Scrubbing floor	4.0
Cooking while standing	1.6	Beating and brushing rugs	4.7
Peeling potatoes	2.9	Vacuum cleaning	3.2
Kneading dough	2.4	Window washing	3.3
Dishwashing	2.6	Washing small things	
Dressing and undressing and		in the kitchen	1.9
washing self	2.1	Hanging out laundry	5.0
Sweeping	3.5	Ironing	2.7

In evaluating individuals engaged in jobs with heavy or moderately heavy physical labor, the sharp variations in work load in the course of a working day must be taken into consideration. Carrying tools and construction materials in such jobs (e.g., carpentry, plumbing, painting) may require more exertion than the job itself. Differences between static and dynamic labor must be borne in mind just as must the effects of temperature and differences between day- and night-shift work. Ergometric testing can in such instances furnish comparative values for the maximal power of healthy persons of the same age, in the form of, say, O_2 consumption or maximal ergostasis, although the direct correlation of these borderline figures is not meaningful in the case of the jobs under consideration.

As already explained, the amount of working energy expended on the job must always be maintained steadily for certain periods of time, say, 30 minutes or more. Even in the most commonly used performance test, that determining maximal ergostasis, the duration of the artificial work load at any given wattage level is only six minutes—considerably shorter than on the job. Nonetheless, it is possible, based on this parameter, to estimate the limitation on long-term performance in a particular case and compare it with the energy exerted on the job in question. Using HR, the most important and the easiest parameter of performance to measure, Lehmann regards a rate of 120 per minute in untrained individuals as the limit of the artificial work load. E. A. Müller and Karrasch report a somewhat lower value, only 30 to 40 beats above the resting pulse. This is preferable for older persons, but may be too high in cases of organic heart damage. On the other hand, in persons who easily become excited, false and exaggerated HRs turn up in unaccustomed circumstances and can be detected least at the lower wattage stages. Therefore it seems more sensible to start from the maximal O_2 consumption, as do Muller and Åstrand, and to regard 40–50% of that as the limit for long-term performance.

Table 65. Energy requirements for various forms of locomotion (after *Spitzer* and *Hettinger*).

	Work kcal/min
Walking on smooth level ground	
4 km/hr	3.1
Same, amputee, 4.2 km/hr	3.4–4.1
Carrying 10 kg load, 4 km/hr	3.6
Mounting stairs 60 steps/min	8.3
Driving a passenger car	
Country road	1.0
City traffic (rush hour)	3.2
Cycling (smooth level street)	
Speed 10 km/hr	2.8
Speed 14 km/hr	4.3
Speed 18 km/hr	6.3

The performance achieved by the wattage-stage procedure at maximal ergostasis amounts to about 70–80% of the maximal working capacity ascertained in the short-run experiment with work load increasing to the point of exhaustion. According to that, the long-term performance is to be thought of as being two-thirds to half the value of the maximal ergostasis. For primarily pulmonary diseases with limited ventilatory and especially respiratory function, the full arterialization that is still possible can under certain circumstances be regarded as the maximal performance. Regarding the clear and continuous decline in arterial O_2 pressure, Hertz therefore suggested >6 mm Hg as a limitation of performance from respiratory causes, and consequently considered the long-term performance capacity to be 40–50% lower.

In cardiac and pulmonary patients it should be remembered that, first, ergometry is as a rule performed under favorable environmental circumstances, which frequently do not represent those found at the subject's place of employment; and that, second, many cases of illness cause considerable variability in performance, for example, emphysema involving various degrees of obstruction or coronary diseases. Third and last, organic cardiac patients with a tendency to grow sicker—for example, those with hemodynamically significant valvular defects, or hypertensive heart trouble with clear signs of hypertrophy of the atrium or ventricle or myogenic dilatation—who experience difficulty even while at rest, are seriously impaired by additional loads put upon them in the course of a job. This applies especially to overloaded hypertensive hearts, and particularly to cases of aortic stenosis. Even with ergometric readings that are still relatively good, the question of requirements, that is, of possible danger inherent in the calculated capacity for long-term performance, is an important problem that cannot be decided on clinical grounds alone. In many of these patients, however, ergometry will be superfluous.

A matter that arises frequently is the diagnosis or classification of pains in the cardiac region. Not infrequently we find in the anamnesis, instead of the characteristic angina resulting from movements or chill, atypical thoracic sensations of discomfort. About a third of all myocardial infarctions occur without any preliminary warning symptoms. Here ergometry can make a great contribution in clearing up the differential diagnosis. Cases of coronary insufficiency, especially, including those following myocardial infarction, can be cited in which there is no pain. The limit to performance in positive cases is due to exhaustion of the coronary reserve, which goes hand in hand with the appearance of ischemic EKG changes during, or sometimes not till after, the work-stress test, with or without typical discomforts. Bachman found that in 46% of his coronary patients the ergometric test had to be interrupted because of ischemic EKG changes signaling a possible anginal attack. The question that is so significant in compensation cases regarding the reliability of ergometric data is not settled with a coronogram. Bachman reports 18% falsely positive and 12% falsely negative results. Krelhaus et al. raised the work load till the heart rate reached 80% of its maximum, but were able to come up with positive findings in only 40% of their cases, admittedly almost exclusively in disease of only one vessel. In multi-vessel situations (stenosis = 50%), 9% were negative. Falsely positive findings occurred in 10% of the cases. In general it is possible to estimate correctness in individually prescribed high work loads at about 80%, with falsely positive findings in about 15% of the cases. (Niederer et al.; Martin et al.) The long-term performance that can be demanded below the ischemic threshold can very seldom be determined schematically. It depends to a considerable extent on the clinical data in the anamnesis and not least on the type of angina pectoris and the psychic stresses in the particular job environment. The classic anamnesis of a case of angina pectoris obviates in many instances the necessity of carrying out a work-load test, even for the purposes of comparing findings or in rehabilitation work. All cardiac infirmities, especially the development of coronaries, should be dealt with under optimal therapy, which of course includes avoidance of possibly incorrect EKG interpretations attributable to digitalis-induced ST changes. In most cases here, that is, pathological work-load EKG without stenocardia, and in the absence of muscular cardiac insufficiency, any medication must be discontinued in advance in accordance with its speed of elimination. If that should not be possible, consider repeating the test after administering nitrate (nitroglycerine or isosorbic dinitrate under the tongue). "Ischemic" ST changes are just as hard to interpret in other respects in cases of left-heart hypertrophy with a tendency to discordance of the repolarization phase, as in left bundle branch block or in Wolff-Parkinson-White syndrome.

In the case of war victims, accident insurance, damage suits and many other forensic matters calling for an expert medical opinion, the most precise possible estimation of the reduction in earning power is demanded of

Table 66. Maximal steady state O_2 consumption pedaling while reclining, 60 rpm (closed system, Fleisch's Metabograph) on the part of normal males (after *Reindell et al.*).

Age group	Number	Weight (kg)	O_2 (cm³)	O_2 (cm³/kg)
10–11	42	35.5	1125.5	31.7
12–13	41	45.0	1430.8	31.8
14–15	42	52.3	1689.9	32.4
16–17	49	63.0	2181.7	34.6
18–19	51	67.5	2668.7	39.6
20–29	50	68.2	2373.0	34.8
30–39	50	70.5	2008.0	28.4
40–49	31	75.0	1847.8	24.6
50–59	30	75.5	1642.6	21.7
60–75	42	74.0	1510.0	20.4

Table 67. Maximal steady state O_2 consumption at pedaling while reclining, 60 rpm (closed system, Fleisch's Metabograph) on the part of normal females (after *Reindell et al.*).

Age group	Number	Weight (kg)	O_2 (cm³)	O_2 (cm³/kg)
10–11	50	33.5	1012	30.2
12–13	50	46.7	1270	27.2
14–15	50	52.7	1448	27.5
16–17	46	56.6	1560	27.6
18–19	50	59.0	1561	26.5
20–29	43	59.1	1627	27.5
30–39	50	59.8	1340	22.4
40–49	22	68.9	1188	17.2
50–59	25	68.1	1144	16.8

the physician. Here ergometry is the method of choice in detecting applicable basic infirmities (in the absence of other disabilities that would render a work-test inadvisable). A prerequisite for any estimate of the reduction in earning power is the establishment of just what is a normal ergometric showing based on age, sex and, at least in the case of more pronounced deviations, also on weight.

If we take the individual ideal values from Tables 66 and 67, either for maximal O_2 consumption or for highest achieved wattage stage in ergostasis, as equal to 100% of the normal performance capacity, then we can estimate the minimal requirement corresponding to the basic metabolism with additional consumption due to digestion and light bodily movements as equal to 10% or about 400–500 ml of O_2 consumption (about 2 to 2.5 kcal). The degree of limitation of performance can then be determined from the ergometric readings, somewhere between these two extremes. Here too we are dealing with a round figure which only too frequently has to be altered considerably, depending on the nature of the clinical diagnosis.

As far as patient safety is concerned, conclusions may be drawn from hundreds of thousands of ergometric examinations. There is exceedingly little risk, even for cardiac patients, when the examination is performed by an experienced physician observing the following guidelines (fewer than one incident per 10,000 tests is a good record!).

2. Appropriate Work Loads and Resuscitation Equipment in Ergometry

1. Facilities for continuous (discontinuous) EKG monitoring recording
2. Discontinuous respiration rate monitoring

3. Defibrillator
4. Equipment for intubation and artificial respiration
5. Oxygen
6. Medicaments: nitroglycerin, antiarrhythmics, noradrenalin, digoxin, lasix, infusion solution

In principle, three work-stressing patterns are employed:

1. Submaximal stressing at a level moderately difficult for the subject, corresponding to a HR of at least 130 per minute (according to Åstrand). The HR and power readings are then extrapolated to a maximal performance capacity or O_2 consumption. Corrective factors are useful in view of age-related decline in maximal HR under work stress.
2. Procedure according to Reindell et al: increasing power while attempting to maintain a relatively steady state, that is, ergostasis, for the most important parameters (HR, O_2 consumption, respiratory time-volume, respiratory rate) until extinction of the steady-state situation. The performance attained is about 75 to 80% of the maximal working capacity obtainable with pattern 3, below.
3. Rapidly increasing power at intervals of one or two minutes, by stages of 25 watts, until the point of exhaustion.

The first of these three methods seems temptingly simple, but is applicable only to those without heart disease, since conclusions based solely on extrapolation of HR to the peak of maximal working capacity are not reliable. Type 3 demands full input of effort on the part of the subject and ignores the possibility of significant organic heart damage. This test, too, is therefore not generally admissible in forensic use.

Type 2, of course, is more time-consuming, but is far less risky because it permits the examiner to recognize without dangerous delay any unexpected performance limitations. Norms are readily available for all age levels apt to be met with (see Tables 66 to 69). Its disadvantage is that the time the procedure takes brings the risk of tiring the peripheral musculature prematurely. This can be compensated for by working at low wattages for only two or three minutes per stage, and trying to achieve ergostasis in only the last two stages. This is very often possible if the examiner already knows from the performance history the performance level expected, and if he monitors any increase in HR and the degree of exertion. Even for confirmation of a coronary insufficiency, small stages of increasing wattage, each lasting about

Table 68. Mean O_2 on bicycle ergometer (following Åstrand, Bühlmann and personal experiments).

Watts	25	50	75	100	125	150	175
O_2 in ml	600	900	1200	1500	1800	2100	2400

Table 69. The maximal HR in ergostasis in normal males and females in the various age brackets (after *Reindell et al.*).

Age in years		10–11	12–13	14–15	16–17	18–19	20–29	30–39	40–49	50–59	60–75
x̄	Men	156	156	158	166	166	163	150	141	121	122
	Women	169	168	162	167	170	160	146	135	130	—
s	Men	16.3	13.3	15.0	11.1	9.2	13.1	8.7	16.7	15.1	16.2
	Women	21.0	13.5	14.0	8.6	12.5	12.6	12.7	12.1	9.1	—
n	Men	38	40	40	45	51	45	38	23	27	42
	Women	50	50	50	54	50	43	50	22	25	—

x̄ = average. s = average quadratic deviation.

two minutes, will suffice. To ascertain capacity for work, however, we prefer a duration of six minutes for the last or last two stages, in order to detect any rise in HR which may occur after the third minute and any ischemia connected with it.

The experienced examiner (the presence of a physician is indispensable, at least in the case of a coronary patient or one with other organic defect) will only very rarely be faced with a dangerous situation if he correctly estimates the overall picture of the case in hand and the subject's performance reserves. He must explain things in detail to the subject and observe with care—and as uninterruptedly as possible—the degree of stress the subject is undergoing and the readings coming out of the examination. The danger inherent in tests verging on maximal performance lies in the well-known discrepancy between performance capacity of diseased hearts and the demand that may be made on them without risk. Only this latter is of forensic interest.

Roskamm (1975) distinguishes four gradually intensifying levels in limitation on a cardiac function. First, there is the organ on stage I, performing unobstrusively in all respects. Even in stage II, the ergometry is unremarkable, even as to cardiac output, but the left ventricular filling pressures are already showing a compensatory increase, detectable only in the pulmonary capillary pressure by means of a catheter. Schmutzler also shows (Chapter XIV) the significance of the central parameters in the example of valve defects, especially in hypertensive hearts. In rare instances, the otherwise loose relationships between performance and ability to withstand workloads split wide open, as Roskamm reports in the case of a 52-year-old who had survived a myocardial infarction with a large parietal aneurysm and occlusion of the anterior descending coronary artery, whose performance data, including capillary pressure and cardiac output, were in the normal range (1974). Particularly in coronary disease, the prognostic estimation of two- and three-vessel involvements (these are the ones most frequently leading to an ischemic reaction) is the integrating component of the examination. Even fresh myocardial infarcts need cause no apparent limitation in performance capacity, as was confirmed by an examination undertaken inadvertently in such a situation years ago by the present writer.

3. Contraindications and Criteria to Stop Testing

The following changes are contraindications against undertaking ergometry or demand its discontinuance if they appear:

1. Fresh myocardial infarct and severe angina pectoris
2. Cardiac insufficiency with signs of decompensation while at rest
3. Obstructive pulmonary emphysema with global hypoventilation
4. Hypertension more serious than degree 2: three diastolic readings of 110–115 mm Hg or greater.

Changes that make discontinuance of ergometry mandatory:

1. Typical stenocardia with or without EKG changes
2. Ischemic EKG changes with or without stenocardia, excluding digitalis (this refers only to horizontal or descending ST-depression of more than 0.1 mV compared to the resting EKG, or to rising ST)
3. Multifocal or clustered extrasystoles or chains of extrasystoles (not isolated extrasystoles and not if they occur similarly as in the resting state); ventricular extrasystoles with R on T phenomenon
4. Paroxysmal tachycardia or attacks of atrial fibrillation
5. Increasing AV interval, especially grade II° or grade III° transmission blockage
6. Broadening of QRS, occurrence of block patterns
7. Rise in systolic blood pressure above 250 (300) mm Hg.
8. Drop in blood pressure
9. Clearly recognizable dyspnea, cyanosis or clamminess with pallor
10. Failure to establish ergostasis or no increase in O_2 pulse between the last two wattage stages
11. Unequivocal and progressive drop in arterial O_2 pressure, especially in the event of primary pulmonary disturbances
12. Respiratory quotient above 1
13. No increase in HR or an inadequate one (sick sinus syndrome)
14. Distinct excess beyond the average maximal HR for the subject's age (i.e., ≈220 minus age in years).

4.   Lack of Cooperation

Willingness on the subject's part to put all he has into performance tests can be taken for granted in sports medicine, but this is hardly the case in compensation cases. Often it is not even genuine faking. The latter is relatively easy to recognize when readings are wide of the mark in control situations, or perhaps even earlier when there is a discrepancy between clinically trivial findings and demonstrated reduction in performance. It is easy to understand a certain lack of effort in a person whose long-dreamed-of compensation or damage payment will be greater if more serious impairment of health can be proved. Certainly, even in older people who are over fifty, it must be borne in mind that years of avoidance of all physical activity or exertion can have a deleterious effect on one's ability to call up performance reserves. The fact remains that, again and again, people faced with a test quit even at low performance levels—at, say, only about double or triple the resting O_2 consumption level, despite the fact that there is no clear-cut or significant indication of any infirmity or disease. Neurotics not infrequently show such behavior, too, even when there are no signs whatever of the above mentioned cardiac or pulmonary insufficiencies, including increased HR. In such situations, however, ergometric data are not without value. It is almost always possible to discount the possibility of disqualifying pulmonary or cardiac conditions as reason for quitting a test, provided none of the contraindications listed above is present.

The suspicion of intentional faking is well-founded if:

1. During previous spirometry with the subject at rest great variations in vital capacity showed up. (Deviations from the average when there is good cooperation amount to about ±8%, according to studies by Larmi.)
2. In the stress test the pretended maximal respiratory time-volume and the HR (which is easy to pin down) differ greatly (more than ±20%) in repeated tests with adequate intervals for recovery.

If these indications are not present, it must remain moot whether there is residual fatigue of the peripheral muscles—as might be seen in 15- or 20-minute tests as a result of long periods of abstinence from physical activity—or an insufficient mustering of willingness to achieve maximal performance. The examiner must then fall back on other clinical findings for a rough estimate of the actual performance level. Here it is just as impossible to arrive at objective results as in cases where, for example, a work has been called off because of shoulder or back pains in a cranking test, or knee-joint arthrosis or claudication while pedaling.

5.   Possibilities of a Simplified Ergometry

To obtain the most exact possible estimate of physical performance capacity, it is necessary to measure numerous parameters with the subject at rest, then during and perhaps also after the exercise. These include respiratory time-volume, O_2 consumption, CO_2 production rate, blood pressure, and perhaps also arterial O_2 pressure and an EKG, to mention only the most important ones. From these can be obtained the O_2 pulse, the respiratory quotient and the respiratory equivalent. The quotient of cardiac volume over O_2 pulse makes possible further insights into functionally or organically caused deviations in the ability to work. To what extent these parameters are necessary for rendering an opinion depends on the examiner's judgment and on the nature of the infirmity being tested for. In a great many cases it will suffice, after previous testing of ventilation by means of vital capacity and forced breathing, to read only HR, blood pressure and EKG, because a similar amount of O_2 is required for interindividually similar effectiveness at the same physical performance level in watts. With relatively slight variations, each wattage stage of a bicycle ergometer (efficiency hardly varies between sitting and reclining postures) can be assigned a definite O_2 consumption and also a corresponding rate of energy consumption in kcal (Table 68). Of course, according to Reindell et al. the values for females between 20 and 30 are about 100 ml below those for men. Sick individuals also have somewhat lower O_2 consumption readings (corresponding to the intensifying O_2 debt) at the maximal wattage level achieved. Maximal HR ergostasis then signals the limit of performance capability. It is possible to calculate the total expenditure of energy (in kcal), maximal O_2 consumption (per kg) and O_2 pulse without too great a margin of error and, if necessary, to include also the cardiac volume. Borderline values in cardiac patients must be considered pathological because the O_2 consumption is always calculated a bit too high. This procedure will almost always indicate whether the condition is worsening or improving. In case of primary pulmonary disturbances, the value obtained ergometrically (under the circumstances as respiratory performance permits) is much more sharply modified by the other clinical data, including spirography with the subject at rest and possibly bronchospirography and mechanical breathing behavior. As with cardiac disturbances, round figures can be obtained in these cases (in principle) through ergometry. Alongside the typical subjective complaints, the EKG is decisively important for the evaluation of coronary diseases. It is usually sufficient to derive the impulses by means of a different electrode in position V_5 against the forehead (CH_5). The same positioning of electrodes must be used before and after the test for purposes of comparison. It is indicative of the test's objectivity—and often surprising—to note with what precision ischemic

EKG changes or stenocardia repeatedly turn up at the same working HR and wattage levels.

If we take into consideration the clinical picture of the disease in each instance and the varying degree of limitation that results, ergometric examination acquires a high level of objectivity for ascertaining round figures on performance capability, as controls prove. Of course, any performance test must fail if proper cooperation is lacking, but even so it will provide some valuable data for drawing conclusions on the problems of forensic medicine.

Ergometric data are naturally more valuable for elaborating a verified clinical diagnosis of, say, a mitral defect than for the precise determination of a reduction in earning capacity. For this reason the medical verdict based on it should not be expressed in too-closely graduated percentages but rather should comprise broader performance brackets. Besides, there are enough uncertainties, even taking into account values based on weight: For example, the performance of a healthy stout person is generally higher than that of a person who weighs the same but is more large-proportioned and muscular. In addition, there is the ticklish problem of taking into account the degree of training. Even medium-heavy physical labor on the job seems not to serve, for example, as training for a higher performance than that of a subject in a sedentary occupation.

A rough estimation of on-the-job capabilities is possible on the basis of subjective data (classification by the New York Heart Association) and the

Table 70. Comparative survey of performance.

Degree of severity (N.Y. Heart Assn)	Ergometric performance (maximal ergostasis)	Ability to work
I No limitation in physical ability to work (at an accustomed physical activity)	125–150 watts ($\gtrsim 1.5$ to $\gtrsim 2$ watts/kg)	All activities with medium-difficult physical exertion (not continuous)
II Minor limitation in physical ability to work. Feels OK while at rest or under light exertion.	75–100 watts ($\gtrsim 1$ to $\gtrsim 1.5$ watts/kg)	Almost all activities without and many with moderate physical exertion, all under favorable environmental conditions.
III Distinct limitation in physical ability to work. In difficulty even at low levels of customary activities.	25–50 watts (< 1 watt/kg)	Ability to work only under favorable working conditions; mostly sedentary occupations
IV No physical activity without distress. Distress in most cases even while at rest.	Can not be subjected to work load	Unable to work

highest ergometric wattage level (steady state for six minutes) achieved without any pathological findings. Those who disagree with this cite data reported by Halhuber (Table 70), which have reference chiefly to males. In the case of females it is necessary, in view of their lower physiological performance capacity, to deduct ten to fifteen percent in performance based on body weight when making comparisons between wattage level achieved and severity of limitation. Work loads on the job must, of course, be evaluated absolutely, that is to say, regardless of sex.

Thus, it is no longer correct to treat ergometry lightly when issuing expert opinions on cardiopulmonary infirmities. With due precautions and observance of contraindications and criteria for mandatory interruption of tests, ergometry is no more dangerous than any exertion (especially those not under medical supervision) in the course of everyday living. Of course, although often decisive, ergometric results are only one element in determining how much physical exertion can be demanded on the job and what limitations exist. Ergometry must always be preceded by a physical and a thorough case history. Only after that, and in full knowledge of other necessary clinical background, should the decision be made as to how much and what kind of ergometric testing is to be used.

References

Åstrand, I.: Acta physiol. scand. 49 (Suppl. 169), 1960.

Åstrand, P. O.: Sportphysiologie, Med. Prisma, Boehringer Sohn, Ingelheim, 1964.

Bachmann, K.: Verh. Dtsch. Ges. Kreislaufforschg. 41, 66 (1975), Dr. D. Steinkopff Verlag, Darmstadt.

Bühlmann, A.: Schweiz. med. Wschr. 92, (1962) 573.

Halhuber, M. I.: Dtsch. med. J. 22, 134 (1971).

Hertz, M. I.: Dtsch. med. J. 22, 134 (1971).

Hertz, C. W.: Dtsch. med. Wschr. 90, (1965) 461.

Hollmann, W.: Der Arbeits- u. Trainingseinfluß auf Kreislauf u. Atmung. Darmstadt: Steinkopff-Verlag, 1959.

König, K., H. Roskamm and H. Reindell: Z. Kreislaufforschg. 57, 713 (1968).

Krelhaus, W., F. Loogen, A. Sewowa and L. Seipel: Verh. Dtsch. Ges. Kreislaufforschg. 41, 190 (1975).

Lange Andersen, K., R. I. Shepard, H. Denolin, E. Varnauskas and R. Masironi: Fundamentals of Exercise Testing. W.H.O. Geneva 1971.

Lehmann, G.: Praktische Arbeitsphysiologie. Stuttgart, Thieme-Verlag, 1962.

Martin, K.-L., R. Hopf and M. Kaltenbach: Z. Kardiol. Suppl. 2, 116 (1975).

Müller, E. A.: 5. Freiburger Symposium, Berlin-Göttingen-Heidelberg: Springer-Verlag, 1958.

Niederer, W., K. Schebelle and M. Petenyi: Z. Kardiol. Suppl. 1, 16 (1974).

Reindell, H.: Herz- Kreislaufkrankheiten u. Sport. München: Barth, 1960.

Reindell, H., K. König and H. Roskamm: Funktionsdiagnostik des gesunden und kranken Herzens. Stuttgart: Thieme-Verlag, 1967.

Roskamm, H.: Herz-Kreislauf, 6, 120 (1974).

Roskamm, H.: Proc. of the Dtsch. Ges. Kreislaufforschg. 41, 35 (1975). Dr. D. Steinkopff-Verlag, Darmstadt 1975.

Roskamm, H., K. König, G. Blümchen and H. Reindell: Z. Kreislaufforschg. 57, 176 (1968).

Spitzer and Hettinger: Tafeln für den Kalorienumsatz bei körperlicher Arbeit. Berlin-Köln-Frankfurt. Beuth-Vertrieb, 1964.

XX. Treadmill vs Bicycle Ergometer

by Vojin N. Smodlaka, M.D., Sc.D.

In the field of stress testing to evaluate the general physical condition and working capacity of a subject (normal or patient) and in the field of training and conditioning normal persons and athletes and reconditioning patients in the process of rehabilitation, we use mostly two kinds of ergometers— treadmills and bicycle ergometers. Each group of ergometers has its own characteristics and advantages which influence investigators and practitioners in their choice of equipment.

In this chapter, we will list the positive and negative characteristics of these ergometers and the differences that occur while exercising on them so that investigators and practitioners can decide which one to use in their particular work.

Treadmills were developed in North America by researchers who were interested in the field of work and sports physiology, studying especially the effects of walking, jogging and running on normal subjects and athletes. The treadmill simulates running, which is performed in place (in human performance laboratories). Extensive research has been done throughout the years. In the beginning, this research was performed on normal subjects, but gradually the interest turned to patients with cardiopulmonary pathologies, especially coronary heart disease. Several models of electrically-driven treadmills have been developed and are in use.

Bicycle ergometers were developed in Europe, where researchers started first with simple mechanical models, switching later to electromagnetic ones, which allowed the expression of resistance (power) in precise units of watts. These ergometers, used as bicycles or cranks, allowed investigators to evaluate the maximal cycling capacity, to compare the results in longitudinal studies and to prescribe a precise power in the process of training, conditioning and reconditioning, which is so important in the pharmacology of exercise because exercise has to be prescribed in precise measure (such as the drug, digitalis).

Technical Differences

Treadmill

Exercise on a treadmill, such as walking, jogging or running, is the most natural way of locomotion for the subjects tested or trained; however, the subject has to be able to walk or run. This is not the case in a very large percentage of patients with a multitude of disabilities, such as geriatric patients with very low cardiopulmonary or muscular reserve, who are unable to stand up or walk, or those with hemiplegia, paraplegia, advanced neurological diseases, severe fractures, etc. For this reason, the treadmill is not a universal ergometer in rehabilitation medicine departments.

The treadmill is a large, electronic device that requires a lot of space. It is heavy, difficult to transport for field investigations, makes a lot of noise and is expensive. The power (work load) cannot be measured directly in kpm or watts but has to be calculated. It is expressed in speed of running and the level of inclination. The smallest power is the slowest speed of walking, which may be very high for patients in poor physical condition or those who are unable to stand or walk due to severe weakness. This makes it difficult to prescribe a precise, low exercise program for these patients. Furthermore, the increments cannot be increased in very small units as is possible with electronic bicycle ergometers.

The work load on the treadmill depends on body weight. In many longitudinal studies, the body weight changes, thus changing the work load for the same stress test. The body weight has a much smaller effect on bicycle ergometer performance. The danger of a fall while running on a treadmill is much greater than cycling the bicycle ergometer. To prevent the fall of a disabled patient, we use the bicycle ergometer and have the patient cycle in the recumbent position.

Bicycle Ergometer

Mechanical or electronic bicycle ergometers are smaller, require less space than treadmills and are lighter and easier to transport, especially the mechanical ones that do not require electricity. They are usually less expensive and make less noise. They may be used in several positions, allowing variations in the process of investigation, testing and training, especially of disabled patients. In addition, bicycle ergometers may be used as follows: as cranks in the standing or sitting positions, cranking one handle with both hands or cranking two pedals, each with one hand; as a bicycle in the sitting or lying position, cycling the pedals with both legs or, as in amputees, with one leg; and adapted for paraplegics to cycle with arms in the sitting position. Testing and reconditioning of many disabled patients is possible only in the sitting or lying positions. For this reason, bicycle ergometers are used as standard equipment in the field of rehabilitation.

The power on bicycle ergometers, especially electronic ones, may be prescribed in precise, small units of 5 watts, starting with zero and increased up to 400 watts and higher in some models. These small power units allow precise measurements of the maximal work load achieved on a maximal stress test and prescription of the exact power in the process of training, conditioning of normal subjects and reconditioning of patients in poor physical condition with low cardiopulmonary reserve (as for patients in hospitals or nursing homes).

Bicycle ergometers also allow us to perform many laboratory tests, especially when the subject cycles in the recumbent position. Catheterization of the heart to study the effect of exercise is performed on x-ray tables using bicycle ergometers with the patient in the recumbent position.

A very common objection to the use of bicycle ergometers is that cycling is not a natural way of exercising, especially for subjects who do not know how to cycle a regular bicycle. This objection, however, applies to all ergometers because every subject has to learn how to perform on them.

Physiological Differences

In this chapter, we will discuss the comparative, physiological studies between parameters registered while exercising the treadmill or bicycle ergometers.

Mellerowicz and Nowacki revealed that exercising on bicycle ergometers in different positions produces varying reactions in spite of using the same power. Figures 7 through 14 in Chapter I of this book demonstrate the differences in the heart rate (HR), VO_2, CO_2 production and respiratory time volume. For these reasons, we always have to use the same tests in the same positions.

Margaria et al., pointed out that walking on a treadmill below 8.5 km/hr is more economical than running and that running about that speed becomes more economical. This should be taken into consideration when testing and retesting. The same authors stated that the mechanical efficiency of running is only 5 to 7% higher in trained athletes than in average subjects. It would be of interest to discover the mechanical efficiency of the trained cyclist versus the average person.

Mellerowicz and Nowacki, Bobbert, Hermansen et al., Åstrand et al., Stenberg et al., Sill and Kirchhoff, Niederberger et al., Wicks et al., Hollmann et al., Faulkner et al., Miyamura et al., Blackburn et al., and Sotobata et al., studied the heart rate (HR) while exercising on ergometers with arms and then with legs at the same VO_2 or same power. The HR was greatest in cranking the bicycle ergometer in the standing position, lower while sitting and lowest while jogging or running on the treadmill.

There may be several reasons for these differences. The first is the difference between the muscle masses and the number and size of involved muscles. The second reason may be the effect of gravity on arterial and venous circulation. The third may be the effect of milking action of the muscles on venous return, which must be different while walking or cycling. The contraction time of the leg muscles while running is shorter than while cycling. Usually the subject performs 190 to 200 steps per minute while running on a treadmill and only 50 to 60 RPM while cycling.

Ventilation

Several authors (Asmussen et al.; Bobbert; Hermansen et al.; Åstrand et al.; Mellerowicz and Nowacki; Stenberg et al.; Sill and Kirchhoff; Hollmann et al.; Niederberger et al.; McKay and Banister) discovered that the respiratory time-volume was higher while cranking the bicycle ergometer at the same VO_2 or power than while cycling with the legs or running on the treadmill. Cranking provokes a degree of hyperventilation, as compared to cycling and walking. The slightly higher respiratory quotient in cranking at each level of VO_2 may be related to this hyperventilation (Bobbert).

Oxygen Consumption

Several authors in different laboratories and with varying techniques found that the VO_2 max was higher on the treadmill while running uphill than on bicycle ergometers while cycling in the sitting position. Hermansen et al. found an increase of 6% VO_2 max; Åstrand and Saltin, 5%; Glassford et al., 8%; Faulkner et al., 11%; Kamon et al., 6% for males and 3.6% for females; McArdle et al., 10.2 to 11.2%; Chase et al., 15%; Niederberger et al., 8%; Wicks et al., 17%; and McKay and Banister, 7.58%. Several others (Wyndham; Hollmann; Miyamura; Valentin and Holzhauser; and Miles, et al.) found an increase also.

The explanation for this phenomenon is that running on a treadmill, especially uphill, involves a larger mass of muscles than does cycling the bicycle ergometer. The smaller mass of muscles used in cycling fatigues faster and prevents the subject from reaching a higher VO_2 max. The greatest sensation of fatigue of the thigh muscles occurs when the subject cycles in the recumbent position. In this position the leg muscles push the pedals without using the body weight, as they do when in the sitting position. At the same time, the effect of gravity on arterial circulation is also eliminated.

Hermansen et al. found a significantly higher cardiac output of 6% during a maximal treadmill test and a higher stroke volume of 5% during submaximal and maximal treadmill tests. Miyamura et al. also found a higher cardiac output during treadmill exercise than during bicycle exercise and a higher $A-VO_2$ difference and higher blood flow in the calves.

Stenberg et al., studying hemodynamic response to work with different muscle groups in the sitting and supine positions, arrived at the following conclusion: During maximal exercise with arms in the sitting position, the cardiac output and VO_2 were only 80 and 66% of the values while working with legs in the sitting position. The stroke volume in the sitting position averaged 68 ml, or 50%, of the stroke volume in male and 56 ml, or 46%, in females. In the supine position, the stroke volume was 103 ml, or 75%, of the maximal in males and 91 ml, or 81%, in females. The higher HR reflects a lower stroke volume during arm work in the sitting position.

The lactic acid in arterial blood was higher during arm work and reflects the more pronounced acidosis which could explain the states of hyperventilation. The higher ventilation, in turn, has an effect on HR and cardiac output and increases both. At a given submaximal VO_2, the intra-arterial blood pressure was higher in arm work.

In comparing treadmill and ergometer tests, Sill and Kirchhoff, and Hollmann et al., discovered a higher O_2 pulse on the treadmill. Wiswell and de Vries concluded that the O_2 pulse tested on the treadmill or bicycle ergometers were practical parameters in the evaluation of physical capacity and cardiorespiratory fitness.

When comparisons were made at the same percentage of VO_2 max on the treadmill and bicycle ergometer, Niederberger et al. discovered higher arterial mean pressure, pressure-rate production, peripheral vascular resistance, pulmonary ventilation and HR during bicycle exercise. In addition, cardiac output was the same and the stroke volume was lower on the bicycle ergometer. They concluded that bicycle exercise constitutes a greater stress on the cardiovascular system. They call for caution while testing patients on a bicycle ergometer after an MI.

Sotobata et. al. concluded that the supine position on the bicycle ergometer imposes greater stress on the heart than the sitting position, using the same external mechanical work.

Our clinical experience in sports medicine, based on observations of athletes during training and competition, taught us that the bicycling sport is a predominantly cardiovascular sport whereas swimming is a predominantly ventilatory sport.

Champion bicyclists have a very slow HR; on some it has been recorded as low as 32 beats/min. Niederberger et al., on the basis of their experiments, arrived at the conclusion that bicycle exercise constitutes a greater stress on the cardiovascular system at any given VO_2 than the treadmill exercise. They concluded that this can have significant implications relative to possible hazards while stress-testing older persons, especially patients with cardiovascular diseases.

We use bicycle ergometers in the process of testing and rehabilitating cardiac patients because of the specific effects of cycling on the cardiovascular system, with due care and precautions.

Body Temperature

It was revealed by Asmussen and Nielsen in 1947 that the rectal temperature was higher in subjects exercising with their legs rather than their arms on bicycle ergometers at a given energy output or at a given heat production. The authors concluded that this was due to a different "setting" of the heat center during work with arms and with legs. Furthermore, they postulated that this was possible because of a different set of nervous impulses reaching the center.

In conclusion, we may say that both ergometers are of practical and theoretical value but neither is of universal use.

The treadmill is recommended for able-bodied subjects who are capable of walking or running on the treadmill, especially for testing the actual maximal VO_2 and for conditioning normal subjects and reconditioning patients. The subject reaches the highest values of VO_2 max on treadmill tests.

On the other hand, bicycle ergometers are recommended for subjects who are unable to walk or run on the treadmills. These disabled subjects may be tested, conditioned and reconditioned in an appropriate position. The subject may crank one handle with both hands in the standing or sitting position, or crank each pedal with one hand in the standing, sitting or lying position. He may also cycle with his legs in the sitting or lying position.

The power on electromagnetic bicycle ergometers may be dosed very precisely in small units of 5 watts and increased by 5 watts up to 400 watts, which is very important for patients in extremely poor physical condition.

References

1. Asmussen, E. and Hemmingsen, I. 1958. Determination of Maximum Working Capacity at Different Ages in Work with the Legs or with the Arms. Scandinav J Clin & Lab Investigation 10:67–71.
2. Asmussen, E. and Nielsen, M. 1947. The Regulation of the Body Temperature During Work Performed with the Arms and with the Legs. Acta Physiol Scand 14:373–382.
3. Åstrand, P.O. 1967. Measurement of Maximal Aerobic Capacity. (Session II: Paper I). Canad Med Assoc J 96:732–734.
4. Åstrand, P.O. and Saltin, B. 1961. Maximal Oxygen Uptake and Heart Rate in Various Types of Muscular Activity. J Appl Physiol 16, 977–981.
5. Blackburn, H. and Winckler, G. et al. 1970. Exercise Tests: Comparison of the Energy Cost and Heart Rate Response to Five Commonly-Used, Single-Stage, Non-Steady State, Submaximal Work Procedures. Medicine and Sport 4:28–36.
6. Bobbert, A.C. 1960. Physiological Comparison of Three Types of Ergometry. J Appl Physiol 15:1007–1014.
7. Faulkner, J.A. and Roberts, D.E., et al. 1971. Cardiovascular Responses to Submaximum and Maximum Effort Cycling and Running. J Appl Physiol 30:4, 457–461.
8. Glassford, R.G. and Baycroft, G.H.Y. et al. 1965. Comparison of Maximal Oxygen Uptake Values Determined by Predicted and Actual Methods. J Appl Physiol 20:509–513.
9. Hermansen, L., Ekblom, G. and Saltin, G. 1970. Cardiac Output During Submaximal and Maximal Treadmill and Bicycle Exercise. J Appl Physiol 29:1, 82–86.
10. Hermansen, L. and Saltin, B. 1969. Oxygen Uptake During Maximal Treadmill and Bicycle Exercise. J Appl Physiol 26:1, 31–37.
11. Hollmann, W., Schmucker, B., et al. 1971. Über das Verhalten Spiroergometrischer Messgrössen bei Radrennfahrern auf dem Laufband und auf dem Fahrraderg ometer. Sportarzt und Sportmedizin 7:153–158.
12. Hollmann, W., Heck, H., et al. 1971. Vergleichende Spiroergometrische Untersuchungen uber den Effekt und die Aussagekraft von Laufband- und Fahrradergometerbelastungen. Sportarzt und Sportmedizin 6:123–134.
13. Kamon, E., Pandolf, K.B. 1972. Maximal Aerobic Power During Laddermill Climbing, Uphill Running and Cycling. J Appl Physiol 32:4, 467–473.
14. Kappagoda, C.T., Linden, R. J. and Newell, J. P. 1979. A Comparison of the Oxygen Consumption/Body Weight Relationship Obtained During Submaximal Exercise on a Bicycle Ergometer and on a Treadmill. Quart J Exper Physiol 64, 205–215.
15. Manca, C., Bianchi, G., et al. 1979. Comparison of Five Different Stress Testing Methods in the ECG Diagnosis of Coronary Artery Disease: Correlation with Coronary Arteriography. Cardiology 64:325–332.
16. Margaria, R., Cerretelli, P., et al. 1963. Energy Cost of Running. J Appl Physiol 18, 367–370.
17. McArdle, W.D., Katch, R.I., and Pechar, G.S. 1973. Comparison of Continuous and Discontinuous Treadmill and Bicycle Tests for Max VO_2. Med Science in Sports 5:3, 156–160.
18. McKay, G.A. and Banister, E.W. 1976. A Comparison of Maximum Oxygen Uptake Determination by Bicycle Ergometry at Various Pedaling Frequencies and by Treadmill Running at Various Speeds. Europ J Appl Physiol 35:191–200.
19. Mellerowicz, H. and Nowacki, P. 1961. Zschr Kreisl Forsch 50:1002.
20. Miles, D.S., Critz, J.B. and Knowlton, R.G. 1980. Cardiovascular, Metabolic and Ventilatory Responses of Women to Equivalent Cycle Ergometer and Treadmill Exercise. Medicine and Science in Sports and Exercise, 12:1, 14–19.
21. Miyamura, M. and Honda, Y. 1972. Oxygen Intake and Cardiac Output During Maximal Treadmill and Bicycle Exercise. J Appl Physiol 32:2, 185–188.
22. Miyamura, M. and Kitamura, K., et al. 1972. Cardiorespiratory Responses to Maximal Treadmill and Bicycle Exercise in Trained and Untrained Subjects. J Sports Med 18:25–32.
23. Niederberger, M. and Bruce, R.A. et al.

1974. Disparities in Ventilatory and Circulatory Responses to Bicycle and Treadmill Exercise. Brit Heart J 36:377–382.

24. Niederberger, M., Gasic, S. and Kummer, F. 1975. Hamodynamische Unterschiede Zwischen Maximaler Laufband- und Fahrradergometrie bei Koronarer Herzkrankheit. Z Kardiol 64:239–245.

25. Sill, V. and Kirchhoff, H.W. 1968. Die Laufbandbelastung als Funktionsprufung von Kreislauf und Atmung. Wehrmed 6:90–101.

26. Shephard, R.J. 1966. The Relative Merits of the Step Test, Bicycle Ergometer and Treadmill in the Assessment of Cardio-Respiratory Fitness. Int Z Angew Physiol 23:219–230.

27. Sotobata, I. and Shino, T., et al. 1979. Work Intensities of Different Modes of Exercise Testing in Clinical Use. Japanese Circulation J 43:161–169.

28. Stenberg, J. and Åstrand, P.O., et al. 1967. Hemodynamic Response to Work with Different Muscle Groups, Sitting and Supine. J Appl Physiol 22:61–70.

29. Valentine, H. and Holzhauser, K.P. 1976. "Laufbandergometer" In: Funktionsprufungen von Herz und Kreislauf. Deutscher Arzte. Verlag, Koln, Chapter 1.4, pp. 330–334.

30. Wicks, J.R. and Sutton, J.R., et al. 1978. Comparison of the Electrocardiographic Changes Induced by Maximum Exercise Testing with Treadmill and Cycle Ergometer. Circulation 57:6, 1066–1070.

31. Wiswell, R.A. and de Vries, H.A. 1979. Time Course of O_2-pulse During Various Tests of Aerobic Power. Eur J Appl Physiol 41:221–232.

32. Wyndham, C.H. and Strydom, N.G., et al. 1966. Studies of the Maximum Capacity of Men for Physical Effort. Part I: A Comparison of Methods of Assessing the Maximum Oxygen Intake. Int Z Angew Physiol Einschl Arbeitsphysiol 22:285–295.

XXI. Summary of Practical Ergometry

1. What is Ergometry?

Ergometry, in literal translation, means the measurement of performance (ergon is Greek for work, labor, performance). In ergometry, unlike any other functional test, the body's performance is precisely measured physically in the current international units of power: kpm/sec or watts (1 kpm/sec = 9.81 watts $\approx$ 10 watts).

Ergometrically measured power can be precisely comparable and reproducible. However, for this to be true, certain internationally defined conditions for the conversion of power (Chapter III, 2) must be adhered to: temperature in the examination room, food intake on the day of the examination, etc.

Among the devices for measuring power, we distinguish between mechanically braked and electromagnetically braked ergometers. The ergometrically measured power is, in both methods, the product of braking force times braking distance in one second; power is, physically speaking, $\dfrac{\text{force} \times \text{distance}}{\text{time}}$. In calibrating the ergometer, power is either indicated on the scales in kpm/sec or in watts, or it is read from tables according to the indicated braking resistance, the revolutions per minute and the time.

Ergometric performance can take the form of hand cranking while standing, or pedaling while seated or reclining. At the same physical power of, say, 100 watts, the biological performance differs a bit among these three forms of exercise. For this reason, comparative or conversion values have been determined (Chapter I, 4).

2. What Regularities Is Ergometry Based on?

Ergometry is based on:

1. The regular relationships between certain performance functions and certain performance parameters (Fig. 220), which are measured precisely using standardized methods
2. A knowledge of the averages and standard deviations of certain performance functions in certain age and sex groups. No data lying outside the $\pm 2\,\sigma$ range can be regarded as normal, by international agreement.

In the $\pm 2\,\sigma$ range lie about 96% of all individual readings in a normal Gaussian distribution.

3. What Does Ergometry Measure?

1. Physical power in kpm/sec or watts
2. HR per minute
3. Arterial pressure in mm Hg or Torr

These three parameters suffice for simple, practical ergometry. In differentiated ergometry, especially for understanding pulmonary performance functions, we also measure the following:

4. Respiratory time-volume in liters per minute
5. O_2 consumption in ml per minute
6. CO_2 production in ml per minute
7. EKG taken during ergometric exercise (ergo-EKG)
8. O_2 saturation of the blood, measured oximetrically:
   P_{O_2}, P_{CO_2}, pH, standard bicarbonate, etc.
9. Intracardial pressures
10. Other functions, such as blood lactate, serum enzymes, etc.

4. How Are Ergometric Data Evaluated?

They are evaluated by comparing the functional parameters measured with the averages and standard deviations ($\pm 1\,\sigma$ and $\pm 2\,\sigma$) of data obtained from healthy age and sex groups to which the subject belongs.

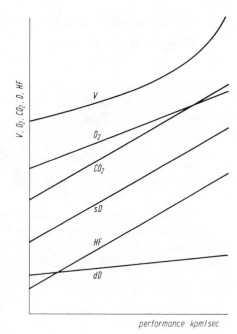

Fig. 220. HR, systolic pressure (sD), diastolic pressure (dD), O_2 consumption, CO_2 production and respiratory time-volume (V), during linearly increased ergometric performance (schematic representation).

In general, it may be said that cardiovascular performance capacity is the greater:

(a) The farther the HR is below average
(b) The greater the systolic performance pressure reserves are. (By systolic performance reserves we mean the difference between the systolic pressure at maximal performance and that taken while at rest.)
(c) The greater the O_2 capacity is (that is, the highest O_2 consumption per minute at maximal ergometric performance).

The performance capacity of the heart and circulation is less:

(a) The farther the HR above the average
(b) The lower the systolic performance reserve
(c) The lower the O_2 capacity.

The performance capacity of the respiratory organs is the greater, the higher the O_2 capacity and the respiratory time-volume are at maximal ergometric power and the smaller the respiratory equivalent is at submaximal ergometric power. The performance capacity of the respiratory organs is the less, the lower the O_2 capacity and the respiratory time-volume are at maximal ergometric power and the greater the respiratory equivalent is at submaximal ergometric power.

5. What Methods Should Be Used in Practical Ergometry?

All ergometric measurements should be performed on a standard ergometer using standardized methods and under defined conditions of performance conversion (see Chapter III).   •

5.1 The Measurement of HR During a Standard Exercise of 1 Watt per kg of Body Weight

The HR during a relatively uniform exercise of one watt per kg of body weight is compared with the averages and standard deviations (Fig. 221). The higher the HR, the lower the cardiocorporeal performance capacity, and the lower the HR the greater the capacity. This simple ergometric method often provides a useful and sufficiently reliable estimate of the cardiocorporeal performance capacity in three to six minutes.

HR is most readily measured by auscultatory or palpatory means with a stopwatch. Between the 50th and 60th second of each minute, the duration of ten heartbeats is timed, and from this is calculated the frequency per minute (Table 71).

The heartbeats or pulse beats during six seconds can also be counted and multiplied by ten to get the rate per minute.

More precise readings are obtained by recording by EKG ten R peaks between the 50th and 60th seconds of each minute and calculating the rate per minute from the time they take.

Table 71. Conversion table for HR per minute from the time taken by ten heartbeats as measured by a stopwatch.

3	200	4	150	5	120	6	100	7	86	8	75	9	67	10	60
3_1	194	4_1	147	5_1	118	6_1	98	7_1	85	8_1	74	9_1	66	10_1	59
3_2	187	4_2	143	5_2	116	6_2	97	7_2	84	8_2	73	9_2	65	10_2	58
3_3	181	4_3	140	5_3	113	6_3	95	7_3	83	8_3	72	9_3	64	10_3	58
3_4	176	4_4	137	5_4	111	6_4	93	7_4	82	8_4	72	9_4	63	10_4	57
3_5	171	4_5	134	5_5	109	6_5	91	7_5	80	8_5	71	9_5	63	10_5	57
3_6	166	4_6	131	5_6	107	6_6	90	7_6	79	8_6	70	9_6	62	10_6	56
3_7	162	4_7	128	5_7	105	6_7	89	7_7	78	8_7	70	9_7	61	10_7	56
3_8	158	4_8	125	5_8	104	6_8	88	7_8	77	8_8	69	9_8	61	10_8	55
3_9	154	4_9	122	5_9	102	6_9	87	7_9	76	8_9	68	9_9	60	10_9	55

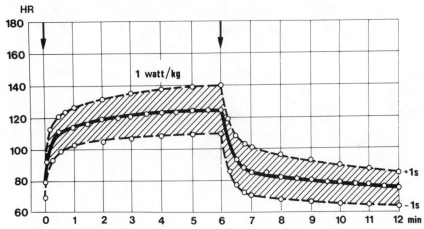

Fig. 221. HR during performance and recovery in 100 men aged 20 to 30 at relatively equal power of 1 watt per kg of body weight (after *Dransfeld and Mellerowicz*).

5.2   Determination of the Pulse Working Capacity 170 (PWC$_{170}$)

The most suitable performance stages are:

(a) 10 watts for one minute
(b) 25 watts for two minutes
(c) 50 watts for three minutes.

The PWC$_{170}$, as determined using these three different stages, comes out approximately the same. The actual differences, even compared with 50-watt stages for six minutes, amount to no more than $\pm4\%$ (Franz and Chintanaseri).

The HR is measured between the 50th and 60th second of each minute in method (a), at the end of each second minute in method (b) and at the end of each third minute in method (c). The HRs as measured are entered on a coordinate system (Fig. 222). Corresponding to the regular linear rise in HR during stepped increase in performance, two, three, four or five data points for HR can be connected by straight lines. The projection of this line cuts the 170-heart-rate ordinate at a definite point which corresponds to the PWC$_{170}$ value on the abscissa. The points on the line should lie within a range of HR of 100 to 170 per minute (or 170 minus ten per decade of age after the 30 to 40 decade). A point falling outside the straight line is to be discarded.

Normal values are:

≈3 watts per kg of body weight (±0.5 watts) for men; ≈2-1/2 watts per kg of body weight (±0.5 watts) for women (see Fig. 223.).

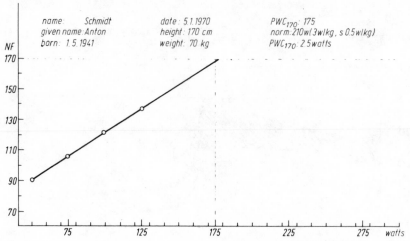

Fig. 222. Example of the determination of the PWC_{170} in stages of 25 watts for two minutes.

During effective rehabilitative training, the absolute PWC_{170} and the relative PWC_{170} in watts per kg of body weight increase. This can be proved by a comparative diagram; the linear rise in HR should become less steep. This is one of the most suitable methods of quantitative objectivization of the success of rehabilitation or of therapeutic measures.

For older individuals (above 40–50), the PWC_{170} is a theoretical figure, since the maximal HR decreases with age. According to the definition of the Rehabilitation Council of the International Society of Cardiology, the HR decreases about ten beats per decade. In making a judgment, it is important to note that although the maximal HR decreases in relation to the increase in age, the theoretical PCW_{170} does not. Therefore, the average of about 3 watts per kg of body weight is also correct for older healthy men and that of 2-1/2 for older healthy women.

5.3   Measuring Arterial Pressure During Ergometric Performance

The arterial pressures are read most practically during pedaling exercise while reclining, using the Riva-Rocci method in stages of 25 watts for two minutes, or, in pathological cases, perhaps of 10 watts for one minute, readings being taken between the 50th and 60th second of the last minute of each stage. (To accomplish this, the blood pressure cuff must be pumped up in readiness between the 30th and 45th seconds.)

The measurement can be concluded in the submaximal or maximal range of cardiocorporeal performance capacity, depending on individual or pathological contingencies of each case.

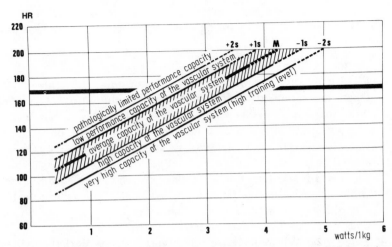

Fig. 223. Averages and standard deviations in HR with increasing performances of 1 watt per kg and 2 watts per kg lasting three minutes each in 100 untrained men aged 20–30 (after *Dransfeld and Mellerowicz*, 1957). With performance stages of 10 watts for one minute or 25 watts for two minutes, no significant differences occur in the determination of PWC_{170}, according to comparative studies by *Franz* (1972).

The systolic performance pressure reserves, as an expression of the maximal pressure performance of the heart, run about 75–100 mm Hg in healthy men aged 20 to 30, in trained individuals >100–150 mm Hg, and in pathological cases, for example, damage to the myocardium, less than about 75 mm Hg.

In the case of serious athero- or arteriosclerotic changes in the arteries, especially the coronaries and carotids, maximal stress loads are contraindicated or may be performed only with caution and with a running EKG monitoring.

5.4 Electrocardiogram During Ergometric Performance (ergo-EKG)

An EKG that is not taken during precisely definable physical exertion is of little value as a cardiological parameter. The margin of error is too great. The differences in physical exertion may be greater than ±50% in, for example, knee bends or step climbing performed under indeterminate conditions and time lapse. An EKG taken after physical exertion is not identical with one taken during it. In preventive and rehabilitative cardiology, it is important to define the degree of physical exercise at which some particular EKG change appears. Therefore, the physical exercise in ergo-electrocardiography must be measured precisely in watts or kpm/sec by means of an ergometer.

In recent years, we have been systematically using different methods in comparative ways. The following ergo-EKG method has proved to be the best:

1. During pedaling while reclining the torso lies at rest (Fig. 224). The EKG is not affected by any muscular currents. The arms are free for taking measurements such as, for example, simultaneous readings of arterial pressure or catheter readings of intracardial pressure, etc.
2. The performance is increased in stages of 10 watts for one minute or 25 watts for two minutes. Stages of greater duration are indicated only in special cases.
3. The EKG is recorded during the last ten seconds of each minute in accordance with the standardization agreements for ergometry. If necessary, the EKG is monitored with an oscilloscope or recorded on a continuous basis (as in the case of extrasystoles).
4. Three to six Wilson leads (or other types of leads, as the individual case calls for) are recorded.
5. The ergo-EKG examination is called off:
   a) If the maximal range of HR ($\pm 2\,\sigma$) and arterial pressure or a respiratory quotient of 1 is reached

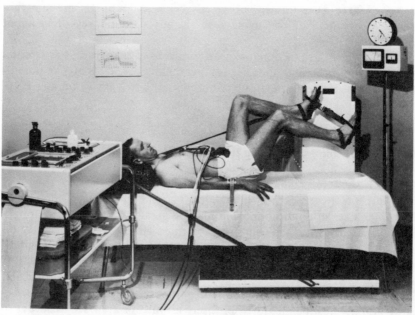

Fig. 224. An ergometric EKG examination in progress (ergo-EKG).

b) If significant ST depression of horizontal or descending type and of more than 0.1 mV occurs

c) In case of extrasystoles, especially multifocal

d) On the appearance of disturbances in conduction

e) If an incipient stenocardia contraindicates further ergometric study.

5.5 Measuring Maximal O_2 Consumption

5.5.1 By an Indirect Method, after Åstrand

On the basis of regular relationships between O_2 consumption and HR during ergometric performance, the maximal O_2 consumption can be recognized by measuring the HR at submaximal performance. The test is carried out on a bicycle ergometer under steady-state conditions. The performance level is to be selected in such a way that the steady-state HR lies between 120 and 160 per minute. If the HR is below 120, the performance level must be increased. HRs are measured during the last ten to thirty seconds of the fourth, fifth and sixth minutes. If the difference in HRs exceeds five beats during the last two minutes, the performance must be prolonged by one or more minutes until a constant HR sets in.

The maximal O_2 consumption can then be derived from Åstrand's tables, corresponding to the HR at a particular submaximal performance level (see Tables 72a and b).

Since the maximal HR decreases with age, the importance of the O_2 consumption obtained in older individuals by this method is in general overestimated. The reading in older people must therefore be corrected through multiplication by an age factor (see Table 72c). Experience shows, however, that in highly trained endurance performers this method gives readings that are too high.

5.5.2 Direct Measurement of the Maximal O_2 Consumption ($\dot{V}_{O_2}$ max)

The performance stages in this method can be either 10 watts for one minute, 25 watts for two minutes or 50 watts for three minutes. Stages of longer duration are not necessary. The total duration of performance should be at least six minutes and should not exceed twelve. Suitable for the first stage are:

a) 25–50 watts for children and teenagers, women and old people

b) 50–100 watts for men aged 20 to 30

c) 50–100 watts for trained women

d) 100–200 watts for trained men.

Table 72a, b, and c. Tables for determining the maximal O_2 consumption from the steady state HR (a: men, b: women, c: correction factor for age) (after *I. Åstrand,* Acta Physiol. Scand. 49, (1960) 45).

Exer-cise HR	Maximal O_2 consumption					Exer-cise HR	Maximal O_2 consumption				
	300 kpm/min	600 kpm/min	900 kpm/min	1200 kpm/min	1500 kpm/min		300 kpm/min	600 kpm/min	900 kpm/min	1200 kpm/min	1500 kpm/min
120	2.2	3.5	4.8			148		2.4	3.2	4.3	5.4
121	2.2	3.4	4.7			149		2.3	3.2	4.3	5.4
122	2.2	3.4	4.6			150		2.3	3.2	4.2	5.3
123	2.1	3.4	4.6			151		2.3	3.1	4.2	5.2
124	2.1	3.3	4.5	6.0		152		2.3	3.1	4.1	5.2
125	2.0	3.2	4.4	5.9		153		2.2	3.0	4.1	5.1
126	2.0	3.2	4.4	5.8		154		2.2	3.0	4.0	5.1
127	2.0	2.1	4.3	5.7		155		2.2	3.0	4.0	5.0
128	2.0	3.1	4.2	5.6		156		2.2	2.9	4.0	5.0
129	1.9	3.0	4.2	5.6		157		2.1	2.9	3.9	4.9
130	1.9	3.0	4.1	5.5		158		2.1	2.9	3.9	4.9
131	1.9	2.9	4.0	5.4		159		2.1	2.8	3.8	4.8
132	1.8	2.9	4.0	5.3		160		2.1	2.8	3.8	4.8
133	1.8	2.8	3.9	5.3		161		2.0	2.8	3.7	4.7
134	1.8	2.8	3.9	5.2		162		2.0	2.8	3.7	4.6
135	1.7	2.8	3.8	5.1		163		2.0	2.8	3.7	4.6
136	1.7	2.7	3.8	5.0		164		2.0	2.7	3.6	4.5
137	1.7	2.7	3.7	5.0		165		2.0	2.7	3.6	4.5
138	1.6	2.7	3.7	4.9		166		1.9	2.7	3.6	4.5
139	1.6	2.6	3.6	4.8		167		1.9	2.6	3.5	4.4
140	1.6	2.6	3.6	4.8	6.0	168		1.9	2.6	3.5	4.4
141		2.6	3.5	4.7	5.9	169		1.9	2.6	3.5	4.3
142		2.5	3.5	4.6	5.8	170		1.8	2.6	3.4	4.3
143		2.5	3.4	4.6	5.7						
144		2.5	3.4	4.5	5.7						
145		2.4	3.4	4.5	5.6						
146		2.4	3.3	4.4	5.6						
147		2.4	3.3	4.4	5.5						

The parameters measured are: HR (see Chapter V, 1), respiratory time-volume (see Chapter X, 1), O_2 consumption and CO_2 production (see Chapters IX, 1 and XII, 1) of the expired air, measured directly during each minute of performance. Measurement can be terminated if the following criteria are attained:

1. If the HR has exceeded the $+2\sigma$ threshold of the maximal values for the subject's age group (see Chapter V, 4.1)
2. If the respiratory quotient has reached or exceeded a value of about 1
3. If the respiratory equivalent exceeds the $+2\sigma$ threshold of the maximal values (see Chapter XI, 2)

Table 72b.

Exercise HR	Maximal O$_2$ consumption					Exercise HR	Maximal O$_2$ consumption				
	300 kpm/min	450 kpm/min	600 kpm/min	750 kpm/min	900 kpm/min		300 kpm/min	450 kpm/min	600 kpm/min	750 kpm/min	900 kpm/min
120	2.6	3.4	4.1	4.8		148	1.6	2.1	2.6	3.1	3.6
121	2.5	3.3	4.0	4.8		149		2.1	2.6	3.0	3.5
122	2.5	3.2	3.9	4.7		150		2.0	2.5	3.0	3.5
123	2.4	3.1	3.9	4.6		151		2.0	2.5	3.0	3.4
124	2.4	3.1	3.8	4.5		152		2.0	2.5	2.9	3.4
125	2.3	3.0	3.7	4.4		153		2.0	2.4	2.9	3.3
126	2.3	3.0	3.6	4.3		154		2.0	2.4	2.8	3.3
127	2.2	2.9	3.5	4.2		155		1.9	2.4	2.8	3.2
128	2.2	2.8	3.5	4.2	4.8	156		1.9	2.3	2.8	3.2
129	2.2	2.8	3.4	4.1	4.8	157		1.9	2.3	2.7	3.2
130	2.1	2.7	3.4	4.0	4.7	158		1.8	2.3	2.7	3.1
131	2.1	2.7	3.4	4.0	4.6	159		1.8	2.2	2.7	3.1
132	2.0	2.7	3.3	3.9	4.5	160		1.8	2.2	2.6	3.0
133	2.0	2.6	3.2	3.8	4.4	161		1.8	2.2	2.6	3.0
134	2.0	2.6	3.2	3.8	4.4	162		1.8	2.2	2.6	3.0
135	2.0	2.6	3.1	3.7	4.3	163		1.7	2.2	2.6	2.9
136	1.9	2.5	3.1	3.6	4.2	164		1.7	2.1	2.5	2.9
137	1.9	2.5	3.0	3.6	4.2	165		1.7	2.1	2.5	2.9
138	1.8	2.4	3.0	3.5	4.1	166		1.7	2.1	2.5	2.8
139	1.8	2.4	2.9	3.5	4.0	167		1.6	2.1	2.4	2.8
140	1.8	2.4	2.8	3.4	4.0	168		1.6	2.0	2.4	2.8
141	1.8	2.3	2.8	3.4	3.9	169		1.6	2.0	2.4	2.8
142	1.7	2.3	2.8	3.3	3.9	170		1.6	2.0	2.4	2.7
143	1.7	2.2	2.7	3.3	3.8						
144	1.7	2.2	2.7	3.2	3.8						
145	1.6	2.2	2.7	3.2	3.7						
146	1.6	2.2	2.6	3.2	3.7						
147	1.6	2.1	2.6	3.1	3.6						

Table 72c.

Age	Factor	HR max.	Factor
15	1.10	210	1.12
25	1.00	200	1.00
35	0.87	190	0.93
40	0.83	180	0.83
45	0.78	170	0.75
50	0.75	160	0.69
55	0.71	150	0.64
60	0.68		
65	0.65		

4. If the subjective complaints occur, for example, stenocardia, the test will be prevented. In patients with a very low working capacity, especially patients with heart disease, the evaluation of maximal oxygen consump-

tion should be performed in step increments of 10 watts of one minute duration with continuous EKG registration.

5. If HbO_2, P_{O_2}, P_{CO_2}, or pH exceed certain thresholds yet to be established (in measurements taken with scientific goals in mind).

6. Contraindications Are:

1. Acute and chronic inflammatory diseases
2. Cardiac insufficiency while at rest and severe performance insufficiency with a low performance reserve ($<\approx 30$ watts)
3. Severe coronary insufficiency with subjective and electrocardiographic indications at physical exertion as low as about 30 watts
4. Tachycardial forms of absolute arrhythmia with atrial fibrillations; multifocal extrasystoles which appear or do not disappear during exertion; disturbances in conduction occurring even at exertions below about 50 watts
5. Myocardial infarction, or being only days or weeks after infarction even though there is early mobilization
6. Severe fixed hypertension ($<\approx 200/120$ mm Hg)
7. Apoplectic insult, and weeks or months thereafter
8. Days or weeks after operation
9. Days or weeks after trauma and healing of wounds
10. Other severe illnesses and infirmities, malignant neoplasms, leukemia, severe anemia, etc.

Appendix

Conversion of Spirographic Values to BTPS (Body Temperature Pressure Saturated) or STPD (Standard Temperature Pressure Dry)

The respiratory volumes are usually determined under ATPS conditions (ambient temperature pressure saturated) when exhaled air is measured in spirometers or gasometers. In closed systems, it is necessary to start with temperature readings at frequent intervals. In measuring inhaled air, we use ambient temperature, ambient pressure and ambient humidity.

To convert to BTPS for tidal volume and respiratory time-volume, which correspond to conditions in the lungs, the room and/or systemic temperature must be measured, and in measuring inhaled air also the relative humidity must be determined and converted to water-vapor pressure (Table 74). For this purpose the gas volumes measured must be multiplied by the factors in Table 73.

If the inhaled air, not fully saturated with water vapor, has been measured, then, especially at high relative humidity, Table 72 can be used with precision sufficient for all practical purposes for conversion to BTPS conditions. A slight methodological error will creep in; in this case, it can be calculated for, but it is reasonable to ignore it. In measuring expired air, too, a small methodological error will be present, since when the volumes of air pass through the gasometer in short puffs the temperature of the instrument and that of the warmer volume of air diverge more or less.

A precise conversion to BTPS conditions can be performed, taking into account room temperature, barometric pressure and relative humidity, by using the following formula from *Handbook of Respiration,* Philadelphia and London: W. B. Saunders Co:

$$\text{Volume (BTPS)} = \text{volume} \times \frac{310}{273t} \times \frac{P_B - p_{H_2O}}{P_B - 47}$$

Table 73. Conversion of spirometrically measured gas volumes (spirometer temperature, water-vapor saturation) to body conditions (37°C, water-vapor saturation) at various barometric pressures (after J. C. Kovach, P. Paulos and C. Arabadjis: J. Thorac. Surg. 29 (1955), 552).

Temp. (°C)	640	650	660	670	680	690	700	710	720	730	740	750	760	770	780
15	1.1388	1.1377	1.1367	1.1358	1.1348	1.1339	1.1330	1.1322	1.1314	1.1306	1.1298	1.1290	1.1283	1.1276	1.1269
16	1.1333	1.1323	1.1313	1.1304	1.1295	1.1286	1.1277	1.1269	1.1260	1.1253	1.1245	1.1238	1.1231	1.1224	1.1217
17	1.1277	1.1268	1.1258	1.1249	1.1240	1.1232	1.1224	1.1216	1.1208	1.1200	1.1193	1.1186	1.1179	1.1172	1.1165
18	1.1222	1.1212	1.1203	1.1194	1.1186	1.1178	1.1170	1.1162	1.1154	1.1147	1.1140	1.1133	1.1126	1.1120	1.1113
19	1.1165	1.1156	1.1147	1.1139	1.1131	1.1123	1.1115	1.1107	1.1100	1.1093	1.1086	1.1080	1.1073	1.1067	1.1061
20	1.1108	1.1099	1.1091	1.1083	1.1075	1.1067	1.1060	1.1052	1.1045	1.1039	1.1032	1.1026	1.1019	1.1014	1.1008
21	1.1056	1.1042	1.1034	1.1027	1.1019	1.1011	1.1004	1.0997	1.0990	1.0984	1.0978	1.0971	1.0965	1.0960	1.0954
22	1.0992	1.0984	1.0976	1.0969	1.0962	1.0954	1.0948	1.0941	1.0935	1.0929	1.0923	1.0917	1.0911	1.0905	1.0900
23	1.0932	1.0925	1.0918	1.0911	1.0904	1.0897	1.0891	1.0884	1.0878	1.0872	1.0867	1.0861	1.0856	1.0850	1.0845
24	1.0873	1.0866	1.0859	1.0852	1.0846	1.0839	1.0833	1.0827	1.0822	1.0816	1.0810	1.0805	1.0800	1.0795	1.0790
25	1.0812	1.0806	1.0799	1.0793	1.0787	1.0781	1.0775	1.0769	1.0764	1.0758	1.0753	1.0748	1.0744	1.0739	1.0734
26	1.0751	1.0746	1.0738	1.0732	1.0727	1.0721	1.0716	1.0710	1.0705	1.0700	1.0696	1.0691	1.0686	1.0682	1.0678
27	1.0688	1.0682	1.0677	1.0671	1.0666	1.0661	1.0656	1.0651	1.0646	1.0641	1.0637	1.0633	1.0629	1.0624	1.0621
28	1.0625	1.0619	1.0614	1.0609	1.0604	1.0599	1.0595	1.0591	1.0586	1.0582	1.0578	1.0574	1.0570	1.0566	1.0563
29	1.0560	1.0555	1.0550	1.0546	1.0548	1.0537	1.0533	1.0529	1.0525	1.0521	1.0518	1.0514	1.0510	1.0507	1.0504
30	1.0494	1.0496	1.0486	1.0482	1.0478	1.0474	1.0470	1.0467	1.0463	1.0460	1.0456	1.0453	1.0450	1.0447	1.0444

Table 74. Pressure of saturated water vapor in mm Hg at temperatures from 0°C to 100°C in mm Hg (from Bartels, Bücherl, Hertz, Rodewald and Schwab: Lungenfunktionsprüfungen. Berlin-Göttingen-Heidelberg: Springer, 1959).

Tens	Units Temperature °C									
	0	1	2	3	4	5	6	7	8	9
0	4.579	4.926	5.294	5.685	6.101	6.543	7.013	7.513	8.045	8.609
10	9.209	9.844	10.518	11.231	11.987	12.788	13.634	14.530	15.477	16.477
20	17.535	18.650	19.827	21.068	22.377	23.756	25.209	26.739	28.349	30.043
30	31.824	33.695	35.663	37.729	39.898	42.175	44.563	47.067	49.692	52.442
40	55.324	58.34	61.50	64.80	68.26	71.88	75.65	79.60	83.71	88.02
50	92.51	97.20	102.09	107.20	112.51	118.04	123.80	129.82	136.08	142.60
60	149.38	156.43	163.77	171.38	179.31	187.54	196.09	204.96	214.17	223.73
70	233.7	243.9	254.6	265.7	277.2	289.1	301.4	314.1	327.3	341.0
80	355.1	369.7	384.9	400.6	416.8	433.6	450.9	468.7	487.1	506.1
90	525.76	546.05	566.99	588.60	610.90	633.90	657.62	682.07	707.27	733.24
100	760.00									

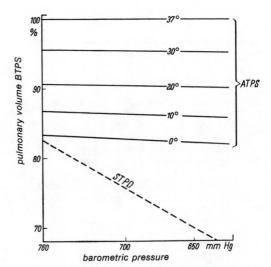

Fig. 225. Diagram for conversion of ATPS to BTPS and STPD for practical purposes (after Rahn, from *Handbook of Respiration,* Philadelphia and London: W. B. Saunders).

where

t	= spirometer temperature in degrees Celsius
P_B	= barometric pressure in mm Hg
P_{H_2O}	= water-vapor pressure at spirometer temperature t
	(can be calculated from relative humidity as measured and Table 73)
47 mm Hg	= water-vapor pressure at saturation and 37°C

The calculated BTPS values can be converted to STPD conditions from Table 75. The figures for O_2 and CO_2 should be given in STPD, in accordance with the report of the commission of the German Society for Internal Medicine on the normalization of nomenclature and symbols for respiratory parameters. In making the calculation, the BTPS figure for respiratory time-volume is multiplied by the volume percent of O_2 (or of CO_2) and the conversion factor for STPD conditions. For practical use, a diagram may be used to calculate the BTPS or STPD from ATPS (Fig. 225).

Table 75. Volume reduction of an ideal gas at 0°, 760 mm Hg, dry (from Bartels, Bücherl, Hertz, Rodewald and Schwab: *Lungenfunktionsprüfungen,* Springer 1959).

Temp. in °C	Barometer 700	701	702	703	704	705	706	707	708	709
10	0.8768	0.8781	0.8794	0.8806	0.8819	0.8832	0.8844	0.8857	0.8870	0.8882
11	0.8729	0.8742	0.8755	0.8767	0.8780	0.8793	0.8805	0.8818	0.8831	0.8843
12	0.8690	0.8703	0.8715	0.8728	0.8741	0.8753	0.8766	0.8778	0.8791	0.8804
13	0.8651	0.8663	0.8676	0.8689	0.8701	0.8714	0.8726	0.8739	0.8751	0.8764
14	0.8611	0.8624	0.8636	0.8649	0.8661	0.8674	0.8686	0.8699	8.8711	0.8724
15	0.8571	0.8584	0.8596	0.8609	0.8621	0.8634	0.8646	0.8659	0.8671	0.8684
16	0.8531	0.8544	0.8556	0.8568	0.8581	0.8593	0.8606	0.8618	0.8631	0.8643
17	0.8491	0.8503	0.8515	0.8528	0.8540	0.8553	0.8565	0.8577	0.8590	0.8602
18	0.8450	0.8462	0.8474	0.8487	0.8499	0.8511	0.8524	0.8536	0.8548	0.8561
19	0.8408	0.8421	0.8433	0.8445	0.8458	0.8470	0.8482	0.8495	0.8507	0.8519
20	0.8367	0.8379	0.8391	0.8404	0.8416	0.8428	0.8440	0.8453	0.8455	0.8477
21	0.8325	0.8337	0.8349	0.8361	0.8374	0.8386	0.8398	0.8410	0.8423	0.8435
22	0.8282	0.8294	0.8307	0.8319	0.8331	0.8343	0.8355	0.8367	0.8380	0.8392
23	0.8239	0.8251	0.8263	0.8276	0.8288	0.8300	0.8312	0.8324	0.8336	0.8348
24	0.8195	0.8208	0.8220	0.8232	0.8244	0.8256	0.8268	0.8280	0.8292	0.8304
25	0.8151	0.8164	0.8176	0.8188	0.8200	0.8212	0.8224	0.8236	0.8248	0.8260
35	0.7672	0.7684	0.7695	0.7707	0.7719	0.7730	0.7742	0.7754	0.7765	0.7777
36	0.7619	0.7631	0.7643	0.7654	0.7666	0.7678	0.7689	0.7701	0.7712	0.7724
37	0.7566	0.7577	0.7589	0.7601	0.7612	0.7624	0.7635	0.7647	0.7659	0.7670
38	0.7511	0.7523	0.7534	0.7546	0.7557	0.7569	0.7580	0.7592	0.7604	0.7615
39	0.7455	0.7467	0.7478	0.7490	0.7501	0.7513	0.7524	0.7536	0.7548	0.7557
40	0.7399	0.7410	0.7421	0.7433	0.7444	0.7456	0.7467	0.7479	0.7490	0.7502

Temp. in °C	Barometer 710	711	712	713	714	715	716	717	718	719
10	0.8895	0.8908	0.8920	0.8937	0.8946	0.8959	0.8971	0.8984	0.8997	0.9009
11	0.8856	0.8868	0.8881	0.8894	0.8906	0.8919	0.8932	0.8944	0.8957	0.8970
12	0.8816	0.8829	0.8841	0.8854	0.8867	0.8879	0.8892	0.8904	0.8917	0.8930
13	0.8776	0.8789	0.8802	0.8814	0.8827	0.8839	0.8852	0.8864	0.8877	0.8890
14	0.8736	0.8749	0.8761	0.8774	0.8786	0.8799	0.8811	0.8824	0.8836	0.8849
15	0.8696	0.8709	0.8721	0.8733	0.8746	0.8758	0.8771	0.8783	0.8796	0.8808
16	0.8655	0.8668	0.8680	0.8693	0.8705	0.8718	0.8730	0.8742	0.8755	0.8767
17	0.8614	0.8627	0.8639	0.8652	0.8664	0.8676	0.8689	0.8701	0.8714	0.8726
18	0.8573	0.8585	0.8598	0.8610	0.8623	0.8635	0.8647	0.8660	0.8672	0.8684
19	0.8532	0.8544	0.8556	0.8568	0.8581	0.8593	0.8605	0.8618	0.8630	0.8642
20	0.8489	0.8502	0.8514	0.8526	0.8538	0.8557	0.8563	0.8575	0.8587	0.8600
21	0.8447	0.8459	0.8471	0.8484	0.8496	0.8508	0.8520	0.8532	0.8545	0.8557
22	0.8404	0.8416	0.8428	0.8440	0.8453	0.8465	0.8477	0.8489	0.8501	0.8513
23	0.8360	0.8373	0.8385	0.8397	0.8409	0.8421	0.8433	0.8445	0.8457	0.8470
24	0.8317	0.8329	0.8341	0.8353	0.8365	0.8377	0.8389	0.8401	0.8413	0.8425
25	0.8272	0.8284	0.8296	0.8308	0.8320	0.8332	0.8344	0.8356	0.8368	0.8380
35	0.7789	0.7800	0.7812	0.7824	0.7835	0.7847	0.7859	0.7870	0.7882	0.7894
36	0.7736	0.7747	0.7759	0.7771	0.7782	0.7794	0.7805	0.7817	0.7829	0.7840
37	0.7682	0.7693	0.7705	0.7716	0.7728	0.7740	0.7751	0.7763	0.7774	0.7786
38	0.7627	0.7638	0.7650	0.7661	0.7773	0.7684	0.7696	0.7708	0.7719	0.7731
39	0.7571	0.7582	0.7594	0.7605	0.7617	0.7628	0.7640	0.7651	0.7663	0.7674
40	0.7513	0.7525	0.7536	0.7548	0.7559	0.7571	0.7582	0.7594	0.7605	0.7617

Table 75, continued.

Temp. in °C	Barometer									
	720	721	722	723	724	725	726	727	728	729
10	0.9022	0.9035	0.9047	0.9060	0.9073	0.9085	0.9098	0.9111	0.9124	0.9136
11	0.8982	0.8995	0.9008	0.9020	0.9033	0.9046	0.9058	0.9071	0.9083	0.9096
12	0.8942	0.8955	0.8967	0.8980	0.8993	0.9052	0.9018	0.9030	0.9043	0.9056
13	0.8902	0.8915	0.8911	0.8940	0.8952	0.8965	0.8977	0.8990	0.9003	0.9015
14	0.8862	0.8874	0.8887	0.8899	0.8912	0.8924	0.8937	0.8949	0.8962	0.8974
15	0.8821	0.8833	0.8846	0.8858	0.8871	0.8883	0.8896	0.8908	0.8921	0.8933
16	0.8780	0.8792	0.8805	0.8817	0.8829	0.8842	0.8854	0.8867	0.8879	0.8892
17	0.8738	0.8751	0.8763	0.8776	0.8788	0.8800	0.8813	0.8825	0.8837	0.8850
18	0.8697	0.8709	0.8721	0.8734	0.8746	0.8758	0.8771	0.8783	0.8795	0.8808
19	0.8655	0.8667	0.8679	0.8691	0.8704	0.8716	0.8728	0.8741	0.8753	0.8765
20	0.8612	0.8624	0.8637	0.8649	0.8661	0.8673	0.8686	0.8698	0.8710	0.8722
21	0.8569	0.8581	0.8594	0.8606	0.8618	0.8630	0.8642	0.8655	0.8667	0.8679
22	0.8526	0.8538	0.8550	0.8562	0.8574	0.8587	0.8599	0.8611	0.8623	0.8637
23	0.8482	0.8494	0.8506	0.8518	0.8530	0.8542	0.8555	0.8567	0.8579	0.8591
24	0.8438	0.8450	0.8462	0.8474	0.8486	0.8498	0.8510	0.8522	0.8534	0.8546
25	0.8393	0.8405	0.8417	0.8429	0.8441	0.8453	0.8465	0.8477	0.8489	0.8501
35	0.7905	0.7917	0.7929	0.7940	0.7952	0.7964	0.7975	0.7987	0.7999	0.8010
36	0.7852	0.7864	0.7875	0.7887	0.7898	0.7910	0.7922	0.7933	0.7945	0.7957
37	0.7798	0.7809	0.7821	0.7832	0.7844	0.7856	0.7867	0.7879	0.7890	0.7902
38	0.7742	0.7754	0.7765	0.7775	0.7788	0.7800	0.7811	0.7823	0.7835	0.7846
39	0.7686	0.7697	0.7709	0.7720	0.7732	0.7743	0.7755	0.7766	0.7778	0.7789
40	0.7628	0.7640	0.7651	0.7662	0.7674	0.7685	0.7697	0.7708	0.7720	0.7731

Temp. in °C	Barometer									
	730	731	732	733	734	735	736	737	738	739
10	0.9149	0.9162	0.9174	0.9187	0.9200	0.9212	0.9225	0.9238	0.9251	0.9263
11	0.9109	0.9121	0.9134	0.9147	0.9159	0.9172	0.9185	0.9197	0.9210	0.9227
12	0.9068	0.9081	0.9093	0.9106	0.9119	0.9131	0.9144	0.9156	0.9169	0.9182
13	0.9028	0.9040	0.9053	0.9065	0.9078	0.9090	0.9103	0.9116	0.9128	0.9141
14	0.8987	0.8999	0.9012	0.9024	0.9037	0.9049	0.9062	0.9074	0.9087	0.9099
15	0.8946	0.8958	0.8970	0.8983	0.8995	0.9008	0.9020	0.9033	0.9045	9.9058
16	0.8904	0.8916	0.8929	0.8941	0.8954	0.8967	0.8979	0.8991	0.9003	0.9016
17	0.8862	0.8875	0.8887	0.8899	0.8912	0.8924	0.8937	0.8949	0.8961	0.8974
18	0.8820	0.8832	0.8845	0.8857	0.8869	0.8882	0.8894	0.8906	0.8919	0.8931
19	0.8778	0.8790	0.8802	0.8814	0.8827	0.8839	0.8851	0.8864	0.8876	0.8888
20	0.8735	0.8747	0.8759	0.8771	0.8784	0.8796	0.8808	0.8820	0.8833	0.8845
21	0.8691	0.8703	0.8716	0.8728	0.8740	0.8752	0.8765	0.8777	0.8789	0.8801
22	0.8647	0.8660	0.8672	0.8684	0.8696	0.8708	0.8721	0.8733	0.8745	0.8757
23	0.8603	0.8615	0.8627	0.8640	0.8652	0.8664	0.8676	0.8688	0.8700	0.8712
24	0.8558	0.8571	0.8583	0.8595	0.8607	0.8619	0.8631	0.8643	0.8655	0.8667
25	0.8513	0.8525	0.8537	0.8549	0.8561	0.8573	0.8585	0.8598	0.8610	0.8622
35	0.8022	0.8034	0.8045	0.8057	0.8069	0.8080	0.8092	0.8103	0.8115	0.8127
36	0.7968	0.7980	0.7991	0.8003	0.8015	0.8026	0.8038	0.8050	0.8061	0.8073
37	0.7914	0.7925	0.7937	0.7948	0.7960	0.7971	0.7983	0.7995	0.8006	0.8018
38	0.7858	0.7869	0.7881	0.7892	0.7904	0.7915	0.7927	0.7938	0.7950	0.7962
39	0.7802	0.7812	0.7824	0.7835	0.7847	0.7858	0.7870	0.7881	0.7893	0.7904
40	0.7743	0.7754	0.7766	0.7777	0.7789	0.7800	0.7812	0.7823	0.7835	0.7846

Table 75, continued.

Temp. in °C	Barometer									
	740	741	742	743	744	745	746	747	748	749
10	0.9277	0.9289	0.9302	0.9314	0.9326	0.9339	0.9351	0.9364	0.9376	0.9389
11	0.9236	0.9248	0.9261	0.9273	0.9285	0.9298	0.9310	0.9323	0.9335	0.9348
12	0.9195	0.9205	0.9218	0.9230	0.9242	0.9255	0.9267	0.9280	0.9293	0.9305
13	0.9154	0.9167	0.9180	0.9192	0.9204	0.9217	0.9229	0.9242	0.9254	0.9267
14	0.9113	0.9126	0.9139	0.9151	0.9163	0.9176	0.9188	0.9201	0.9213	0.9226
15	0.9071	0.9084	0.9097	0.9109	0.9121	0.9134	0.9146	0.9159	0.9171	0.9184
16	0.9029	0.9042	0.9055	0.9067	0.9079	0.9092	0.9104	0.9117	0.9128	0.9142
17	0.8987	0.9000	0.9013	0.9025	0.9037	0.9050	0.9062	0.9075	0.9087	0.9100
18	0.8945	0.8958	0.8971	0.8983	0.8995	0.9008	0.9020	0.9033	0.9045	0.9058
19	0.8902	0.8915	0.8927	0.8939	0.8951	0.8964	0.8976	0.8989	0.9001	0.9012
20	0.8859	0.8872	0.8884	0.8896	0.8908	0.8921	0.8933	0.8946	0.8958	0.8971
21	0.8818	0.8830	0.8843	0.8855	0.8867	0.8886	0.8892	0.8905	0.8916	0.8930
22	0.8771	0.8783	0.8795	0.8807	0.8819	0.8832	0.8844	0.8857	0.8869	0.8882
23	0.8726	0.8738	0.8750	0.8762	0.8774	0.8787	0.8799	0.8812	0.8824	0.8837
24	0.8681	0.8693	0.8706	0.8718	0.8730	0.8743	0.8755	0.8768	0.8780	0.8793
25	0.8635	0.8647	0.8659	0.8671	0.8683	0.8696	0.8708	0.8721	0.8733	0.8746
35	0.8141	0.8152	0.8164	0.8176	0.8187	0.8198	0.8210	0.8222	0.8234	0.8245
36	0.8079	0.8091	0.8103	0.8114	0.8126	0.8137	0.8149	0.8161	0.8172	0.8183
37	0.8030	0.8041	0.8053	0.8064	0.8076	0.8088	0.8099	0.8111	0.8123	0.8134
38	0.7969	0.7981	0.7993	0.8004	0.8016	0.8027	0.8039	0.8050	0.8062	0.8073
39	0.7921	0.7932	0.7944	0.7955	0.7967	0.7979	0.7990	0.8002	0.8013	0.8024
40	0.7861	0.7872	0.7884	0.7896	0.7907	0.7919	0.7930	0.7942	0.7953	0.7965

Temp. in °C	Barometer									
	750	751	752	753	754	755	756	757	758	759
10	0.9404	0.9416	0.9429	0.9442	0.9454	0.9466	0.9479	0.9492	0.9505	0.9518
11	0.9363	0.9375	0.9388	0.9401	0.9413	0.9425	0.9438	0.9451	0.9464	0.9477
12	0.9318	0.9331	0.9343	0.9456	0.9368	0.9380	0.9394	0.9407	0.9420	0.9433
13	0.9280	0.9292	0.9304	0.9317	0.9326	0.9341	0.9355	0.9368	0.9381	0.9394
14	0.9238	0.9250	0.9262	0.9276	0.9288	0.9300	0.9313	0.9326	0.9339	0.9352
15	0.9196	0.9208	0.9220	0.9233	0.9245	0.9257	0.9271	0.9284	0.9297	0.9310
16	0.9154	0.9166	0.9178	0.9191	0.9203	0.9215	0.9228	0.9241	0.9254	0.9267
17	0.9111	0.9123	0.9135	0.9148	0.9160	0.9172	0.9185	0.9198	0.9211	0.9224
18	0.9068	0.9080	0.9092	0.9105	0.9118	0.9130	0.9142	0.9155	0.9168	0.9181
19	0.9025	0.9037	0.9049	0.9062	0.9074	0.9086	0.9099	0.9112	0.9125	0.9138
20	0.8981	0.8993	0.9005	0.9017	0.9029	0.9041	0.9053	0.9065	0.9077	0.9089
21	0.8940	0.8952	0.8964	0.8977	0.8989	0.9001	0.9013	0.9026	0.9039	0.9052
22	0.8890	0.8902	0.8914	0.8929	0.8941	0.8953	0.8966	0.8979	0.8992	0.9005
23	0.8847	0.8859	0.8871	0.8884	0.8896	0.8908	0.8920	0.8933	0.8946	0.8959
24	0.8801	0.8813	0.8825	0.8838	0.8850	0.8862	0.8875	0.8888	0.8901	0.8914
25	0.8757	0.8769	0.8781	0.8793	0.8805	0.8817	0.8829	0.8842	0.8855	0.8868
35	0.8257	0.8269	0.8281	0.8292	0.8304	0.8316	0.8327	0.8339	0.8351	0.8362
36	0.8195	0.8207	0.8219	0.8230	0.8242	0.8254	0.8265	0.8277	0.8288	0.8300
37	0.8146	0.8157	0.8169	0.8180	0.8181	0.8203	0.8215	0.8227	0.8238	0.8249
38	0.8085	0.8097	0.8108	0.8120	0.8131	0.8143	0.8154	0.8166	0.8177	0.8189
39	0.8036	0.8048	0.8059	0.8071	0.8082	0.8094	0.8105	0.8117	0.8148	0.8140
40	0.7976	0.7987	0.7999	0.8010	0.8022	0.8033	0.8045	0.8056	0.8068	0.8079

Table 75, continued.

Temp. in °C	Barometer 760	761	762	763	764	765	766	767	768	769
10	0.9530	0.9543	0.9556	0.9568	0.9580	0.9593	0.9606	0.9618	0.9631	0.9644
11	0.9489	0.9502	0.9515	0.9527	0.9535	0.9552	0.9565	0.9577	0.9590	0.9603
12	0.9444	0.9457	0.9470	0.9482	0.9494	0.9507	0.9519	0.9531	0.9544	0.9557
13	0.9405	0.9418	0.9431	0.9443	0.9455	0.9468	0.9481	0.9493	0.9506	0.9519
14	0.9362	0.9376	0.9384	0.9401	0.9413	0.9426	0.9438	0.9450	0.9463	0.9476
15	0.9320	0.9333	0.9346	0.9358	0.9370	0.9382	0.9395	0.9407	0.9420	0.9432
16	0.9278	0.9291	0.9304	0.9316	0.9328	0.9340	0.9352	0.9364	0.9377	0.9389
17	0.9235	0.9247	0.9260	0.9272	0.9285	0.9297	0.9309	0.9321	0.9334	0.9346
18	0.9192	0.9204	0.9217	0.9229	0.9242	0.9254	0.9266	0.9278	0.9291	0.9303
19	0.9148	0.9160	0.9172	0.9184	0.9197	0.9209	0.9222	0.9234	0.9247	0.9259
20	0.9104	0.9116	0.9128	0.9140	0.9152	0.9165	0.9177	0.9189	0.9202	0.9214
21	0.9062	0.9074	0.9086	0.9098	0.9111	0.9123	0.9135	0.9147	0.9160	0.9172
22	0.9014	0.9026	0.9038	0.9050	0.9063	0.9075	0.9087	0.9099	0.9112	0.9124
23	0.8969	0.8980	0.8992	0.9004	0.9017	0.9029	0.9041	0.9053	0.9066	0.9078
24	0.8932	0.8934	0.8946	0.8958	0.8971	0.8983	0.8995	0.9007	0.9020	0.9032
25	0.8879	0.8889	0.8901	0.8913	0.8926	0.8938	0.8950	0.8962	0.8974	0.8986
35	0.8374	0.8386	0.8397	0.8409	0.8421	0.8432	0.8444	0.8456	0.8467	0.8479
36	0.8312	0.8324	0.8335	0.8347	0.8358	0.8370	0.8382	0.8393	0.8405	0.8416
37	0.8261	0.8273	0.8286	0.8296	0.8308	0.8319	0.8331	0.8342	0.8354	0.8366
38	0.8200	0.8212	0.8224	0.8235	0.8247	0.8258	0.8270	0.8281	0.8293	0.8304
39	0.8151	0.8162	0.8174	0.8186	0.8197	0.8208	0.8220	0.8232	0.8243	0.8255
40	0.8091	0.8102	0.8114	0.8125	0.8137	0.8148	0.8160	0.8171	0.8183	0.8194

Temp. in °C	Barometer 770	771	772	773	774	775	776	777	778	779	780
10	0.9657	0.9670	0.9683	0.9696	0.9708	0.9721	0.9733	0.9746	0.9759	0.9771	0.9784
11	0.9616	0.9628	0.9641	0.9634	0.9666	0.9679	0.9691	0.9701	0.9717	0.9729	0.9742
12	0.9570	0.9582	0.9595	0.9608	0.9620	0.9633	0.9645	0.9658	0.9671	0.9683	0.9696
13	0.9531	0.9543	0.9556	0.9569	0.9581	0.9594	0.9606	0.9619	0.9632	0.9644	0.9657
14	0.9488	0.9501	0.9513	0.9526	0.9538	0.9551	0.9563	0.9575	0.9588	0.9600	0.9613
15	0.9444	0.9458	0.9470	0.9483	0.9496	0.9508	0.9520	0.9532	0.9545	0.9557	0.9570
16	0.9401	0.9414	0.9426	0.9439	0.9452	0.9464	0.9476	0.9488	0.9501	0.9513	0.9526
17	0.9358	0.9371	0.9383	0.9396	0.9409	0.9421	0.9433	0.9445	0.9458	0.9470	0.9483
18	0.9315	0.9327	0.9339	0.9352	0.9365	0.9377	0.9389	0.9401	0.9414	0.9426	0.9439
19	0.9271	0.9283	0.9295	0.9308	0.9320	0.9332	0.9344	0.9356	0.9369	0.9381	0.9394
20	0.9226	0.9238	0.9250	0.9263	0.9275	0.9288	0.9300	0.9312	0.9325	0.9337	0.9350
21	0.9184	0.9196	0.9208	0.9221	0.9233	0.9245	0.9257	0.9269	0.9282	0.9294	0.9307
22	0.9136	0.9148	0.9160	0.9172	0.9184	0.9197	0.9209	0.9221	0.9234	0.9246	0.9260
23	0.9090	0.9102	0.9114	0.9126	0.9138	0.9151	0.9163	0.9175	0.9188	0.9200	0.9213
24	0.9044	0.9056	0.9068	0.9080	0.9092	0.9104	0.9116	0.9128	0.9140	0.9152	0.9165
25	0.8998	0.9009	0.9021	0.9033	0.9045	0.9057	0.9069	0.9081	0.9093	0.9105	0.9117
35	0.8491	0.8502	0.8514	0.8526	0.8537	0.8549	0.8561	0.8572	0.8584	0.8596	0.8607
36	0.8428	0.8440	0.8451	0.8463	0.8475	0.8486	0.8498	0.8509	0.8521	0.8533	0.8544
37	0.8377	0.8389	0.8401	0.8412	0.8425	0.8435	0.8447	0.8458	0.8470	0.8481	0.8493
38	0.8316	0.8328	0.8339	0.8351	0.8362	0.8374	0.8385	0.8397	0.8408	0.8420	0.8431
39	0.8266	0.8278	0.8289	0.8301	0.8313	0.8324	0.8336	0.8347	0.8359	0.8370	0.8382
40	0.8206	0.8217	0.8229	0.8240	0.8251	0.8263	0.8274	0.8286	0.8297	0.8309	0.8320

Index